Workbook and Licensure Exam Prep

RADIOGRAPHY ESSENTIALS FOR LIMITED SCOPE

Workbook and Licensure Exam Prep

RADIOGRAPHY ESSENTIALS FOR LIMITED SCOPE

Seventh Edition

Eugene D. Frank, MA, FASRT, FAEIRS
RT(R) (ARRT) (Retired)
Associate Professor Emeritus
Mayo Clinic College of Medicine
Rochester, Minnesota

Ruth Ann Ehrlich, RT(R) (ARRT)
Senior Instructor in Radiology (Retired)
University of Western States
Portland, Oregon

Editorial Intern
Eva G. Pankratz, BS
University of Northwestern—St. Paul
English-Writing, Spanish
St. Paul, Minnesota

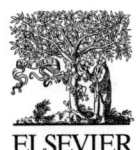

ELSEVIER

Elsevier
3251 Riverport Lane
St. Louis, Missouri 63043

WORKBOOK AND LICENSURE EXAM PREP FOR
RADIOGRAPHY ESSENTIALS FOR LIMITED SCOPE, SEVENTH EDITION

ISBN: 978-0-323-93622-4

Notice

Practitioners and researchers must always rely on their own experience and knowledge in evaluating and using any information, methods, compounds or experiments described herein. Because of rapid advances in the medical sciences, in particular, independent verification of diagnoses and drug dosages should be made. To the fullest extent of the law, no responsibility is assumed by Elsevier, authors, editors or contributors for any injury and/or damage to persons or property as a matter of products liability, negligence or otherwise, or from any use or operation of any methods, products, instructions, or ideas contained in the material herein.

Senior Content Strategist: Luke Held
Content Development Manager: Danielle M. Frazier
Publishing Services Manager: Deepthi Unni
Senior Project Manager: Manchu Mohan

Printed in India.

Last digit is the print number: 9   8   7   6   5   4   3   2   1

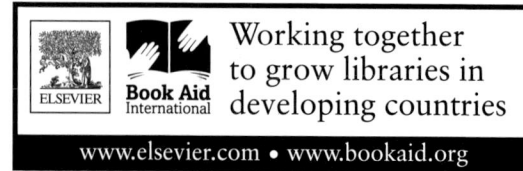

Contents

Section One   Learning Activities, **1**

1 Role of the Limited X-ray Machine Operator, **1**
2 Introduction to Radiographic Equipment, **5**
3 Basic Mathematics for Limited Operators, **11**
4 Basic Physics for Radiography, **31**
5 X-ray Production, **39**
6 X-ray Circuit and Tube Heat Management, **47**
7 Principles of Exposure and Image Quality, **55**
8 Digital Imaging, **67**
9 Scatter Radiation and Its Control, **81**
10 Formulating X-ray Techniques, **89**
11 Radiobiology and Radiation Safety, **97**
12 Introduction to Anatomy, Positioning, and Pathology, **111**
13 Upper Limb and Shoulder Girdle, **121**
14 Lower Limb and Pelvis, **139**
15 Spine, **161**
16 Bony Thorax, Chest, and Abdomen, **175**
17 Skull, Facial Bones, and Paranasal Sinuses, **189**
18 Radiography of Pediatric and Geriatric Patients, **207**
19 Image Evaluation, **213**
20 Ethics, Legal Considerations, and Professionalism, **217**
21 Safety and Infection Control, **225**
22 Assessing Patients and Managing Acute Situations, **235**
23 Medications and Their Administration, **241**
24 Medical Laboratory Skills, **245**
25 Additional Procedures for Assessment and Diagnosis, **249**
26 Bone Densitometry, **257**

Answers to Section One, 271

Section Two   Preparation Guide Limited Scope
of Practice in Radiography Examination, **347**

Section Three   Preparation Guide Bone Densitometry
Equipment Operator Examination, **385**

1 Role of the Limited X-ray Machine Operator

EXERCISE 1

Answer the following questions by selecting the best choice.

1. X-rays were discovered by:
   A. Eastman.
   B. Crookes.
   C. Edison.
   D. Roentgen.

2. The Joint Review Committee on Education in Radiologic Technology (JRCERT) is the:
   A. organization that accredits schools for radiologic technologists.
   B. organization that accredits schools for limited operators.
   C. professional organization for radiologic technologists.
   D. professional organization for limited operators.

3. Another term that has the same meaning as a *practical radiographer* is:
   A. radiologic technologist.
   B. medical assistant.
   C. limited operator.
   D. imaging specialist.

4. (True/False) To determine the credentials needed for you to practice limited radiography, you should contact the appropriate state agency.

5. The term limited operator is used because:
   A. scope of practice is limited.
   B. salaries are limited.
   C. opportunities are limited.
   D. radiographer's competence is limited.

6. *Reciprocity* means that:
   A. special credentials are required.
   B. credentials issued in one area are recognized in another.
   C. an application has been made for a license or permit, but the license or permit has not been granted.
   D. there is freedom to practice without a license or permit.

7. Which of the following physicians has received extensive additional training and would be considered a specialist?
   1. Radiologist
   2. Obstetrician
   3. Pediatrician
   A. 1 and 2
   B. 1 and 3
   C. 2 and 3
   D. 1, 2, and 3

8. A specialist who interprets radiographs and performs special imaging procedures is called:
   A. a radiologic technologist.
   B. a chiropractor.
   C. a primary care physician.
   D. a radiologist.

9. An order for an x-ray examination is issued by:
   A. a physician.
   B. a nurse.
   C. a radiologic technologist.
   D. a medical assistant.

10. Which of the following are considered duties of a limited operator?
    1. Determine what examination should be performed.
    2. Explain the procedure and the preparation to the patient.
    3. Position the patient correctly in relation to the image receptor and the x-ray tube.
    A. 1 and 2
    B. 1 and 3
    C. 2 and 3
    D. 1, 2, and 3

11. The largest professional organization for radiologic technologists is the:
    A. ARRT.
    B. ASRT.
    C. JRCERT.
    D. ASSRT.

12. The curriculum for limited x-ray machine operators is published by the:
   A. ARRT.
   B. ASRT.
   C. JRCERT.
   D. ASSRT.

13. An organization that now provides accreditation for limited x-ray schools is the:
   A. ARRT.
   B. ASRT.
   C. JRCERT.
   D. ASSRT.

14. A podiatrist diagnoses and treats disorders and diseases of:
   A. the chest.
   B. the feet.
   C. children.
   D. the nervous system.

15. Bone densitometry is a specialized x-ray machine and procedure that measures:
   A. bone growth.
   B. bone mineral content.
   C. bone aging.
   D. bone blood flow.

16. Which of the following documents cites information that is "mandatory and enforceable"?
   A. ARRT Code of Ethics
   B. ARRT Rules of Ethics
   C. ARRT Handbook
   D. ARRT Standard of Ethics

17. (True/False) Limited operators can perform the same x-ray examinations that radiographers can.

18. (True/False) Credentials for limited operators vary greatly from state to state.

EXERCISE 2

Answer the following questions.

1. When, where, and by whom were x-rays discovered?

   _____

   _____

2. What is the purpose of the ARRT? Why might this organization be important to a limited x-ray machine operator?

   _____

   _____

   _____

3. List the possible consequences of practicing radiography outside the limitations imposed by local regulations.

   _____

   _____

   _____

   _____

   _____

4. What professional credential is used by radiologic technologists after passing the ARRT examination in radiography, and what does it stand for?

   _____

   _____

5. Explain what is meant by *reciprocity*.

_____

_____

6. List three activities that might take place in the "front office" of a clinic and four that typically occur in the "back office."

   Front office:

   1. _____

   2. _____

   3. _____

   Back office:

   1. _____

   2. _____

   3. _____

   4. _____

7. List five typical duties of a limited x-ray machine operator.

   1. _____

   2. _____

   3. _____

   4. _____

   5. _____

8. The official term for people who perform limited x-ray procedures is limited x-ray machine operator. Name at least three other terms that may be used in some states.

   1. _____

   2. _____

   3. _____

9. A bone densitometry machine is used to measure:

_____

EXERCISE 3

Match the following terms with their definitions.

1. _____ Angiography

2. _____ Computed tomography

3. _____ Positron emission tomography

4. _____ Mammography

5. _____ Sonography

6. _____ Nuclear medicine

7. _____ Radiation therapy

8. _____ Magnetic resonance imaging

A. Treatment of malignant disease using radiation

B. Computerized imaging system that uses a powerful magnetic field and radiofrequency pulses to produce images of the body

C. Imaging of soft tissue structures using sound echoes

D. Imaging of blood vessels with the injection of special compounds called *contrast media*

E. Imaging of the breast using a special x-ray machine

F. Injection or ingestion of radioactive materials and the recording of their uptake in the body using a gamma camera

G. Computerized x-ray system that provides axial images (transverse "slices") of all parts of the body

H. A highly sophisticated computerized form of nuclear medical imaging

EXERCISE 4

Match the following healthcare specialties with their definitions.

1. _____ Anesthesiologist

2. _____ Geriatrician

3. _____ Obstetrician

4. _____ Oncologist

5. _____ Pediatrician

6. _____ Radiologist

7. _____ Orthopedist

8. _____ Thoracic specialist

9. _____ Podiatrist

10. _____ Chiropractor

A. Diagnoses and treats disorders and diseases of the spine

B. Specializes in problems and diseases of the elderly

C. Treats and diagnoses disorders and diseases in children

D. Specializes in diagnosis by means of medical imaging

E. Specializes in tumor identification and treatment

F. Administers anesthetics and monitors patients during surgery

G. Specializes in problems of the chest

H. Diagnoses and treats problems of the musculoskeletal system

I. Diagnoses and treats disorders and diseases of the feet

J. Specializes in pregnancy, labor, delivery, and postpartum care

2 Introduction to Radiographic Equipment

EXERCISE 1

Answer the following questions by selecting the best choice.

1. The x-ray room has an area that protects the limited operator from scatter radiation. This area is called:
   A. control console.
   B. transformer.
   C. control booth.
   D. radiation field.

2. The mechanism on the x-ray tube crane that provides "stops" in a specific location is the:
   A. control console.
   B. transformer.
   C. tube port.
   D. detent.

3. The image that has been exposed on the image receptor (IR) but has not been processed is called:
   A. remnant radiation.
   B. scatter radiation.
   C. latent image.
   D. visible image.

4. The absorption of x-rays by matter is called:
   A. fog.
   B. attenuation.
   C. remnant radiation.
   D. exit radiation.

5. The IR system may consist of the following:
   A. Control console and transformer
   B. X-ray tube and tube stand
   C. Tube locks and detent
   D. Cassette and phosphor plate

6. A line that is perpendicular to the long axis of the x-ray tube and that is in the center of the x-ray beam is called the:
   A. central ray.
   B. scatter radiation.
   C. x-ray tube.
   D. primary x-ray beam.

7. The device that protects the IR from being fogged by scatter radiation is called a:
   A. detent.
   B. grid or Bucky.
   C. cassette.
   D. collimator.

8. The device that allows the limited operator to vary the size of the radiation field is called:
   A. collimator.
   B. tube port.
   C. control console.
   D. detent.

9. The purpose of a safety check performed before making an exposure is to:
   A. ensure a quality radiographic image.
   B. prevent a radiation hazard to oneself.
   C. prevent accidental exposure of coworkers.
   D. protect the patient from unnecessary exposure.

10. A radiation hazard exists in the x-ray room:
    A. throughout the room during an exposure.
    B. only in the path of the primary x-ray beam during an exposure.
    C. throughout the room at all times.
    D. throughout the room during exposure and for several minutes afterward.

11. A type of filmless x-ray system that produces digital images is called:
    A. a remnant system.
    B. mobile radiography.
    C. an IR.
    D. computed radiography (CR).

12. Digital images produced using the CR systems use a(n) _____ to process the image.
    A. darkroom and chemical processor
    B. image reader device
    C. computer with an SSD hard drive
    D. special high-capacity computer

13. The most frequent adverse incident that occurs in a radiology department is:
    A. bleeding.
    B. pinching of fingers.
    C. falling.
    D. back pain.

14. After the x-rays have gone into the patient, and some have been attenuated, the x-rays will exit the patient. This exit radiation is now called:
    A. remnant radiation.
    B. primary radiation.
    C. scatter radiation.
    D. quality radiation.

15. The part or area of the x-ray tube where the x-rays exit is termed the:
    A. Bucky.
    B. central ray.
    C. tube housing.
    D. tube port.

16. The square area of the x-ray beam that strikes the patient is the:
    A. central ray.
    B. collimator light.
    C. tube port.
    D. radiation field.

EXERCISE 2

Answer the following questions.

1. How can you determine the location of the central ray?

   _____

   _____

2. What is the location of remnant or exit radiation?

   _____

   _____

3. What is meant by *attenuation*?

   _____

   _____

4. What component of the x-ray machine is located in the control booth?

   _____

   _____

5. What should you do before attempting to move x-ray equipment?

   _____

   _____

6. Where would you look to find a collimator?

   _____

   _____

7. How might you determine the size of the radiation field without actually measuring it?

_____

_____

8. List the four steps in a preexposure safety check.

    1. _____

    2. _____

    3. _____

    4. _____

9. How soon is it safe to reenter the x-ray room after an exposure?

_____

_____

10. Define the difference between primary and remnant radiation.

_____

_____

_____

_____

11. What are the common sizes of CR plates?

_____

12. Describe the Trendelenburg position.

_____

_____

13. Describe the latent image.

_____

_____

14. Many x-ray projections are done with the patient standing or sitting upright using what device?

_____

7

Match the following terms with their descriptions.

1. _____ Tube housing

2. _____ Tube port

3. _____ X-ray tube

4. _____ Scatter radiation

5. _____ Radiation fog

6. _____ Computed radiography (CR)

7. _____ Image receptor (IR)

A. Source of the x-rays

B. Unwanted image exposure that is caused by scattered x-rays

C. Surrounds the x-ray tube and is lined with lead

D. Filmless x-ray system that uses a digital format to produce images

E. Receives the energy of the x-ray beam and forms the image of the body part

F. Opening where the x-rays exit the tube

G. The x-rays that strike the patient and travel in all directions, inside and outside the body

CHALLENGE EXERCISE

This exercise does not have to be completed at the same time as the other exercises in this workbook chapter. The exercise is designed to assess the retention of the essential information contained in the corresponding textbook chapter. It is recommended that you complete this exercise when you begin to study for the state limited licensure examination. This will help determine what you know and which information should be further reviewed.

1. X-rays exit the tube port through an opening called the:

   _____.

2. The x-ray tube is surrounded by a lead-lined device called the:

   _____.

3. The invisible imaginary line in the center of the x-ray beam that is used for centering is called the:

   _____.

4. The square lighted area on the patient and table where the x-rays strike is called the:

   _____.

5. What is the name of the radiation that exits the patient?

   _____.

6. The unseen image contained within the plate phosphor is called the:

   _____.

7. The x-ray beam that leaves the tube is called:

   _____.

8. The absorption of x-rays by the human body is called:

   _____.

9. The primary source of scatter radiation is the:

   _____.

10. Primary beam x-rays that leave the body and travel in all directions are called:

    _____.

11. What is the difference in energy between the primary beam radiation and the scattered radiation?

    _____.

12. The unwanted radiation exposure on the x-ray image caused by scatter radiation is called:

    _____.

13. Scatter radiation exits the patient in which direction?

    _____.

14. In the radiology department, the IR consists of what two components?

    _____.

15. Which digital imaging system do most limited operators use?

    _____.

16. What is the name of the device that accepts the CR plate and scans it?

    _____.

17. The most frequent adverse incident that occurs in the radiology department is:

    _____.

18. Name several key safety precautions that should occur when moving x-ray equipment.

1._____.

2._____.

19. What is the name of the movable device under the x-ray table that contains a grid and holds the IR?

_____.

20. The device that allows x-rays to be taken in the upright position is called the:

_____.

21. Lowering the head on the x-ray table at least 15 degrees is termed:

_____.

22. Name several important preexposure safety checks:

_____.

3 Basic Mathematics for Limited Operators

EXERCISE 1

Match the following terms with their definitions.

1. _____ Sum

2. _____ Difference

3. _____ Product

4. _____ Dividend

5. _____ Divisor

6. _____ Quotient

7. _____ Remainder

A. The number that is "left over" when the dividend cannot be evenly divided by the divisor

B. The answer to a multiplication problem

C. Total, the answer to an addition problem

D. The number by which the dividend is divided

E. The answer to a division problem

F. The answer to a subtraction problem

G. In a division problem, the number that is divided

EXERCISE 2

Answer the following questions.

1. The lower number of a fraction is called the _____.

2. The upper number of a fraction is called the _____.

3. A mixed number consists of a(n)_____ and a(n)_____.

4. To multiply a whole number by a fraction, multiply the whole number by

   _____ and then divide the product by

   _____.

5. Calculate the value of the following fractions of whole numbers.

   A. $\frac{1}{10} \times 80$ _____

   B. $\frac{1}{10} \times 200$ _____

   C. $\frac{2}{5} \times 150$ _____

   D. $\frac{1}{4} \times 300$ _____

   E. $\frac{7}{10} \times 80$ _____

6. Reduce the following fractions to the lowest terms.

A. $^4/_{10}$ _____

B. $^3/_{12}$ _____

C. $^6/_{18}$ _____

D. $^{12}/_{20}$ _____

E. $^8/_{24}$ _____

F. $^{15}/_{25}$ _____

G. $^6/_8$ _____

EXERCISE 3

Answer the following questions.

1. In a decimal, numerals to the left of the decimal point represent _____.

2. The first place to the right of the decimal point represents _____, the second place represents ____

_____, and the third place represents _____.

3. (True/False) 0.7 = 0.700.

4. (True/False) 3.3 = 3.03.

5. Set up the problems and calculate the sums of the following decimals.

A. 21.7 + 5.39 = _____

B. 33.06 + 30.2 = _____

C. 14.911 + 208.7 = _____

D. 29.844 + 3.3 + 27.6 = _____

E. 285.2 + 46.91 + 11.402 = _____

6. Set up the problems and calculate the differences for the following decimals.

A. $335.65 - 46.23 =$ _____

B. $456.33 - 3.87 =$ _____

C. $39.8 - 6.323 =$ _____

D. $21 - 7.51 =$ _____

E. $19.042 - 4.12 =$ _____

7. How do you determine where to place the decimal point in a problem that involves multiplication of decimals?

_____

_____

8. Set up the problems and calculate the products in the following problems involving multiplication of decimals.

A. $29.5 \times 5 =$ _____

B. $17.6 \times 40 =$ _____

C. $341.225 \times 48.33 =$ _____

D. $0.2213 \times 82.7 =$ _____

E. $83.22 \times 906.1 =$ _____

9. Set up the problems and calculate the quotients in the following problems involving division of decimals.

A. $34.5 \div 5 =$ _____

B. $720.35 \div 10 =$ _____

C. $29 \div 2.5 =$ _____

D. $284.31 \div 4.05 =$ _____

E. $609.56 \div 6.22 =$ _____

10. To convert a fraction to a decimal, divide the _____ by the _____.

11. Convert the following fractions and mixed numbers to decimals.

    A. $\frac{1}{8}$ _____

    B. $\frac{3}{8}$ _____

    C. $\frac{1}{60}$ _____

    D. $\frac{2}{5}$ _____

    E. $11\frac{1}{4}$ _____

12. *(Circle the correct phrase.)* When rounding off a decimal, drop the excess numerals from (left to right/right to left).

13. When rounding off a decimal, if the last numeral dropped is _____ or greater, increase the final remaining numeral by one; if the last numeral dropped is _____ or less, no change is necessary.

14. Round off the following decimals to the number of decimal places indicated in parentheses.

    A. 1.66666 (2) _____

    B. 0.74139 (4) _____

    C. 0.2509 (2) _____

    D. 3.2551 (3) _____

    E. 10.4444 (2) _____

15. Perform the indicated calculations in the following problems by first converting the fractions to decimals. If the decimals in this exercise have four or more decimal places, round them off to three decimal places.

    A. $\frac{1}{4} + \frac{1}{20} + \frac{2}{3} =$ _____

    B. $\frac{3}{10} + \frac{1}{5} + \frac{1}{2} =$ _____

    C. $\frac{3}{4} - \frac{3}{8} =$ _____

    D. $\frac{2}{15} \times 200 =$ _____

    E. $\frac{3}{5} \div \frac{1}{2} =$ _____

EXERCISE 4

Answer the following questions.

1. (True/False) When adding or subtracting two percentages, the percentages must be converted to decimals.

2. (True/False) When multiplying or dividing percentages, or when performing calculations involving percentages and whole numbers, the percentages must be converted to decimals.

3. Convert the following percentages to decimals.

   A. 20% _____

   B. 71.3% _____

   C. 85% _____

   D. 69% _____

   E. 172% _____

   F. 800% _____

4. Convert the following decimals to percentages.

   A. 0.33 _____

   B. 0.4 _____

   C. 0.06 _____

   D. 1.89 _____

   E. 2.3 _____

   F. 6.0 _____

5. Perform the following calculations involving percentages.

   A. $73\% + 27\% = $ _____

   B. $50\% + 25\% = $ _____

   C. $30\% - 3\% = $ _____

   D. $20\% \times 60\% = $ _____

   E. $79\% \times 30\% = $ _____

   F. $25\% \div 10\% = $ _____

   G. $48\% \div 2\% = $ _____

6. Calculate the values of the following percentages up to two decimal places.

   A. $30\% \text{ of } 27 = $ _____

   B. $95\% \text{ of } 320 = $ _____

C. 50% of 31 = _____.

D. 170% of 60 = _____.

e. 200% of 20 = _____.

7. Determine the following percentages. Express your answers to the nearest tenth of a percent.

A. 11 = _____% of 64

B. 71 = _____% of 90

C. 50 = _____% of 300

D. 40 = _____% of 200

E. 70 = _____% of 35

8. Calculate the solutions to the following problems that involve increasing and decreasing numbers by a percentage.

   A. Increase 75 by 15%.

   B. Increase 30 by 100%.

   C. Increase 12 by 20%.

   D. Decrease 85 by 10%.

   E. Decrease 50 by 12%.

Answer the following questions.

1. A declaration that two mathematical statements (groups of numbers, together with their operational signs or mathematical functions) are equal to each other is called a(n) _____.

2. (True/False) The same symbols for mathematical operations used in arithmetic are also used in algebra.

3. *(Circle the correct word.)* The slanted line between the x and the 3 in the equation $x/3 = 6$ means that x is (multiplied/ divided) by 3.

4. (True/False) When an equation consists of two fractions, you can eliminate the denominators from consideration by using cross multiplication.

5. 3:4 is an example of a(n)_____.

6. 3:4::6:8 is an example of a(n)_____.

7. Determine the value of x up to three decimal places in each of the following equations.

   A. $2x + 9 = 11 + 3$

   B. $\frac{16}{x} = 12 - 4$

   C. $x - 61 = 12$

   D. $45 = 4x - 15$

   E. $3x = \frac{9}{3}$

   F. $64 = 8x$

G. $\frac{25}{x} = \frac{10}{2}$

H. $\frac{x}{3} = \frac{48}{12}$

I. $\frac{72}{8} = \frac{80}{x}$

J. $\frac{10}{x} = \frac{4}{6}$

EXERCISE 6

Answer the following questions.

1. Write the expression that indicates four cubed. _____

2. Write the expression that indicates five to the fifth power. _____

3. Calculate the values of the following exponential numbers.

A. $3^2 =$ _____.

B. $3^3 =$ _____.

C. $2^4 =$_____.

D. $9^2 =$ _____.

E. $40^2 =$ _____.

4. Calculate the square roots in the following problems.

   A. $\sqrt{9} =$ _____.

   B. $\sqrt{16} =$ _____.

   C. $\sqrt{25} =$ _____.

   D. $\sqrt{81} =$ _____.

   E. $\sqrt{144} =$ _____.

EXERCISE 7

1. Match the metric prefixes with their meanings.

1. _____ Kilo-	A. 10
2. _____ Nano-	B. 100
3. _____ Milli-	C. 1000
4. _____ Deci-	D. $\frac{1}{10}$ (0.1)
5. _____ Hecto-	E. $\frac{1}{100}$ (0.01)
6. _____ Centi-	F. $\frac{1}{1000}$ (0.001)
7. _____ Micro-	G. $\frac{1}{1,000,000}$ (0.000001)
8. _____ Deca-	H. $\frac{1}{1,000,000,000}$ (0.000000001)

2. Fill in the blanks in these statements of English measurement equivalents.

   A. One yard = _____ feet.

   B. One foot = _____ inches.

   C. One pint = _____ ounces.

   D. One ton = _____ pounds.

   E. One pound = _____ ounces.

3. Fill in the blanks in these statements of metric equivalents.

    A. 1 meter = _____ centimeters.

    B. 1 kilogram = _____ grams.

    C. 1 liter = _____ milliliters.

    D. 1 millisecond = _____ second.

4. Convert the following metric measurements from one unit to another.

    A. Convert 70 kilovolts to volts.

    B. Convert 5 meters to centimeters.

    C. Convert 30 milliliters to liters.

    D. Convert 100 grams to kilograms.

    E. Convert 2 milligrams to grams.

5. Convert the following measurements from one English unit to another.

    A. Convert 18 inches to yards.

    B. Convert 2 quarts to fluid ounces.

    C. Convert 68 inches to feet.

D. Convert 20 quarts to gallons.

E. Convert 3.5 pounds to ounces.

6. Calculate the following conversions between English and metric units. Limit your answers to no more than four decimal places.

A. Convert 5 fluid ounces to milliliters.

B. Convert 100 pounds to kilograms.

C. Convert 14 inches to meters.

D. Convert 50 millimeters to inches.

E. Convert 100 grams to ounces.

7. Calculate the following time and temperature conversions.

A. Convert $\frac{1}{60}$ second to milliseconds.

B. Convert 260 seconds to hours.

C. Convert 2.4 days to hours.

D. Convert 75°F to the Celsius scale.

E. Convert 25°C to the Fahrenheit scale.

EXERCISE 8

Answer the following questions.

1. Milliampere-seconds (mAs) is a useful unit in radiography because it indicates _____.

2. State the formula for determining mAs. _____

3. When both mA and mAs are known, the formula for determining the exposure time is _____

_____.

4. Calculate the mAs for the following exposures.

A. 200 mA, 0.05 second

B. 300 mA, 0.25 second

C. 100 mA, 0.7 second

D. 500 mA, $\frac{1}{20}$ second

E. 50 mA, 0.3 second

F. 150 mA, $1\frac{1}{4}$ seconds

G. 400 mA, 2 milliseconds

5. Calculate the exposure time for the following exposures. Round any extended decimals to three decimal places.

   A. 50 mA, 10 mAs

   B. 200 mA, 40 mAs

   C. 300 mA, 6 mAs

   D. 100 mA, 2 mAs

   E. 400 mA, 75 mAs

EXERCISE 9

Answer the following questions.

1. Write the formula for changing mAs to compensate for a change in source-image receptor distance (SID).

   _____

2. Solve the following problems involving changes in SID.

   A. What is the relative change in radiation intensity when the distance changes from 40 inches SID to 80 inches SID?

B. What is the relative change in radiation intensity when the distance is changed from 60 inches SID to 40 inches SID?

C. A satisfactory radiograph is made using 25 mAs at 40 inches SID. How many mAs are needed to produce a similar radiograph at 48 inches SID?

D. A satisfactory radiograph is made using 30 mAs at 72 inches SID. How many mAs are needed to produce a similar radiograph at 84 inches SID?

E. A satisfactory radiograph is made using 12 mAs at 40 inches SID. How many mAs are needed to produce a similar radiograph at 72 inches SID?

EXERCISE 10

Answer the following questions.

1. Below 85 peak kilovoltage (kVp), an adjustment of _____ kVp/cm will compensate for small changes in part

   size. Above 85 kVp, a change of _____ kVp/cm is necessary.

2. To compensate for a 2-cm *increase* in part size using mAs, increase the original mAs by _____%. To compen

   sate for a 2-cm *decrease* in part size using mAs, decrease the original mAs by _____%.

3. Solve the following problems involving changes in patient part size.

   A. A satisfactory radiograph is made using 90 kVp on a patient part measuring 24 cm. Adjust the kVp to compensate for a patient part size decrease to 21 cm.

   B. A satisfactory radiograph is made using 72 kVp on a patient part measuring 16 cm. Adjust the kVp to compensate for a patient part size increase to 19 cm.

27

C. A satisfactory radiograph is made using 20 mAs on a patient part measuring 22 cm. Adjust the mAs to compensate for a patient part size decrease to 20 cm.

D. A satisfactory radiograph is made using 50 mAs on a patient part measuring 26 cm. Adjust the mAs to compensate for a patient part size increase to 30 cm.

E. A satisfactory radiograph is made using 15 mAs on a patient part measuring 13 cm. Adjust the mAs to compensate for a patient part size increase to 15 cm.

4. *(Circle the correct word.)* When using the 15% rule to increase kVp, you must (multiply/divide) the mAs by 2.

EXERCISE 11

Answer the following questions.

1. Write the formula used for determining the volume of medication that will deliver a specific dose. _____

_____

2. The prescribed dose is 60 mg. The available stock is in the form of 15-mg tablets. How many should be given?

_____

3. The prescribed dose is 150 mg. The available stock has a strength of 50 mg/mL. How much should be given?

_____

4. The prescribed dose is 80 mcg. The available stock has a strength of 20 mcg/mL. How much should be given?

_____

5. The prescribed dose is 2 mg. The available stock has a strength of 1 mg per tablet. How much should be given?

_____

6. A toddler got into the medicine cabinet and ate four acetaminophen (Tylenol) tablets. The tablet strength is 500 mg. What dose did the child receive?

_____

7. A physician prescribed a dose of 2 mg/kg of body weight for a child. The child weighs 40 pounds. The drug is available in a strength of 4 mg/mL. How many milliliters should the child receive?

_____

CHALLENGE EXERCISE

This exercise does not have to be completed at the same time as the other exercises in this workbook chapter. The exercise is designed to assess the retention of the essential information contained in the corresponding textbook chapter. It is recommended that you complete this exercise when you begin to study for the state limited licensure examination. This will help determine what you know and which information should be further reviewed.

1. The answer to a division problem is called the _____.

2. Calculate the result when 85 is increased by 15%. _____

3. If the mAs is increased from 20 to 30, what is the percentage of the increase? _____

4. The factor that indicates the total quantity of radiation in an exposure is the _____.

5. An exposure is made using 500 mAs and 3 msec. Calculate the mAs for this exposure.

_____

6. How many milliliters are contained in a liter? _____

7. The prescribed dose of a drug is 120 mcg. The available stock has a strength of 20 mcg/mL. What quantity should be given?

_____

8. State the formula for determining the new mAs to compensate for a change in SID.

_____

4 Basic Physics for Radiography

Answer the following questions by selecting the best choice.

1. Which of the following would be considered a basic form of matter?
   1. Solid
   2. Liquid
   3. Mass
   A. 1 and 2
   B. 1 and 3
   C. 2 and 3
   D. 1, 2, and 3

2. Electromagnetic energy occurs in the form of a:
   A. photon.
   B. atom.
   C. sinusoidal wave.
   D. wavelength.

3. Which of the following is located in an orbit around the nucleus of an atom?
   A. Photon
   B. Electron
   C. Neutron
   D. Positron

4. Which of the following has a negative (−) electrical charge?
   A. Neutron
   B. Proton
   C. Electron
   D. Positron

5. The negative effects of radiation that occur for humans are due to:
   A. rectification.
   B. ionization.
   C. wavelength of the photon.
   D. frequency of the photon.

6. When a neutral atom gains or loses an electron, the atom is said to be:
   A. radioactive.
   B. unstable.
   C. ionized.
   D. neutral.

7. The force or speed of the electron flow in the current is measured using the:
   A. wavelength.
   B. frequency.
   C. ampere.
   D. volt.

8. X-rays consist of:
   A. electromagnetic energy.
   B. potential energy.
   C. chemical energy.
   D. thermal energy.

9. X-rays with greater energy have shorter _____ and are more penetrating.
   A. frequencies
   B. velocity
   C. wavelength
   D. potential difference

10. Of the following types of electromagnetic energy, which has the shortest wavelength?
    A. Radio waves
    B. Diagnostic rays
    C. Microwaves
    D. Ultraviolet light

11. Which of the following are accurate statements regarding the characteristics of x-rays?
    1. They are highly penetrating and invisible.
    2. They cause certain crystals to fluoresce.
    3. They travel in straight lines at the speed of light.
    A. 1 and 2
    B. 1 and 3
    C. 2 and 3
    D. 1, 2, and 3

12. The smallest possible unit of electromagnetic energy is the:
    A. photon.
    B. atom.
    C. nuclear energy.
    D. matter.

13. The term for a continuous path for the flow of electrical charges from the power source through one or more electrical devices and back to the source is:
    A. electrical circuit.
    B. voltage.
    C. frequency.
    D. resistance.

14. The common unit of measure for the potential difference across an x-ray tube is the:
    A. ampere.
    B. milliampere.
    C. volt.
    D. ohm.

15. The rate or volume of the electron flow in a current is measured using the:
    A. ohm.
    B. hertz.
    C. volt.
    D. ampere.

16. The purpose of a transformer is to:
    A. convert alternating current (AC) into direct current (DC).
    B. convert DC into AC.
    C. increase or decrease voltage.
    D. reduce the resistance in a circuit.

17. Which electron shell in the atom is most important for the production of x-rays?
    A. N
    B. M
    C. L
    D. K

18. If a conductor (wire) is moved in and out of a magnetic field, what will flow in the circuit?
    A. Voltage
    B. Electricity or current
    C. Milliamperage
    D. Hertz

19. When a current is flowing through a circuit, it creates a magnetic field surrounding the conductor. This magnetic field can be used to _____current to flow in another conductor.
    A. induce
    B. increase
    C. decrease
    D. change AC to DC

20. The process of converting AC current to DC current is called:
    A. conduction.
    B. transformation.
    C. induction.
    D. rectification.

21. One of the most important elements in radiology that is used to create x-rays is:
    A. calcium.
    B. tungsten.
    C. carbon.
    D. lead.

22. (True/False) X-rays cause ionization in the human body. This has a negative effect on the body.

23. (True/False) When a step-up transformer increases voltage from the primary side to the secondary side of a transformer, amperage is increased.

24. (True/False) If a transformer has 100 turns on the primary side and 25 turns on the secondary side, it is a step-down transformer.

25. (True/False) Electromagnetic energy has both electric and magnetic properties.

26. (True/False) X-rays with greater energy have a lower frequency.

27. (True/False) X-rays can cause cancer.

EXERCISE 2

Answer the following questions.

1. Describe *rectification.*

   _____

2. Name the electron orbit shell nearest the nucleus of an atom.

   _____

3. Name two forms of electromagnetic radiation that have a longer wavelength than diagnostic x-rays.

1. _____

2. _____

4. How does wavelength affect the usefulness of an x-ray beam?

_____

_____

5. What is meant by *ionization,* and what determines the ionizing capability of electromagnetic radiation?

_____

_____

_____

_____

_____

6. List at least six characteristics of x-rays.

1. _____

2. _____

3. _____

4. _____

5. _____

6. _____

7. What is the velocity of x-rays? Are they faster or slower than visible light?

_____

_____

_____

_____

8. State the units used to measure current and potential difference.

_____

_____

_____

9. Voltage in an x-ray machine is increased to the kilovoltage level by which device?

_____

10. An x-ray tube cannot produce x-rays unless the circuit is:

_____

11. What is meant by electromagnetic *induction?*

_____

_____

12. What is the primary purpose of a transformer?

_____

_____

_____

EXERCISE 3

Match the following terms with their definitions.

1. _____ Electromagnetic induction   A. Quantity of electrons flowing in a circuit

2. _____ Sine wave   B. Unit to measure the rate of current flow in a circuit

3. _____ Transformer   C. Equal to 1000 V

4. _____ Alternating current   D. Equal to 0.001 A ($\frac{1}{1000}$ A)

5. _____ Kilovolt (kV)   E. Current changes polarity from negative to positive at regular intervals

6. _____ Rectification   F. Increases or decreases voltage by a fixed amount (AC only)

7. _____ Ampere (A)   G. Using a magnet and conductor to create electric current

8. _____ Milliampere (mA)   H. Process of changing AC to DC

9. _____ Volt (V)   I. The shape or form of electric energy

10. _____ Current   J. Unit to measure potential difference

CHALLENGE EXERCISE

This exercise does not have to be completed at the same time as the other exercises in this workbook chapter. The exercise is designed to assess retention of the essential information contained in the corresponding textbook chapter. It is recommended that you complete this exercise when you begin to study for the state limited licensure examination. This will help determine what you know and which information should be further reviewed.

1. Name the three basic forms of matter.

   _____.

2. The smallest possible unit of electromagnetic energy is called the:

   _____.

3. What is the atomic name of the particles that circle the nucleus of the atom?

   _____.

4. What is the name of the innermost shell of an atom that is important in radiology?

   _____.

5. Electrons are held in place in their shell by a(n):

   _____.

6. One of the most important elements used in the production of an x-ray is:

   _____.

7. When an electron is removed from an atom in the human body, the process is termed:

   _____.

8. What is the official name of the type of x-ray energy that occurs in a high-frequency sine wave?

   _____.

9. In a sine wave, the name given to the distance from one crest of the wave to another crest is the:

   _____.

10. The velocity of electromagnetic radiation is the product of:

    _____.

11. Why is *ionization* very important in the field of radiology?

    _____.

12. Diagnostic x-rays consist of what type of radiation on the electromagnetic spectrum?

_____.

13. What type of wavelength do x-rays have?

_____.

14. What type of frequency do x-rays have?

_____.

15. Name at least five characteristics of x-rays.

_____

_____

16. Current is the quantity of electrons flowing in an electrical circuit. This current is measured in:

_____

_____.

17. Potential difference is the force behind the current in an electrical circuit. This force is measured in:

_____.

18. A typical x-ray tube operates in what kilovoltage range?

_____.

19. A typical x-ray tube operates in what milliamperage range?

_____.

20. What type of current is delivered to homes in the United States and Canada?

_____.

21. The process of changing AC to DC is called:

_____.

22. High-frequency x-ray generators can change the standard electrical frequency (Hertz [Hz]) to as high as:

_____.

23. When an electrical current uses its magnetic field to create a secondary current, the process is called:

_____.

24. What is the name of the device that produces the high voltage needed for x-ray production?

_____.

25. Name the two types of x-ray transformers that can raise or lower the voltage.

_____.

26. Explain electromagnetic *induction*.

_____

5 X-ray Production

EXERCISE 1

Answer the following questions by selecting the best choice.

1. The target angle affects the x-ray tube's:
   1. heat capacity.
   2. spatial resolution.
   3. maximum size of the x-ray beam.
   A. 1 and 2
   B. 1 and 3
   C. 2 and 3
   D. 1, 2, and 3

2. An "electron cloud" surrounding the filament of the cathode is referred to as a:
   A. space charge.
   B. photon.
   C. filament.
   D. focusing cup.

3. Free electrons for x-ray production come from the:
   A. filament.
   B. target.
   C. anode.
   D. focusing cup.

4. The creation of the space charge in the x-ray tube produces:
   A. resistance.
   B. variable resistance.
   C. conductivity.
   D. thermionic emission.

5. The majority of photons in the x-ray beam are created by which process?
   A. Characteristic interactions
   B. Bremsstrahlung interactions
   C. Magnetic induction
   D. Space charge

6. More than 99% of the energy of the electron stream is converted into:
   A. bremsstrahlung photons.
   B. characteristic photons.
   C. secondary radiation.
   D. heat.

7. The high-speed rotation (10,000 rpm) of the anode enables:
   A. generation of a larger space charge.
   B. production of a greater number of electrons.
   C. greater dissipation of heat from high technical factors.
   D. focusing of the electron stream on a smaller area of the target.

8. The degree of angulation of the x-ray tube target will determine the:
   A. heat capacity of the tube.
   B. shape of the x-ray beam.
   C. size of the actual and effective focal spot.
   D. number of photons in the x-ray beam.

9. A dual-focus x-ray tube has:
   1. two filaments.
   2. two focal spot sizes.
   3. two anodes.
   A. 1 and 2
   B. 1 and 3
   C. 2 and 3
   D. 1, 2, and 3

10. The anode heel effect is a phenomenon of x-ray production that results in:
    A. dissipation of anode heat.
    B. uneven distribution of radiation within the x-ray field.
    C. filtration of the long x-ray wavelengths in the x-ray beam.
    D. production of characteristic radiation.

11. To take advantage of the anode heel effect when making a radiograph of the femur for an AP projection on a 14 × 17-in. IR at a 40-inch SID, the patient should be placed so that the:
    A. head is toward the anode end of the tube.
    B. head is toward the cathode end of the tube.

12. The penetrating power of the x-ray beam is controlled by varying the:
    A. milliamperes (mA).
    B. peak kilovoltage (kVp).
    C. anode speed.
    D. exposure time.

13. The rate of current flow across the x-ray tube is measured in:
    A. ohms.
    B. kilovolts.
    C. roentgens.
    D. mA.

14. Doubling the mA will result in:
    1. increased patient dose.
    2. twice as many photons in the x-ray beam.
    3. increased radiographic density.
    A. 1 and 2
    B. 1 and 3
    C. 2 and 3
    D. 1, 2, and 3

15. The unit used to indicate the total quantity of x-ray exposure is:
    A. mA.
    B. seconds (of exposure time).
    C. kilovolts.
    D. milliampere-seconds (mAs).

16. An x-ray exposure is made using the following factors: 200 mA, 0.02 sec., 70 kVp, 40 in. SID. The value of the mAs for this exposure is:
    A. 0.04
    B. 0.4
    C. 4.0
    D. 40.0

17. The device for removing long-wavelength low-energy radiation from the primary x-ray beam is the:
    A. transformer.
    B. filter.
    C. rheostat.
    D. rectifier.

18. X-ray equipment capable of producing 70 kVp or more is required to have total filtration of at least:
    A. 0.5 mm aluminum equivalents (Al equiv).
    B. 1.5 mm Al equiv.
    C. 2.0 mm Al equiv.
    D. 2.5 mm Al equiv.

19. The purpose of rotating the anode of the x-ray tube is to:
    A. increase the heat capacity of the anode.
    B. increase the production of x-ray photons.
    C. decrease resistance in the circuit.
    D. decrease the size of the focal spot.

20. Spatial resolution is determined by the:
    A. size of the electron stream.
    B. size of the actual focal spot.
    C. size of the effective focal spot.
    D. speed of rotation.

21. Above 70 kVp, what percentage of photons is created by the bremsstrahlung process?
    A. 15%
    B. 30%
    C. 85%
    D. 100%

22. The amount of detail seen in the x-ray image is referred to as:
    A. density.
    B. contrast.
    C. the line focus principle.
    D. spatial resolution.

23. The amount of radiation absorbed in the body during an x-ray exposure is referred to as the:
    A. kVp.
    B. dose.
    C. exposure.
    D. penetrating power.

24. Which of the following are part of the inherent filtration in the x-ray tube?
    1. Oil
    2. Aluminum filter
    3. Pyrex glass envelope
    A. 1 and 2
    B. 1 and 3
    C. 2 and 3
    D. 1, 2, and 3

25. Characteristic radiation is only produced above what kVp?
    A. 65
    B. 70
    C. 75
    D. 80

Answer the following questions.

1. Describe the element tungsten. List two reasons why it is a good material for x-ray tube targets and at least one reason why it is used for x-ray tube filaments.

_____

_____

_____

Tube targets:

1. _____

2. _____

Tube filaments:

1. _____

2. What is meant by *thermionic emission*, and what is its purpose in the x-ray tube?

_____

_____

3. What is meant by the term *heterogeneous*, and what type of target interaction produces heterogeneous radiation?

_____

_____

4. What does a dual-focus tube have that a single-focus tube does not?

_____

5. How much target angulation is needed in a general-purpose tube? Why?

_____

_____

6. What is the effect on the x-ray beam if the kVp is increased?

_____

7. Why might it be desirable to increase mA? Why might it be undesirable?

_____

_____

8. An exposure is made using 100 mA and 0.25 sec. What is the value of the mAs? State another combination of mA and time that will produce the same quantity of exposure.

_____

_____

9. If the x-ray tube has 0.5 mm Al equiv inherent filtration, and the collimator provides an additional 1.25 mm Al equiv, how much additional filtration must be added to meet minimum safety requirements?

_____

10. What is the standard rotation speed of the x-ray tube's anode?

_____

11. What is the percentage of characteristic radiation that is produced below 70 kVp?

_____

12. What is the difference in radiation intensity between the anode and cathode ends of the x-ray beam when a 14- × 17-inch IR is used at a 40-inch SID (state in percentage)?

_____

13. The primary purpose of filtration is to:

_____

14. Name the three components of the x-ray tube that contribute to the inherent filtration.

1. _____

2. _____

3. _____

15. If a patient has a body part that has a very thick portion and a very thin portion, which aspect of the x-ray tube should be placed over the thinnest area?

_____

16. Describe *dose* as it applies to x-rays.

_____

EXERCISE 3

Label the following drawings.

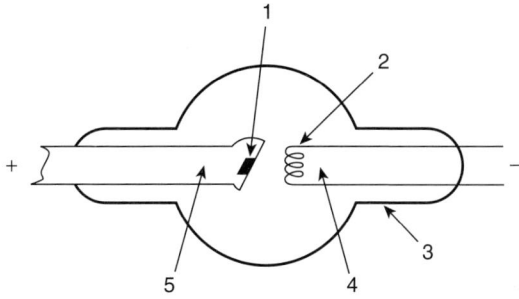

Fig. 5.1 Simple x-ray tube.

1. _____

2. _____

3. _____

4. _____

5. _____

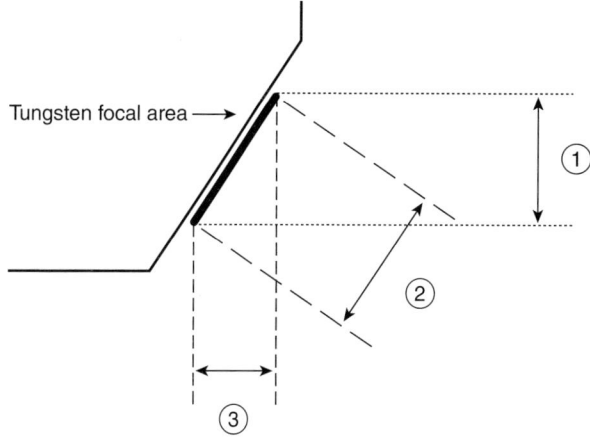

Tungsten focal area

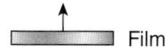

Film

Fig. 5.2 Effective focal spot.

1. _____

2. _____

3. _____

EXERCISE 4

Find the mAs for each of the technical factors below.

1. 20 mA × 1.00 sec = _____ mAs

2. 10 mA × 0.50 sec = _____ mAs

3. 100 mA × 0.75 sec = _____ mAs

4. 50 mA × 1.50 sec = _____ mAs

Determine the mA for each of the mAs values below.

5. 100 mAs = _____ mA × 2.00 sec

6. 200 mAs = _____ mA × 0.50 sec

7. 300 mAs = _____ mA × 1.50 sec

8. 75 mAs = _____ mA × 0.75 sec

Find the seconds for each of the mAs and mA values below.

9. 100 mAs = 100 mA × _____ sec

10. 200 mAs = 400 mA × _____ sec

11. 500 mAs = 250 mA × _____ sec

12. 300 mAs = 400 mA × _____ sec

CHALLENGE EXERCISE

This exercise does not have to be completed at the same time as the other exercises in this workbook chapter. The exercise is designed to assess the retention of the essential information contained in the corresponding textbook chapter. It is recommended that you complete this exercise when you begin to study for the state limited licensure examination. This will help determine what you know and which information should be further reviewed.

1. Of what material is the filament made?

   _____

2. Of what material is the target/anode made?

   _____

3. What is added to the port to remove the long-wavelength radiation?

   _____

4. What is the term used to describe the heating of an element to a hot temperature and the expanding of the electrons in the atom?

   _____

5. Is the cathode side of the x-ray tube positive or negative?

   _____

6. Is the anode side of the x-ray tube positive or negative?

   _____

7. What is the purpose of having a "high-speed" anode?

   _____

8. What are the two rotation speeds for the anode?

   _____

9. What type of radiation production makes up the greatest portion of the x-ray beam bremsstrahlung or characteristic?

_____

10. Characteristic radiation is not produced below which kVp level?

_____

11. The majority of the energy in the x-ray tube is converted to:

_____

12. What is the name of the radiation produced when an incoming electron into the anode is suddenly braked and deviated?

_____

13. The degree of angulation of the x-ray tube target (anode) will determine the:

_____.

14. How is the volume or intensity of x-rays affected by the heel effect?

_____

15. To take advantage of the heel effect on a body part that has both a thick area and a thin area, where should the cathode be placed?

_____

16. The power and speed of the electrons inside the x-ray tube and the energy of the x-rays that emerge are controlled by the:

_____.

17. The current, or volume, of x-ray production is measured in units of:

_____.

18. The mA or mAs used for an exposure determines the:

_____.

19. The penetrating power of the x-ray beam is controlled by the:

_____.

20. Name two characteristics of tungsten.

_____

21. How much aluminum filtration must be in the x-ray tube to meet government standards?

_____

22. What is the advantage of using aluminum filtration in the port of the x-ray tube?

_____

23. Name the three components that make up the inherent filtration.

_____

24. The amount of detail or resolution seen in the radiographic image is referred to as:

_____.

25. What type of motor is used to turn the anode inside the x-ray tube?

_____

26. When is the large focal spot used?

_____

27. The anode heel effect is most pronounced when using which size of IR?

_____

28. The target angle directly affects the:

_____.

6 X-ray Circuit and Tube Heat Management

Answer the following questions by selecting the best choice.

1. When using automatic exposure control (AEC), the density of the image can be adjusted up or down using which of the following devices?
   A. Density control
   B. Anatomically programmed radiography (APR)
   C. Milliamperage button
   D. Backup timer

2. The autotransformer's primary purpose is to vary the:
   A. voltage.
   B. amperage.
   C. exposure time.
   D. high frequency.

3. Which transformer is located in the filament circuit?
   A. Rectifier
   B. Step-up transformer
   C. Step-down transformer
   D. Autotransformer

4. The primary purpose of the filament circuit is to:
   A. control the exposure time.
   B. supply voltage to the x-ray tube.
   C. heat the x-ray tube filament for thermionic emission.
   D. supply power to the autotransformer.

5. A timer that is capable of producing ultrashort exposure times is typical of a(n):
   A. electronic timer.
   B. synchronous timer.
   C. mechanical timer.
   D. phototimer.

6. The primary purpose of a rectifier in an x-ray circuit is to:
   A. vary the peak kilovoltage (kVp).
   B. vary the milliamperes (mA).
   C. measure current in the x-ray tube.
   D. change alternating current (AC) into direct current (DC).

7. The primary purpose of the high-voltage circuit is to:
   A. vary the kVp in the x-ray tube.
   B. supply the x-ray tube with voltage high enough to produce x-rays.
   C. change AC into DC.
   D. increase the frequency from 60 hertz (Hz) to 6000 Hz.

8. The advantages of using a high-frequency (HF) generator are they:
   1. produce x-rays more efficiently.
   2. require less exposure time to produce a given amount of exposure.
   3. produce the greatest amount of x-rays for the same exposure technique.
   A. 1 and 2
   B. 1 and 3
   C. 2 and 3
   D. 1, 2, and 3

9. When using AEC, the *backup timer* must be set to:
   1. maintain an optimal density image.
   2. not overexpose the patient.
   3. prevent damage to the x-ray tube.
   A. 1 and 2
   B. 1 and 3
   C. 2 and 3
   D. 1, 2, and 3

10. AEC automatically varies the:
    A. mA.
    B. kVp.
    C. exposure time.
    D. mA and kVp.

11. Public Law 90-602 states that x-ray generators must terminate the exposure at _____ for exposures above 50 kVp.
    A. 200 mAs
    B. 600 mAs
    C. 1.0 sec
    D. 2.5 sec

12. Which of the following steps should be used to extend x-ray tube life?
    1. Warm up the anode.
    2. Use high mA settings.
    3. Do not make repeated exposures near the tube limits.
    A. 1 and 2
    B. 1 and 3
    C. 2 and 3
    D. 1, 2, and 3

13. How many heat units (HUs) are generated using a high-frequency generator at 200 mA, 0.10 sec, and 85 kVp?
    A. 1700 HUs
    B. 2295 HUs
    C. 2380 HUs
    D. 3640 HUs

14. For which type of x-ray exposure system can the technical factors be programmed into the system?
    A. Manual exposure techniques
    B. Automatic exposure control
    C. APR
    D. High-frequency system

15. Which transformer is located in the high-voltage circuit?
    A. Step-down transformer
    B. Step-up transformer
    C. Autotransformer
    D. Rectifier

16. The *backup timer* must be set at _____ of the anticipated x-ray exposure.
    A. 25%
    B. 50%
    C. 75%
    D. 150%

17. In a high-frequency x-ray generator, the standard 60-Hz frequency is increased to about:
    A. 1000 Hz.
    B. 3000 Hz.
    C. 6000 Hz.
    D. 7000 Hz.

18. The anode in the x-ray tube can crack if one of the following occurs:
    A. the mAs is too high.
    B. the kVp is too high.
    C. the tube is not warmed up properly.
    D. exposures are made too fast.

19. (True/False) There are three detectors in an AEC system.

20. (True/False) The *backup timer* should be set to 0.50 sec.

21. (True/False) The shortest exposure times are obtained using high-frequency generators.

22. (True/False) The heat unit (HU) formula for a high-frequency (HF) x-ray generator is:

$$HU = mA \times Time \times kVp \times 1.40$$

23. (True/False) The exposure switch should be mounted to the generator with a minimum two-foot cord.

EXERCISE 2

Match the components listed below with one of the three following circuits.

1. Low-voltage circuit

2. Filament circuit

3. High-voltage circuit

A. _____ Rectifier unit   D. _____ X-ray tube

B. _____ AC power supply   E. _____ Step-down transformer

C. _____ Step-up transformer   F. _____ Autotransformer

Answer the following questions.

1. Name at least five ways that x-ray tube life can be extended.

    1. _____

    2. _____

    3. _____

    4. _____

    5. _____

2. What is the primary purpose of the autotransformer?

    _____

    _____

    _____

3. State two reasons a *backup timer* is needed on the x-ray generator.

    1. _____

    2. _____

4. What is the range of kVp values used in x-ray generators?

    _____

5. List two advantages of using a high-frequency (HF) x-ray generator.

    1. _____

    2. _____

6. State, in order, the four steps for making an x-ray exposure after the control panel has been set.

    1. _____

    2. _____

    3. _____

    4. _____

7. Name two things that occur when the rotor switch is activated.

    1. _____

    2. _____

8. Name at least three features of an x-ray tube that are designed for handling high heat.

    1. _____

    2. _____

    3. _____

9. To ensure that x-ray tubes will last a long time, the maximum heat capacity should remain below:

    _____.

10. Public Law 90-602 states x-ray generators must terminate the exposure at:

    _____.

11. Where is the center automatic exposure control (AEC) detector located on a three-detector system?

    _____

12. The small focal spot is used when mA stations below _____ mA are used.

13. Name the three transformers in an x-ray machine.

    1. _____

    2. _____

    3. _____

14. Name at least five technical factors that are automatically set when using APR.

    1. _____

    2. _____

    3. _____

    4. _____

    5. _____

15. What is the purpose of the *backup timer*?

    _____

16. What will happen if there is an excessive exposure on a cold x-ray tube?

    _____

17. How many exposures should be made to adequately warm up the x-ray tube?

    _____

18. When using an AEC system for the exposure technique, positioning to the wrong anatomy or overcollimating can lead to:

    _____.

19. When using an AEC system for exposure technique, what must be absolutely accurate to avoid a repeat x-ray?

    _____

CHALLENGE EXERCISE

This exercise does not have to be completed at the same time as the other exercises in this workbook chapter. The exercise is designed to assess retention of the essential information contained in the corresponding textbook chapter. It is recommended that you complete this exercise when you begin to study for the state limited licensure examination. This will help determine what you know and which information should be further reviewed.

1. What are the names of the three x-ray circuits?

   _____

   _____

   _____

2. What is the purpose of the autotransformer?

   _____

3. What is the purpose of the filament circuit?

   _____

4. What is the purpose of the high-voltage circuit?

   _____

5. Name the three transformers used in the x-ray circuit.

   _____

   _____

   _____

51

6. In which circuit is the step-down transformer located?

_____

7. In which circuit is the step-up transformer located?

_____

8. The process of changing AC current to DC current is called:

_____.

9. How many exposures should be made to adequately warm up an x-ray tube?

_____

10. What will happen if there is an excessive exposure to a cold x-ray tube?

_____

11. Name the three types of x-ray generators.

_____

_____

_____

12. What is the purpose of the *backup timer*?

_____

13. How many detectors are there in an AEC system?

_____

14. The most common x-ray generator used today is the:

_____.

15. Which x-ray generator is considered the most efficient at producing x-rays?

_____

16. The standard 60-Hz frequency of an electric current is brought up to what level in a high-frequency x-ray generator?

_____

17. Name four advantages of using high-frequency (HF) generators.

_____

_____

_____

_____

18. The most common type of x-ray exposure timer is the:

_____.

19. Which exposure control system requires that the kVp, mA, and exposure time be individually selected?

_____

20. With automatic exposure control, which technical factor is automatically selected?

_____

21. When using automatic exposure control (AEC) for the exposure, what must be absolutely accurate to ensure that a correct exposure will occur?

_____

22. If overcollimation occurs when using automatic exposure control, and the primary beam reaches the detector without going through the body part, the resultant image will be:

_____.

23. When using anatomically programmed radiography (APR) for the exposure technique, what technical factors are automatically set?

_____

24. According to the Federal law, x-ray exposures must be terminated at:_____

_____.

25. What is the formula for determining a heat unit (HU)?

_____

26. Calculate a HU for an x-ray technique of 300 mA, 65 kVp, 0.10 sec for a high-frequency generator.

_____

27. X-ray tubes will last longer if they are operated at what capacity or less?

   _____

28. The electronic timers used today can make exposure times as low as:

   _____.

29. Describe how warm-up x-ray exposures should be made.

   _____

30. List five recommendations for prolonging x-ray tube life.

   1. _____

   2. _____

   3. _____

   4. _____

   5. _____

31. When using an AEC system for exposure technique, what must be absolutely accurate to avoid a repeat x-ray?

   _____

7 Principles of Exposure and Image Quality

EXERCISE 1

Answer the following questions by selecting the best choice.

1. The unit used to indicate the total quantity of x-rays in an exposure is:
   A. milliampere-seconds (mAs).
   B. seconds (sec).
   C. peak kilovoltage (kVp).
   D. milliamperes (mA).

2. Which of the following will result in increased radiographic brightness (density)?
   1. Increased mA
   2. Increased exposure time
   3. Decreased source-image receptor distance (SID)
   A. 1 and 2
   B. 1 and 3
   C. 2 and 3
   D. 1, 2, and 3

3. The mass density of the body part is referred to as:
   A. tissue density.
   B. radiographic density.
   C. radiographic contrast.
   D. subject contrast.

4. The primary controller of radiographic density is:
   A. SID.
   B. object-image receptor distance (OID).
   C. mAs.
   D. kVp.

5. The difference in radiographic density between any two adjacent portions of the image is called:
   A. tissue density.
   B. spatial resolution.
   C. contrast.
   D. distortion.

6. The primary factor controlling radiographic contrast and x-ray penetration is:
   A. mA.
   B. exposure time.
   C. mAs.
   D. kVp.

7. High contrast produced by using low kVp results in an image with:
   A. a long scale of contrast.
   B. a short scale of contrast.
   C. overpenetration.
   D. unsharpness.

8. Generalized unwanted exposure on the image is called:
   A. overexposure.
   B. overpenetration.
   C. fog.
   D. a long scale of contrast.

9. A decrease in SID will result in:
   A. increased magnification.
   B. underexposure.
   C. loss of contrast.
   D. decreased radiographic density.

10. A misrepresentation in the size or shape of the structure being examined is called:
    A. fog.
    B. distortion.
    C. unsharpness.
    D. spatial resolution.

11. The "fuzzy" unsharpness at the edges of structures or body parts is called:
    A. fog.
    B. distortion.
    C. umbra.
    D. penumbra.

12. The smaller the effective focal spot, the _____ the penumbra, and the _____ the spatial resolution.
    A. less, less
    B. less, greater
    C. greater, greater
    D. greater, less

13. When a large OID is used, spatial resolution can be improved by:
    1. decreasing the SID.
    2. increasing the SID.
    3. maintaining the small focal spot.
    A. 1 and 2
    B. 1 and 3
    C. 2 and 3
    D. 1, 2, and 3

14. Fog affects radiographic quality by causing:
    A. decreased contrast.
    B. underexposure.
    C. increased contrast.
    D. distortion.

15. Motion of the patient, either voluntary or involuntary, during the exposure will result in decreased:
    A. contrast.
    B. distortion.
    C. radiographic density.
    D. spatial resolution.

16. A term used to describe a grainy or mottled image is:
    A. umbra.
    B. distortion.
    C. quantum mottle.
    D. penumbra.

17. One means of controlling distortion is by controlling the:
    A. focal spot.
    B. motion.
    C. part position.
    D. quantum mottle.

18. The factors that affect the quantity of x-rays in the x-ray beam are:
    1. mAs.
    2. kVp.
    3. APR.
    A. 1 and 2
    B. 1 and 3
    C. 2 and 3
    D. 1, 2, and 3

19. Which of the following will affect the quality of the x-ray beam?
    A. mAs
    B. kVp
    C. APR.
    D. automatic exposure control.

20. If the mAs is doubled, the dose to the patient will:
    A. increase by 10%.
    B. double.
    C. increase by a factor of 4.
    D. remain the same.

21. According to the inverse square law, if the SID is doubled (e.g., 40 to 80 inches), the intensity or quantity of x-rays will:
    A. double.
    B. increase by 50%.
    C. be cut in half.
    D. decrease to one-fourth of the original intensity.

22. The principal means of controlling involuntary motion is to:
    A. increase the mA.
    B. increase the kVp.
    C. use a short exposure time.
    D. use a long exposure time.

23. Which one of the following could you use to control spatial resolution?
    A. kVp
    B. Focal spot
    C. Part position
    D. CR angle

24. All of the following are photographic or geometric factors that affect how the x-ray image looks on the monitor, *except*:
    A. kilovoltage.
    B. contrast.
    C. density.
    D. spatial resolution.

25. (True/False) A doubling in kVp would result in four times more x-rays being emitted from the tube.

26. (True/False) If the SID is increased or decreased, the density on the image is not changed.

27. (True/False) If the SID is reduced in half (e.g., 40 to 20 inches), the intensity or quantity of x-rays will increase by four times.

28. (True/False) The contrast on the viewing monitor is adjusted by controlling the window level.

29. (True/False) The sharpness of the radiographic image is referred to as spatial resolution.

30. (True/False) Increased quantum mottle will result in increased spatial resolution.

Match the following terms with the corresponding definitions or descriptions.

1. _____ OID   A. Source-image receptor distance

2. _____ Penumbra   B. Intensity is inversely proportional to the square of the distance

3. _____ Inverse square law   C. Object-image receptor distance

4. _____ SID   D. Result of unequal magnification

5. _____ Size distortion   E. Overall blackness on the image

6. _____ Elongation   F. Magnification of a part

7. _____ Shape distortion   G. Unsharp edges

8. _____ Foreshortening   H. Difference in density between adjacent structures

9. _____ Brightness (density)   I. Object appears shorter

10. _____ Long-scale contrast   J. Object appears longer

11. _____ Contrast   K. Produced by low kVp

12. _____ Short-scale contrast L. Produced by high kVp

13. _____ Quantum mottle   M. Grainy or mottled image

EXERCISE 3

Answer the following questions.

1. Which of the prime factors of exposure are directly proportional to the quantity of exposure?

   _____

2. What unit is used to indicate the total quantity of exposure?

   _____

3. If an exposure is made using 300 mA, 0.3 sec, 85 kVp, and 40-inch SID, what is the value of the mAs?

   _____

4. If the radiographic image is too dark, which exposure factor(s) would you change to solve the problem?

   _____

5. When the goal is to differentiate between tissues that have very similar densities, is a long or short scale of contrast most desirable? Why?

_____

_____

6. What should you do if motion is anticipated in advance of making the exposure?

_____

_____

_____

7. List two possible causes when a radiographic image appears gray and "flat."

    1. _____

    2. _____

8. If a large OID produces an unacceptable loss of spatial resolution, what other factors can be changed to improve the image?

_____

_____

9. When an overall radiographic image appears blurred, what aspect of image quality is affected? Which exposure factor might be changed to solve this problem?

_____

_____

10. List at least three measures that should be taken to prevent voluntary motion during radiography.

    1. _____

    2. _____

    3. _____

11. List at least three factors that will affect radiographic contrast.

    1. _____

    2. _____

    3. _____

12. List the five factors that will affect distortion.

   1. _____

   2. _____

   3. _____

   4. _____

   5. _____

13. List at least five factors that will increase spatial resolution in the radiographic image.

   1. _____

   2. _____

   3. _____

   4. _____

   5. _____

14. Name the four prime factors of radiographic exposure:

   1. _____

   2. _____

   3. _____

   4. _____

15. The digital imaging term for *density* is:

   _____.

16. The brightness of the viewing monitor in digital imaging is adjusted by the:

   _____.

17. Which photographic factor makes the anatomy in the image visible?

   _____

18. What is the name of the tool that is used to simulate different densities on a radiograph?

   _____

19. High contrast can also be called:

   _____.

20. Low contrast can also be called:

   _____.

21. Which two factors affect the subject contrast?

   1. _____

   2. _____

22. Unwanted exposure in the radiographic image is called:

   _____.

23. Radiographic distortion can be categorized in which two ways?

   1. _____

   2. _____

24. Size distortion can be controlled by keeping _____ as low as possible.

25. Unequal magnification of a body part is referred to as:

   _____.

26. What are the two terms used to describe shape distortion?

   1. _____

   2. _____

27. Quantum mottle occurs when:

   _____.

28. Name the four photographic and geometric factors that affect how the x-ray image looks on the computer screen.

   1. _____

   2. _____

   3. _____

   4. _____

CHALLENGE EXERCISE

This exercise does not have to be completed at the same time as the other exercises in this workbook chapter. The exercise is designed to assess retention of the essential information contained in the corresponding textbook chapter. It is recommended that you complete this exercise when you begin to study for the state limited licensure examination. This will help determine what you know and which information should be further reviewed.

1. Name the four "prime" factors of radiographic exposure.

   1. _____

   2. _____

   3. _____

   4. _____

2. Which factors affect x-ray quantity?

   _____

3. Which factors affect x-ray quality?

   _____

4. Milliamperage (mA) affects the:

   _____

5. If the mA, exposure time, or mAs doubles, the number of photons will:

   _____

6. If the mA, exposure time, or mAs doubles, the dose to the patient will:

   _____

7. The unit used to indicate the total quantity of x-rays in an exposure is:

   _____

8. How is the energy of the x-ray beam affected when the kVp is adjusted?

   _____

9. Which technique factors, if adjusted upward, will increase density?

   _____

10. The primary controller of radiographic density is:

    _____

11. A doubling in kVp will result in how many more photons being emitted?

_____

12. Which factor is the primary controller of penetration?

_____

13. Which factor is the primary controller of radiographic contrast?

_____

14. What is the distance between the tube target and the image receptor (IR) called?

_____

15. The inverse square law tells us the relationship between which two factors?

_____

16. If the SID is doubled, what will happen to x-ray intensity or quantity?

_____

17. If the SID is reduced by 50%, what will happen to x-ray intensity or quantity?

_____

18. The typical SIDs used in radiology departments today are:

_____.

19. Define density.

_____

20. Define contrast.

_____

21. Define distortion.

_____

22. Define spatial resolution.

_____

23. The term used to describe a dark image is:

_____.

24. The term used to describe a light image is:

_____.

25. Tissue density refers to:

_____.

26. What is the term used to describe density in the digital environment?

_____

27. How does a decrease in kVp affect contrast? An increase in kVp?

_____

28. What is a penetrometer?

_____

29. Describe short-scale contrast and long-scale contrast.

_____

30. The densities of the tissues within the patient are referred to as:

_____.

31. Contrast is influenced by:

_____.

32. Describe the term *fog*.

_____

33. How does collimation affect fog?

_____

34. When contrast needs to be altered on the viewing monitor, which control is adjusted?

_____

35. Low kVp produces an image with what type of contrast?

_____

36. High kVp produces an image with what type of contrast?

_____

37. Another name for size distortion is:

_____.

38. The distance between the body part and the IR is called the:

_____.

39. Define *elongation*.

_____

40. Define *foreshortening*.

_____

41. What are the five factors that affect spatial resolution?

_____

_____

_____

_____

_____

42. Having unsharp or fuzzy edges of structures in an image is called:

_____.

43. Changing from the small to the large focal spot results in:

_____.

44. An increase in the OID will result in:

_____.

45. Motion of the patient, tube, or IR during the exposure results in:

_____.

46. If an x-ray image is blurred or has motion, which exposure factors are used to correct this?

_____

47. Patient motion can be categorized in what two ways?

_____

_____

48. The first step in avoiding motion is to use:

_____.

49. The principal method of reducing involuntary motion is to:

_____.

50. The technical term for a grainy or spotty image is:

_____.

51. What causes an image to have a grainy appearance?

_____

52. What are two ways to minimize shape distortion?

_____

_____

53. Name three things that will increase spatial resolution.

_____

_____

_____

54. There are four photographic and geometric factors that affect how the x-ray image looks on the computer screen. Those factors are:

_____.

_____.

_____.

_____.

8 Digital Imaging

EXERCISE 1

Match the following terms with their descriptions.

1. _____ Digital imaging

2. _____ Computed radiography (CR)

3. _____ Photostimulable storage phosphor (PSP)

4. _____ Digital radiography (DR)

5. _____ Indirect conversion

6. _____ Direct conversion

7. _____ Postprocessing

A. A "cassette-less" digital x-ray system

B. A "cassette-based" digital x-ray system

C. Means for adjusting any image of a body part with computer software

D. Process in which detectors convert x-ray energy directly into an electrical signal

E. General term for the process of acquiring images of the body using x-rays, displaying them digitally, and viewing and storing them on computers

F. Two-step process in which x-ray energy is converted to light and then to an electrical signal

G. Stores the image of the body part

EXERCISE 2

Match the following terms with their descriptions.

1. _____ Brightness

2. _____ Contrast resolution

3. _____ Quantum mottle

4. _____ Matrix

5. _____ Pixel

6. _____ Spatial resolution

7. _____ Window level

8. _____ Window width

A. Describes x-ray images that are grainy or mottled (spotty), caused when not enough photons reach the detector

B. Ability to distinguish anatomic structures of similar subject contrast

C. A control that adjusts the density in the image

D. A series of thousands of small squares that make up the viewing monitor's active area

E. A control that adjusts the contrast in the image

F. The amount of detail or sharpness of an image as seen on the viewing monitor

G. Used in place of "density" in digital imaging

H. An individual square or picture element in the monitor's active area

67

Answer the following questions by selecting the best choice.

1. Which of the following modalities in radiology produces digital images that can be sent through a computer network?
   1. Computed tomography
   2. Magnetic resonance imaging
   3. Conventional radiography
   A. 1 and 2
   B. 1 and 3
   C. 2 and 3
   D. 1, 2, and 3

2. Which of the following is used in CR to store a digital image?
   A. Laser light
   B. PSP plate
   C. Flat-panel detector
   D. Film or screen cassette

3. Which of the following describes the manual blackening out of the white borders on an image?
   A. Smoothing
   B. Edge enhancement
   C. Modulation transfer function (MTF)
   D. Electronic cropping

4. Which of the following is/are necessary to process a CR image?
   1. Darkroom
   2. CR reader unit
   3. Computer systems with monitors
   A. 1 and 2
   B. 1 and 3
   C. 2 and 3
   D. 1, 2, and 3

5. After an imaging plate is scanned by the CR reader unit, it is erased with:
   A. laser light.
   B. white light.
   C. red light.
   D. fluorescent light.

6. One of the most important aspects of setting the exposure technique when using digital imaging systems is to ensure that which of the following is correctly set on the generator?
   A. kVp
   B. Source-image receptor distance
   C. mA
   D. Exposure time

7. Which of the following is a true statement regarding the use of collimation with digital systems?
   A. At least two sides of collimation should be seen on the image.
   B. No collimation edges should be seen on the image.
   C. At least 1 cm of collimation should be seen on all four sides.
   D. At least 2 cm of collimation should be seen on two of the sides.

8. The erasure process will begin if a CR cassette is opened and the plate is exposed for:
   A. 5 sec.
   B. 10 sec.
   C. 15 sec.
   D. 20 sec.

9. The photoconductor used in DR flat-panel detectors is:
   A. amorphous selenium and silicon.
   B. barium fluorohalide.
   C. solidified copper.
   D. carbon fiber.

10. A major advantage of CR and DR digital imaging systems is:
    A. elimination of repeat images.
    B. higher-contrast images.
    C. the ability to see images very fast.
    D. a lower dose o the patient.

11. The viewing monitor's active area is made up of thousands of small squares called the:
    A. flat panel.
    B. dynamic range.
    C. pixels.
    D. matrix.

12. How many pixels are there in a 1650×1800 viewing monitor?
    A. 2,500
    B. 2,900
    C. 2,500,000
    D. 2,970,000

13. Which matrix below will provide the greatest spatial resolution?
    A. 800×1200
    B. 1650×1800
    C. 1800×2250
    D. 2000×2500

14. The response of the detector to different levels of radiation exposure is termed:
    A. spatial resolution.
    B. the dynamic range.
    C. masking.
    D. the signal-to-noise ratio.

15. The ability of a digital system to convert the x-ray input electrical signal into a useful radiographic image is termed the:
    A. contrast resolution.
    B. spatial resolution.
    C. dynamic range.
    D. signal-to-noise ratio.

16. With direct-conversion DR, the x-ray energy is directly converted to:
    A. light.
    B. light and then an electrical signal.
    C. an electrical signal.
    D. an electrical signal and then a capacitor.

17. Which of the following takes the stored charge in the flat-panel detector and converts it into digital value?
    A. Charged coupled device (CCD)
    B. Analog-to-digital converter (ADC)
    C. Complementary metal oxide semiconductor (CMOS)
    D. Smoothing processor

18. The universally accepted standard for exchanging medical images is termed:
    A. DICOM.
    B. PACS.
    C. SNL.
    D. ALARA.

19. The image management system used in a digital radiology department is called:
    A. PSP.
    B. SNL.
    C. PACS.
    D. DICOM.

20. When using a CR plate, how much of the energy of the latent image is lost if the plate is not processed within 8 hours?
    A. 5%
    B. 10%
    C. 15%
    D. 25%

21. Which of the following will be seen in the x-ray image if either the kVp or the mA is set too low for the projection?
    A. Quantum mottle
    B. Low-contrast resolution
    C. Greater brightness
    D. High signal-to-noise ratio

22. What is the name of the processing technique by which x-ray images can be made sharper and have greatly increased contrast?
    A. Smoothing
    B. Edge enhancement
    C. Shuttering
    D. Rescaling

23. Which of the following artifacts appear along the length of travel on the image due to dust on the light guide?
    A. Fogging
    B. Moiré pattern
    C. Phantom
    D. White line

24. If the image plate is not erased completely, which artifact will appear?
    A. Phantom
    B. Fogging
    C. Light spots
    D. Extraneous line patterns

25. All of the following are digital-related artifacts, *except*:
    A. white line.
    B. phantom.
    C. equalization.
    D. Moiré pattern.

26. A characteristic of the imaging plate (IP) is that it will absorb low-energy scatter radiation. This will result in:
    A. deal pixels.
    B. unwanted radiation fog on the image.
    C. increased contrast in the image.
    D. an increased fill factor.

27. Which of the following properties of DR is superior to CR?
    A. Spatial resolution
    B. Decreased radiation dose
    C. Improved MTF
    D. Improved postprocessing

28. Which of the following are indirect DR detectors?
    1. CCD
    2. CMOS
    3. ADC
    A. 1 and 2
    B. 1 and 3
    C. 2 and 3
    D. 1, 2, and 3

29. Small-size pixels will have decreased pixel pitch. This will result in:
    A. less contrast resolution.
    B. greater artifacts.
    C. greater dynamic range.
    D. improved spatial resolution.

30. All of the following would be quality control procedures, *except*;
    A. image receptor (IR) inspection and cleaning.
    B. a second CR plate erasure.
    C. monitor cleaning.
    D. flat-panel detector calibration.

31. The SMPTE or AAPM test pattern used to check the monitor can detect which of the following problems?
    1. Dynamic range
    2. Geometric distortion
    3. Spatial resolution
    A. 1 and 2
    B. 1 and 3
    C. 2 and 3
    D. 1, 2, and 3

32. Which of the following would *not* be a software system used to store records in a hospital?
    A. RIS
    B. ADC
    C. HIS
    D. EMR

33. When anatomy is too large to fit on one 14 x 17-in IR, multiple images can be made. What processing function can merge these images seamlessly into one image?
    A. Smoothing
    B. Image annotation
    C. Stitching
    D. Electronic cropping

EXERCISE 4

Fill in the blanks with the correct word or words.

1. With CR digital systems, the imaging plate is scanned with a(n) _____ after being inserted into the reader device.

2. The phosphor plate inside the CR cassette can be used _____ times before it needs to be replaced.

3. The phosphor that absorbs the x-ray energy in a(n) _____ system is called a *flat-panel detector*.

4. Name at least two major advantages of using CR and DR systems.

    1. _____

    2. _____

5. _____ will occur in digital systems if there are too few photons reaching the IR.

6. In digital imaging environments, the abbreviation *PACS* stands for _____

    _____.

7. _____ should be used for body parts that have extreme differences in tissue density.

8. Because of the wider dynamic range of digital systems, a *slightly* higher _____ setting may be acceptable for radiography projections done using a grid or Bucky.

9. If a CR plate is divided in half and used for two separate exposures, the side not receiving the exposure must always

be _____.

10. The storage phosphors in CR plates are sensitive to _____.

11. With DR, images can be processed and seen in _____ seconds.

12. In digital imaging, unwanted graininess in the image is called _____.

13. With DR indirect conversion, _____ steps are required to process the image.

14. Two postprocessing techniques are:

   1. _____

   2. _____

15. The method for calibrating a particular display system for the purpose of presenting images consistently on different viewing monitors and printers is called the:

   _____.

16. Name at least six artifact patterns seen in digital imaging.

   1. _____

   2. _____

   3. _____

   4. _____

   5. _____

   6. _____

17. The technique that can be useful in viewing very small structures and the fine details of bone is called

   _____.

18. When the x-ray exposure is greater or less than what is needed to produce an image, automatic _____ occurs.

19. Name two types of indirect DR conversion detectors that convert light to an electrical signal.

_____

_____

20. Define "sampling frequency."

_____

21. What is the advantage of having a high "fill factor"?

_____

22. What does the "modulation transfer function" measure?

_____

23. Define "histogram."

_____

24. Define "look-up table" (LUT).

_____

25. Electronic cropping is not a substitute for:

_____.

26. Define the "white line artifact."

_____

27. The amount of x-rays that can be captured by a detector element (DEL) is known as the:

_____.

28. Dust or a foreign material will cause which artifact?

_____

29. Extraneous lines in an x-ray image are caused by electronic noise in the:

_____.

30. Histogram analysis is also used to maintain consistent image brightness despite over- or underexposure to the IR. This is known as:

_____.

31. A negative aspect of using an IP is that it will absorb low-energy scatter radiation. This will create_____ on the x-ray image.

32. Stitching is most commonly done with which x-ray examination?

_____

EXERCISE 5

Fill in the blanks with T or F to indicate whether each of the following statements is true or false.

1. _____ An exposure technique chart is not necessary when using digital imaging systems.

2. _____ With direct-conversion DR, the x-ray energy is converted directly into an electrical signal.

3. _____ Subtraction and contrast enhancement are postprocessing techniques.

4. _____ CR imaging plates should never be split to enable two separate exposures on one plate.

5. _____ CR imaging plates are more sensitive to scatter radiation both before and after exposure to x-rays.

6. _____ When there is a high signal-to-noise ratio, the least amount of information is captured.

EXERCISE 6

Match the following terms with their descriptions.

1. _____ Analog-to-digital converter (ADC)

2. _____ Dead pixels

3. _____ Rescaling

4. _____ Smoothing

5. _____ Edge enhancement

6. _____ Dynamic range

A. A processing technique in which each pixel's frequency is averaged with the surrounding tissue's pixel values. This is done to remove noise, which can be bothersome to the radiologist.

B. Takes the stored charge from the detector and converts it into a digital value.

C. When the x-ray exposure is greater or less than what is needed to produce an image, this processing system is engaged. It is designed to display all the pixels in the area of interest with uniform density and contrast.

D. The response of the detector to different levels of radiation exposure.

E. Occurs when there may be a defect in a component of the computer screen matrix. This may cause a loss of patient information.

F. A processing technique in which images can be made sharper and have greatly increased contrast; however, it does introduce some noise and loss of detail.

CHALLENGE EXERCISE

This exercise does not have to be completed at the same time as the other exercises in this workbook chapter. The exercise is designed to assess retention of the essential information contained in the corresponding textbook chapter. It is recommended that you complete this exercise when you begin to study for the state limited licensure examination. This will help determine what you know and which information should be further reviewed.

1. What is the name of the cassette-based digital imaging system?

   _____

2. The PSP in the CR imaging plate is:

   _____.

3. Imaging plates from digital CR are processed in a(n):

   _____.

4. How many times can a CR imaging plate be used?

   _____

5. How does scatter radiation affect the CR imaging plate?

   _____

6. What type of light source is used in the CR reader unit to release the stored x-ray energy?

   _____

7. What type of light source is used to erase the stored image in a CR imaging plate?

   _____

8. The cassette-less digital imaging system is called:

   _____.

9. A flat-panel detector is used in which digital imaging system?

   _____

10. What is the "white line artifact"?

    _____

11. What is the size of the flat-panel detector in the table of a DR imaging system?

    _____

12. What are the two categories of DR imaging systems?

1. _____

2. _____

13. How long does it take to process a CR or DR image using a general digital system?

_____

14. One of the major advantages of digital imaging systems is the ability to:

_____.

15. What are the two steps in processing an indirect-conversion DR image?

1. _____

2. _____

16. With direct-conversion DR systems, the x-ray energy is converted directly to:

_____.

17. On a digital viewing monitor, the active area of the monitor is called the:

_____.

18. On a digital viewing monitor, each individual picture element square is called a(n):

_____.

19. The amount of detail or sharpness in a digital image is termed:

_____.

20. How many pixels are there in a 1200×1200-matrix viewing monitor?

_____

21. How do smaller pixels affect spatial resolution?

_____

22. How will a larger matrix affect the pixels?

_____

23. The ability of a digital system to distinguish anatomic structures that have a similar subject contrast is termed:

_____.

24. The number of gray shades that an imaging system can produce is termed:

_____.

25. "Noise" in the digital image is referred to as:

_____.

26. The ability of a digital system to convert the x-ray-input electrical signal into a useful image is termed:

_____.

27. How does a greater electrical signal in a digital imaging system affect noise and image quality?

_____

28. What adjustment controls the density or brightness of the digital image on the viewing monitor and printed image?

_____

29. What adjustment controls the contrast of the digital image on the viewing monitor and printed image?

_____

30. What two entities require that exposure technique charts be placed in every radiography room?

1. _____

2. _____

31. The acronym for maintaining optimal image quality and low radiation exposure to the patient is:

_____.

32. One of the most important aspects of setting the exposure technique in digital imaging systems is to ensure that which factor is set correctly?

_____

33. What is the name of the device that takes the stored charge in the detector and converts it into digital values?

_____

34. What are the names of the two types of indirect-conversion flat-panel detectors?

_____

35. The further adjustment of a digital image after it is processed is termed:

_____.

36. The universally accepted standard for exchanging medical images and viewing images from different manufacturers is termed:

_____.

37. The method of calibrating a digital display system so that all images are presented consistently is termed:

_____.

38. Two common postprocessing techniques are:

_____.

39. What causes the quantum mottle artifact in the digital image?

_____

40. What causes the moiré pattern artifact in the digital image?

_____

41. What causes the phantom or ghost image artifact in the digital image?

_____

42. What causes the fogged image artifact in the digital image?

_____

43. What causes extraneous line pattern artifacts in the digital image?

_____

44. The management system used in digital imaging to store and view images is termed:

_____.

45. What types of patient information must be included on every digital image?

_____

46. What technical exposure adjustment can be made to reduce radiation exposure to the patient?

_____

47. What device should be used when imaging body parts that have widely different thicknesses of structures?

_____

48. What types of images from a radiology department are stored in a PACS system?

_____

49. Where should the body part be ideally placed on a CR plate?

_____

50. What device should be available if one CR plate is divided in half for two images?

_____

51. If a digital image appears on the viewing monitor as overexposed or underexposed, what should be checked?

_____

52. How many margins of the collimator should ideally be seen on a digital image?

_____

53. With CR imaging plates, how much of the energy of the x-ray image in the phosphor is lost in 8 hours?

_____

54. Defective pixels are caused by:

_____.

55. What is the name of the processing technique by which images can be made sharper and have greatly increased contrast?

_____

56. What is the name of the technique in which each pixel's frequency is averaged with the surrounding tissue's pixel values in an effort to reduce noise in the image?

_____

57. What is the name of the processing technique that allows x-ray images to be produced with uniform density and contrast, regardless of the amount of exposure?

_____

58. Define "look-up table" (LUT).

_____

59. Define "modulation transfer function" (MTF).

_____

60. What is the "white line artifact"?

_____

61. What is a "histogram analysis error"?

_____

62. Define "electronic cropping."

_____

9 Scatter Radiation and Its Control

EXERCISE 1

Answer the following questions by selecting the best choice.

1. Radiation produced by the photoelectric effect is called:
   A. scattered radiation.
   B. the Compton effect.
   C. secondary radiation.
   D. coherent scattering.

2. Scattered radiation affects the radiographic image by causing:
   1. fog.
   2. reduced contrast.
   3. reduced recorded detail.
   A. 1 and 2
   B. 1 and 3
   C. 2 and 3
   D. 1, 2, and 3

3. Which of the following factors will affect the quantity of scattered radiation fog on a radiograph?
   1. Peak kilovoltage (kVp)
   2. Computed radiography plate
   3. Field size
   A. 1 and 2
   B. 1 and 3
   C. 2 and 3
   D. 1, 2, and 3

4. The most effective method of reducing scattered radiation fog on a radiograph is to:
   A. decrease the object-image receptor distance.
   B. decrease the source-image receptor distance (SID).
   C. increase the kVp.
   D. use a grid or Bucky.

5. As the kVp is increased, the photoelectric effect:
   A. is decreased.
   B. is increased.
   C. remains the same.
   D. remains the same if the kVp is less than 60.

6. As the kVp is increased, the Compton effect:
   A. is decreased.
   B. is increased.
   C. remains the same.
   D. remains the same if the kVp is less than 60.

7. On a radiograph, the appearance of decreased density on the side of the image is most likely caused by the:
   A. grid motion.
   B. grid cutoff.
   C. grid ratio.
   D. grid frequency.

8. A moving grid may be part of a radiographic table or upright unit and is called a:
   A. Bucky grid.
   B. cross-hatch grid.
   C. focused grid.
   D. linear grid.

9. What effect does a thicker or larger body part have on scatter radiation?
   A. There will be greater scatter.
   B. There will be less scatter.
   C. Scatter will remain the same.
   D. Scatter can increase or decrease depending on the atomic number of the part.

10. The central ray alignment quality control (QC) test must show that the alignment is within _____ degree(s) of perpendicular.
    A. 1
    B. 2
    C. 3
    D. 4

11. When a body part is dense or has a greater atomic number scatter radiation:
    A. is increased.
    B. is decreased.
    C. remains the same.
    D. remains the same if the kVp is greater than 60.

12. Which of the following will reduce scatter radiation?
    A. Increase the kVp
    B. Use a smaller field size
    C. Increase the SID
    D. Decrease the milliampere-seconds (mAs)

13. In the diagnostic range of kVp settings (45 to 125 kVp), the majority of scattered radiation will be from which interaction with matter?
    A. Compton effect
    B. Coherent scattering
    C. Photoelectric effect
    D. Characteristic radiation

14. Total absorption of an x-ray photon by the atom of the body part is termed:
    A. the Compton effect.
    B. coherent scattering.
    C. the photoelectric effect.
    D. characteristic radiation.

15. The majority of photons that are scattered will scatter in which direction?
    A. Toward the head
    B. Toward the feet
    C. Back toward the x-ray tube
    D. In a forward direction toward the image receptor (IR)

16. The control limit for the QC test of the collimator on the x-ray tube is:
    A. ±2% of the SID.
    B. ±3% of the SID.
    C. ±4% of the SID.
    D. ±5% of the SID.

17. The principal source of scatter radiation is the:
    A. tabletop.
    B. patient.
    C. grid.
    D. IR.

18. A grid is used when the body part becomes larger than:
    A. 5 cm.
    B. 8 cm.
    C. 10 to 12 cm.
    D. 12 to 14 cm.

19. All of the following factors affect the quantity of scatter, *except*:
    A. volume of tissue
    B. field size
    C. kilovoltage
    D. SID

20. Grid cutoff will occur when the:
    1. tube is off-center.
    2. tube is tilted.
    3. SID is too great.
    A. 1 and 2
    B. 1 and 3
    C. 2 and 3
    D. 1, 2, and 3

21. When performing the QC test of the central ray's beam alignment, the x-ray tube must be within:
    A. 1 degree of perpendicular.
    B. 2 degrees of perpendicular.
    C. ±2% of the SID.
    D. ±3% of the SID.

22. A scattered photon has _____ energy than the incoming primary beam photon.
    A. less
    B. more
    C. less, if the kVp is over 80
    D. more, if the kVp is over 80

23. At what kVp level(s) do Compton interactions occur?
    A. 45 kVp
    B. 50 kVp
    C. 80 to 125 kVp
    D. 45 to 125 kVp

24. If the size of the x-ray field increases, what happens to scatter radiation fog?
    A. It increases.
    B. It decreases.
    C. It remains the same.
    D. It contributes to the dose to the patient.

25. Scatter radiation that is directed from the patient back toward the x-ray tube is called:
    A. backscatter.
    B. forward scatter.
    C. side scatter.
    D. Compton scatter.

26. The number of lead strips per inch is called:
    A. grid radius.
    B. grid ratio.
    C. focal range.
    D. grid frequency.

EXERCISE 2

Fill in the blanks with T or F to indicate whether each of the following statements is true or false.

1. _____ Higher kVp results in more scattered radiation fog.

2. _____ The QC test of the collimator field and x-ray field must show that the two fields are within 2% of the SID.

3. _____ As the kVp is increased, the Compton effect is decreased.

4. _____ As the kVp is increased, the photoelectric effect is increased.

5. _____ The production of scatter results in fog on the radiograph.

6. _____ As collimation is increased, or made larger, scatter radiation fog is decreased.

7. _____ The atomic number of the body part influences the quantity of scatter radiation fog.

8. _____ ↑ *Tissue thickness* = ↑ interactions = ↑ scatter = ↑ fog.

9. _____ The patient is the principal source of scattered radiation in radiography.

10. _____ A grid is placed between the patient and the IR.

11. _____ Compton scatter travels in a forward direction only.

12. _____ Scatter radiation fog reduces the visibility of detail.

13. _____ The standard control limit for the x-ray tube's central ray alignment is that the tube must be mounted so that the beam is within 1 degree of perpendicular.

14. _____ The collimator and the beam alignment must be checked using two separate QC tests.

15. _____ High-ratio grids will require a decrease in exposure technique compared to low-ratio grids or no grids.

EXERCISE 3

Answer the following questions.

1. Which type of radiation interaction produces scattered radiation that is characteristic of the subject irradiated?

   _____

   _____

2. List the two factors that affect the volume of tissue irradiated.

   1. _____

   2. _____

3. When the kVp is increased, will the quantity of scatter radiation fog be increased or decreased? Why?

   _____

   _____

4. What is the principal source of scattered radiation that causes fog in radiography?

_____

_____

5. State the four factors that directly affect the quantity of scatter radiation fog.

1. _____

2. _____

3. _____

4. _____

6. The *primary* scatter consideration is the:

_____.

7. Why is there less scatter radiation with a body part that is more dense or has a higher atomic number?

_____

8. One of the most important things a limited operator can do to control scatter radiation is to:

_____.

9. What are the names of the two test tools used to perform a QC check of the collimator and the central ray alignment?

_____

_____

10. What happens to the incoming x-ray photon when the Compton effect is occurring?

_____

11. What happens to the incoming x-ray photon during the photoelectric effect?

_____

12. What prevents the lead strips in the grid from showing on the x-ray image?

_____

13. As the kVp is increased, the photoelectric effect will:

_____.

14. A grid must be used when the kVp set on the generator is greater than:

_____.

15. If the volume of tissue increases, the amount of scatter radiation fog will:

_____.

16. Grids with lead strips that are aligned to coincide with the primary beam angle are called:

_____.

17. What effect do grids have on dose to the patient?

_____

CHALLENGE EXERCISE

This exercise does not have to be completed at the same time as the other exercises in this workbook chapter. The exercise is designed to assess retention of the essential information contained in the corresponding textbook chapter. It is recommended that you complete this exercise when you begin to study for the state limited licensure examination. This will help determine what you know and which information should be further reviewed.

1. The two main types of interactions that occur when radiation is absorbed by matter are:

   1. _____.

   2. _____.

2. Compton scatter leaves the body in what directions?

   _____

3. Scatter radiation that is directed back toward the x-ray tube is termed:

   _____.

4. Most of the photons that scatter will scatter in which specific direction?

   _____

5. What happens to the x-ray photon during the Compton effect?

   _____

6. What happens to the x-ray photon during the photoelectric effect?

   _____

7. What happens to the energy of the photon when it is scattered?

_____

8. When the kVp is increased, the Compton scatter is:

_____.

9. When the kVp is increased, the photoelectric effect is:

_____.

10. The production of scatter radiation during an exposure results in what effect on the x-ray image?

_____

11. Name the four primary factors that directly affect the quantity of scatter radiation fog:

   1. _____

   2. _____

   3. _____

   4. _____

12. The primary consideration that affects the volume of scatter radiation is the:

_____.

13. How is scatter affected when the body part is thicker or larger?

_____

14. Fog on the radiograph becomes objectionable when the body part size is larger than:

_____.

15. What is the effect of increased kVp on scatter radiation fog?

_____

16. How is scatter affected when a body part is very dense or has a high atomic number?

_____

17. One of the most important things a limited operator can do to control scatter radiation is:

    _____.

18. The principal method of reducing scatter radiation fog is to use which device?

    _____

19. Name three strategies that can be used to reduce scatter radiation fog.

    1. _____

    2. _____

    3. _____

20. A grid is typically used when the body part size and kVp reach:

    _____.

21. What does decreasing collimation do to the contrast in the image?

    _____

22. When fog prevents specific details from being seen in the image, what type of image may be requested?

    _____

23. Name the two QC tests that are done regularly to check the collimator's light field size and the central ray alignment.

    1. _____

    2. _____

24. Name the test tools used to check the collimator's light field and also the central ray alignment.

    1. _____

    2. _____

25. The control limit for the collimator's light field and the actual radiation field must be within:

    _____.

26. The control limit for the x-ray tube's beam alignment is that the beam must be within:

    _____.

10 Formulating X-ray Techniques

EXERCISE 1

Answer the following questions by selecting the best choice.

1. A technique chart provides the following information:
   1. Milliamperage (mA).
   2. Peak kilovoltage (kVp).
   3. Source-image receptor distance (SID).
   A. 1 and 2
   B. 1 and 3
   C. 2 and 3
   D. 1, 2, and 3

2. Which of the following methods is an effective way to obtain a technique chart?
   1. Have each x-ray operator write down the techniques for 1 week.
   2. Request assistance from the imaging manufacturer's technical representative.
   3. Hire a radiologic technologist who can provide technique chart preparation.
   A. 1 and 2
   B. 1 and 3
   C. 2 and 3
   D. 1, 2, and 3

3. Technique charts are based on patient part measurements obtained using an x-ray caliper. These measurements are expressed as:
   A. depth, in inches.
   B. circumference, in inches.
   C. thickness, in centimeters.
   D. diameter, in millimeters.

4. The kVp that is sufficient to penetrate the body part adequately without excess exposure to the patient is called:
   A. fixed kVp.
   B. optimum kVp.
   C. variable kVp.
   D. manual kVp.

5. Which statement regarding technique charts is true? Technique charts are:
   A. the same for every radiology department.
   B. the same for every x-ray machine within a radiology department.
   C. unique, depending on the image receptor used, the grid ratio, and the SID.
   D. unique to each x-ray machine and each facility.

6. Which of the following may be a cause of technique chart failure?
   A. Incorrect mA station selection
   B. Excessive exposure time
   C. Insufficient exposure time
   D. kVp level not optimum to penetrate the part

7. The advantages of using a variable kVp (fixed mA) technique chart are:
   1. lower subject contrast.
   2. improved visibility of the spatial resolution.
   3. the ability to make small incremental changes in exposure technique.
   A. 1 and 2
   B. 1 and 3
   C. 2 and 3
   D. 1, 2, and 3

8. How much of a change in mAs is needed if there is a 2-cm increase in the part size?
   A. 20%
   B. 25%
   C. 30%
   D. 40%

9. When an image is too light, what is usually the best technique adjustment for the repeat image?
   A. Double the mAs (100% increase)
   B. Reduce the mAs (reduce 50%)
   C. Increase the kVp 15%
   D. Decrease the kVp 15%

10. Which technical factor should be used to correct problems with radiographic brightness (density)?
    A. mA
    B. kVp
    C. mAs
    D. Exposure time

11. The official organization that accredits hospitals and clinics and requires technique charts is:
    A. the Joint Commission.
    B. the American Registry of Radiologic Technologists.
    C. the American Society of Radiologic Technologists.
    D. the State Hospital Association.

12. When the kVp is adjusted what characteristic is primarily seen in the radiographic image?
    A. Density
    B. Contrast
    C. Spatial resolution
    D. Distortion

13. How much does the mAs have to be changed to see a visible shift in the image brightness (density)?
    A. 5%
    B. 10%
    C. 25%
    D. 30%

14. All of the following x-ray projections can benefit from the use of compensating filters, *except*:
    A. AP thoracic spine.
    B. Axiolateral hip.
    C. AP skull.
    D. AP foot.

15. Which type of technique chart has a specific mAs value for each projection and uses small changes in kVp to compensate for variances in the patient's part size?
    A. Fixed kVp (variable mAs)
    B. Variable kVp (fixed mAs)
    C. Fixed SID
    D. Variable SID

16. If the kVp is increased using the "15% rule," an 80-kVp exposure would be changed to which of the following?
    A. 68 kVp
    B. 92 kVp
    C. 105 kVp
    D. 160 kVp

17. Which of the following body parts would benefit from the use of a compensating filter?
    A. AP thoracic spine
    B. AP abdomen
    C. AP cervical spine
    D. AP skull

18. Which category of patients seldom requires a compensating filter for general imaging?
    A. Geriatric
    B. Pediatric
    C. Age 18 to 30
    D. Age 30 to 60

19. What is the major limitation in obtaining images of obese patients?
    A. A strong enough table to hold the patient
    B. Reduced resolution due to motion
    C. Inadequate penetration of the body part
    D. Inability to adjust the mAs high enough

20. An major advantage of using a compensating filter for some x-ray projections is that it:
    A. prevents taking two x-rays of the same body part.
    B. reduces contrast in dense body parts.
    C. increases contrast in dense body parts.
    D. saves time in producing the image.

21. When taking an x-ray of a patient with a plaster cast, how should the technique be adjusted?
    A. Double the mAs
    B. Add 10 kVp
    C. Measure the thickness of the cast and add 5 kVp
    D. Measure the thickness of the cast and use the technique from the chart based on the cast measurement

22. If the digital exposure indicator (EI) indicates the exposure is out of range, the repeat image should be made with which of the following changes?
    1. If the exposure is low, double the mAs
    2. If the exposure is high, halve the mAs
    3. If the exposure is either low or high, use the 15% Rule and adjust up or down accordingly
    A. 1 and 2
    B. 1 and 3
    C. 2 and 3
    D. 1, 2, and 3

23. (True/False) Once established on the technique chart, the kVp should never be changed unless the contrast needs to be changed.

24. (True/False) If a compensating filter is used with a body part that has significantly varying tissue density, such as the shoulder in an AP projection, two separate exposures will still have to be made.

25. (True/False) The use of compensating filters can help reduce the entrance skin exposure.

26. (True/False) The major limitation in obtaining images of obese patients is inadequate penetration of the body part.

27. (True/False) The most important adjustment that can be made on an obese patient is the mA.

EXERCISE 2

Indicate the correct mAs for the new SID to maintain brightness (density).

1. If 25 mAs is used at 40 inches, calculate the mAs at 80 inches.

2. If 30 mAs is used at 60 inches, calculate the mAs at 30 inches.

EXERCISE 3

Label the following with an up arrow (↑) to indicate the need for increased technique or a down arrow (↓) to indicate the need for decreased technique.

1. _____ Paget disease

2. _____ Edema

3. _____ Bowel obstruction

4. _____ Pneumonia

5. _____ Ascites

6. _____ Pneumothorax

7. _____ Malignancy

8. _____ Advanced age

9. _____ Degenerative arthritis

10. _____ Gout

11. _____ Atelectasis

12. _____ Chronic obstructive pulmonary disease (COPD)

13. _____ Metastases

14. _____ Pleural effusion

EXERCISE 4

Answer the following questions.

1. What is the definition of "optimum kVp"?

   _____

   _____

2. Which tool and which units are used to measure body part thickness for radiography?

   _____

3. Name two advantages of a variable kVp (fixed mA) technique chart.

   1. _____

   2. _____

4. Name two advantages of using a fixed kVp (variable mA) technique chart

   1. _____

   2. _____

5. When imaging a patient, the general rule of thumb for making changes in mAs is to make the adjustments:

   _____.

6. You are about to take a radiograph that requires 10 mAs, and you have decided to use 100 mA. What should the exposure time setting be?

   _____

7. List two pathologic conditions that require an exposure increase and two that require a decrease.

   Increase:

   1. _____

   2. _____

   Decrease:

   1. _____

   2. _____

8. An acceptable radiograph is made using 200 mA, 0.3 sec, and 70 kVp. Calculate a new exposure technique that will provide lower contrast and less patient dose for the same examination on the same patient.

   _____

9. If a satisfactory radiograph is made using 20 mAs at 40 inches of SID, how many mAs would be necessary to produce a similar radiograph at 72 inches of SID?

   _____

   _____

10. Name three reasons why an exposure technique chart may not work properly.

    1. _____

    2. _____

    3. _____

11. If the mAs has to be changed when an image is too light or too dark the adjustments should be made in increments of:

    _____.

12. When using the "15% rule," a 15% change in kVp will produce approximately the same changes in radiographic brightness (density) as:

    _____.

13. When are compensating filters of value in taking an x-ray of a body part?

_____

14. Name three body parts that have significantly varied tissue density and would benefit from using a compensating filter?

    1. _____

    2. _____

    3. _____

15. What are the particular advantages of using a compensating filter for standing full-spine radiography?

_____

16. Why must you use caution when mounting a compensating filter on the x-ray tube?

_____

17. How is the exposure technique adjusted for a patient with a plaster cast?

_____

CHALLENGE EXERCISE

This exercise does not have to be completed at the same time as the other exercises in this workbook chapter. The exercise is designed to assess retention of the essential information contained in the corresponding textbook chapter. It is recommended that you complete this exercise when you begin to study for the state limited licensure examination. This will help determine what you know and which information should be further reviewed.

1. A listing of the examinations and the exposure factors used for those examinations that must be placed in every room is called the:

_____.

2. What is the name of the organization that provides accreditation for hospitals and clinics?

_____

3. Name several technical factors that must be included on an exposure technique chart.

_____

_____

4. A technique chart that requires every factor to be set individually is called a(n):

_____.

5. An exposure technique chart may not need to be posted for the _____ type of exposure control system.

6. What is the name of the device or tool used to measure patient part size?

_____

7. The kVp can be determined for a technique chart using what two types of kVp settings?

   1. _____

   2. _____

8. What does "optimal kVp" mean?

_____

9. What does the "15% rule" mean?

_____

10. If the digital exposure indicator (EI) indicates the exposure is out of range, the repeat image should be made with which of the following changes?

_____

11. When there is a likelihood of motion in a radiograph, how should the mA and exposure time be set?

_____

12. Name two ways in which an exposure technique chart can fail.

   1. _____

   2. _____

13. Name at least four pathologic conditions that would require an *increase* in exposure factors.

   1. _____

   2. _____

   3. _____

   4. _____

14. Name at least four pathologic conditions that would require a *decrease* in exposure factors.

    1. _____

    2. _____

    3. _____

    4. _____

15. Specialty exposure technique charts must be provided for which two diverse groups of patients?

    1. _____

    2. _____

16. The major limitation in imaging obese patients is:

    _____.

17. What is the most important technical factor adjustment that should be made when imaging obese patients?

    _____

18. What is the minimum change in mAs that will prompt a visible change in image brightness (density)?

    _____

19. When a radiograph needs to be repeated because the original image was too dark or too light, what is the minimum change in mAs that should be made in each case?

    _____

20. What is the formula used if the mAs has to be adjusted because of a change in SID?

    _____

21. What type of body part will require a compensating filter?

    _____

22. Name at least four body parts or x-ray projections for which a compensating filter will help obtain a radiograph of more even density.

1. _____

2. _____

3. _____

4. _____

23. Where are compensating filters placed?

_____

11 Radiobiology and Radiation Safety

EXERCISE 1

Answer the following questions by selecting the best choice.

1. The International System of Units (SI) unit for measuring the *absorbed dose* in the patient is the:
   A. roentgen (R).
   B. gray-$_t$ (Gy-$_t$).
   C. gray-$_a$ (Gy-$_a$).
   D. sievert (Sv).

2. The measuring unit of *exposure* in the SI system is the:
   A. roentgen (R).
   B. gray-$_t$ (Gy-$_t$).
   C. gray-$_a$ (Gy-$_a$).
   D. sievert (Sv).

3. The SI unit used to report the *equivalent dose*, or occupational dose, to radiation workers in the United States is the:
   A. roentgen (R).
   B. gray-$_t$ (Gy-$_t$).
   C. gray-$_a$ (Gy-$_a$).
   D. sievert (Sv).

4. According to the law of Bergonié-Tribondeau, which of the following types of cells would be most radiosensitive?
   A. Skin cells
   B. Nerve and muscle cells
   C. Embryonic tissue
   D. Cortical bone

5. *Short-term* effects of radiation are typically observed within:
   A. 1 day.
   B. 3 days.
   C. 1 month.
   D. 3 months.

6. Which of the following is considered an observable *short-term* effect of radiation exposure?
   A. Cataractogenesis
   B. Carcinogenesis
   C. Mutations
   D. Erythema

7. The reduction of a limited operator's exposure to ionizing radiation can be accomplished by:
      1. decreasing the time in the radiation field.
      2. increasing the distance from the radiation source and scatter.
      3. using exposure techniques with a low—kVp.
   A. 1 and 2
   B. 1 and 3
   C. 2 and 3
   D. 1, 2, and 3

8. The annual *effective dose* limit for a whole-body dose of occupational radiation for nonpregnant workers over the age of 18 is:
   A. 50 mSv.
   B. 500 mSv.
   C. 50 mGy-$_a$.
   D. 500 mGy-$_a$.

9. Which of the following are considered low-dose techniques?
      1. Increasing kVp, decreasing mAs
      2. Using low mA settings
      3. Using a minimum SID of 40 inches
   A. 1 and 2
   B. 1 and 3
   C. 2 and 3
   D. 1, 2, and 3

10. Which of the following changes will decrease the patient dose?
    A. Using low-mA settings
    B. Decreasing the filtration
    C. Using high-kVp techniques
    D. Using a 36-inch SID

11. When radiation exposure occurs during pregnancy, the greatest risk of birth defects occurs when the dose to the uterus exceeds:
    A. 5 mGy-$_t$.
    B. 10 mGy-$_t$.
    C. 15 mGy-$_t$.
    D. 150 mGy-$_t$.

12. All of the following are true about an individual's personal dosimeter, *except* it:
    A. should be worn in the region of the collar.
    B. should be worn inside a lead apron.
    C. should be worn outside a lead apron.
    D. should be worn on the anterior surface of the body.

13. The *radiation weighting factor* for x-ray photons is:
    A. 1.
    B. 2.
    C. 3.
    D. 5.

14. An equivalent *dose* of 0.400 Sv would be converted to _____ mSv.
    A. 4.0
    B. 40
    C. 400
    D. 4000

15. In our everyday work, the *equivalent dose* is used for:
    A. air radiation measurements.
    B. measurements of the x-ray room.
    C. radiation protection purposes.
    D. pregnant occupational workers.

16. The greatest cause of unnecessary radiation exposure to patients that can be controlled by the limited operator is:
    A. motion.
    B. repeat exposures.
    C. use of high-kVp techniques.
    D. use of high-mA techniques.

17. Whenever the gonads are within _____ of the margin of the radiation field, the gonadal dose will be significantly reduced by shielding.
    A. 2 cm
    B. 4 cm
    C. 5 cm
    D. 6 cm

18. A pregnant radiation worker's monthly *equivalent dose* limit is:
    A. 0.3 mSv.
    B. 0.5 mSv.
    C. 1.0 mSv.
    D. 1.5 mSv.

19. A 33-year-old radiation worker would have a *cumulative effective dose* limit of:
    A. 3 mSv.
    B. 30 mSv.
    C. 33 mSv.
    D. 330 mSv.

20. An *erythema* can develop in a patient if the radiation dose to the skin reaches:
    A. 100 mSv.
    B. 1000 mSv.
    C. 2000 mSv.
    D. 2500 mSv.

21. When the dose to the patient is clarified by the *type and energy* of the radiation, it is termed the:
    A. exposure.
    B. absorbed dose.
    C. equivalent dose.
    D. effective dose.

22. Patient dose in radiography is most often calculated according to the exposure level at the:
    A. skin.
    B. gonads.
    C. collar.
    D. exit of the body part.

23. *Short-term* effects of radiation will occur at doses greater than:
    A. 50 mGy-$_t$.
    B. 100 mGy-$_t$.
    C. 250 mGy-$_t$.
    D. 500 mGy-$_t$.

24. In diagnostic radiology, we are most concerned about which effect of radiation exposure?
    A. Somatic effect
    B. Genetic effect
    C. Long-term effect
    D. Short-term effect

25. The LD 50/30, or the lethal dose that would be fatal to 50% of the irradiated population within 30 days, is:
    A. 500 mGy-$_t$.
    B. 2000 mGy-$_t$.
    C. 3000 to 4000 mGy-$_t$.
    D. 5000 to 7000 mGy-$_t$.

26. The greatest percentage of *long-term* effects from radiation exposure will occur:
    A. at 5 years.
    B. at 10 years.
    C. at between 10 and 15 years.
    D. at between 12 and 20 years.

27. Which of the following would be considered a *long-term* effect of radiation exposure?
    1. Cataracts
    2. Life span shortening
    3. Leukemia
    A. 1 and 2
    B. 1 and 3
    C. 2 and 3
    D. 1, 2, and 3

28. When a person becomes sick very fast due to a whole-body dose of radiation in a short period of time, this is referred to as:
    A. linear energy transfer (LET).
    B. acute radiation syndrome (ARS).
    C. somatic effect.
    D. lethal dose.

29. What is the SI unit term for radiation *exposure*?
    A. Effective dose
    B. Dose equivalent
    C. Absorbed dose
    D. Air kerma

30. Which x-ray examinations below would require a gonadal dose?
    1. C-spine
    2. L-spine
    3. Abdomen
    A. 1 and 2
    B. 1 and 3
    C. 2 and 3
    D. 1, 2, and 3

31. The sum of the air kerma over the exposed area of the patient during an x-ray exam is called the:
    A. DAP.
    B. LET.
    C. OER.
    D. ESE.

32. How much of an average annual effective dose of radiation does an individual in the USA receive each year?
    A. 0.2 mSv
    B. 5.5 mSv
    C. 6.3 mSv
    D. 7.0 mSv

33. All of the following will reduce radiation exposure to the patient, *except*:
    A. reduce repeats.
    B. use the smallest radiation field.
    C. use optimal kVp.
    D. use of a grid.

34. (True/False) The standard lead equivalency of the lead aprons used in the radiology department should be a minimum of 0.75-mm lead.

35. (True/False) Radiographers should perform lead apron and glove inspection every 6 months.

36. (True/False) A human who receives an acute whole-body exposure of 6.0 Sv will die.

37. (True/False) The earliest biologic effect that will be seen in the human body after exposure to radiation is nausea and vomiting.

38. (True/False) In diagnostic radiology, the absorbed dose and the equivalent dose are always the same value.

39. (True/False) Younger cells are no more sensitive to radiation than adult cells.

40. (True/False) Long-term effects from radiation exposure are not predictable.

41. (True/False) The greatest risk to a fetus is during the last 3 months of pregnancy.

42. (True/False) LET is the amount of x-ray energy transferred on average, per the length of passage through the tissue.

43. When there is more oxygen in the tissues, they are more sensitive to radiation compared to tissues with low oxygen.

EXERCISE 2

Match the following terms with their definitions or descriptions.

1. _____ Effective dose

2. _____ Gray-t

3. _____ Long-term somatic

4. _____ Air kerma

5. _____ Equivalent dose

6. _____ Carcinogenesis

7. _____ ALARA

8. _____ Mutation

9. _____ Gonad shield

10. _____ Erythema

11. _____ Entrance skin exposure

A. Radiation burn

B. Upper limit of occupational exposure permissible

C. Genetic changes or effects

D. Device to prevent unnecessary radiation to reproductive organs

E. An effect that is not predictable

F. SI unit used to measure absorbed dose

G. Term used to describe absorbed dose based on type and energy of x-ray

H. SI unit of radiation exposure

I. Radiation exposure should be limited to the lowest possible levels

J. Development of malignant disease

K. Exposure at the skin level

EXERCISE 3

Answer the following questions.

1. Name at least four methods that limited operators can use to reduce radiation exposure to patients.

   1. _____

   2. _____

   3. _____

   4. _____

2. A gonad shield must have a lead equivalency of at least:

   _____.

3. The two radiology procedures with the greatest risk for occupational exposures are those involving:

   1. _____

   2. _____

4. Explain the differences between the long-term and short-term somatic effects of radiation.

_____

_____

_____

_____

_____

5. The three principal methods used to protect limited operators from unnecessary radiation exposure are:

1. _____

2. _____

3. _____

6. At what radiation dose level would you see the first signs of a biologic effect? What would that effect be?

_____

_____

_____

_____

7. Name three reasons why the optically stimulated luminescence (OSL) personal dosimeter is the most commonly used dosimeter.

1. _____

2. _____

3. _____

8. What should a limited operator do to minimize the need for repeat examinations?

_____

_____

_____

_____

_____

_____

_____

9. What is meant by low-dose technique?

_____

_____

_____

_____

10. What is the limited operator's responsibility for ensuring that an embryo is not inadvertently exposed to x-rays?

_____

_____

_____

_____

_____

11. What is the primary method used to provide radiation safety for limited operators?

_____

_____

12. What is the lead equivalency of aprons and gloves worn by limited operators?

1. Aprons: _____

2. Gloves: _____

13. What does ALARA mean?

_____

14. Define ionizing *radiation*.

_____

_____

_____

15. Define radiation *protection*.

_____

_____

_____

16. Where should the radiation badge be worn?

_____

_____

17. Genetic effects and mutations are the results of radiation to which part of the body?

_____

18. The average person living in the United States is exposed to an annual dose of how much radiation?

_____

19. Describe the purpose of the control badge that comes with the personal dosimeters.

_____

20. When the genetic effects of radiation occur in a patient, they can potentially be seen in:

_____

_____

21. The largest amount of the annual radiation received from medical examinations comes from:

_____

22. List two x-ray examinations that will give a pregnant woman a higher amount of fetal dose.

_____

23. A pregnant radiation worker should be given a second personal dosimeter. Where should it be worn?

_____

24. If a baby is born with a mutation from having a large amount of radiation while in the mother's womb, the mutation could potentially be:

_____

CHALLENGE EXERCISE

This exercise does not have to be completed at the same time as the other exercises in this workbook chapter. The exercise is designed to assess retention of the essential information contained in the corresponding textbook chapter. It is recommended that you complete this exercise when you begin to study for the state limited licensure examination. This will help determine what you know and which information should be further reviewed.

1. The unit of _radiation exposure_ is the:

_____.

2. The amount of x-rays absorbed by the irradiated tissue, or patient, is called the:

_____.

3. The absorbed dose in the body based on the type and energy of matter is called the:

_____.

4. X-ray photons have a radiation weighting factor of:

_____.

5. The measurement units of *exposure*, *absorbed dose*, and *equivalent dose* are:

    Exposure: _____

    Absorbed dose: _____

    Equivalent dose: _____

6. Convert 0.10 Gy_a to mGy_a.

_____

7. In our everyday work, the *equivalent dose* is used for:

_____.

8. Describe ESE.

_____.

9. The law of Bergonié-Tribondeau tells us what radiation exposure is about?

_____.

10. Name the four characteristics of the law of Bergonié-Tribondeau.

    1. _____

    2. _____

    3. _____

    4. _____

11. Describe the radiation sensitivity difference between a younger patient's cells and an older patient's cells.

_____

12. Describe the radiation sensitivity difference between simple cells and highly complex cells.

   _____

13. Name several cells in the body that would be very sensitive to radiation.

   _____

14. Name several cells in the body that would *not* be very sensitive to radiation.

   _____

15. Name four ways in which radiation effects in the body are classified.

   1. _____

   2. _____

   3. _____

   4. _____

16. Which radiation effect would be seen in about 3 months?

   _____

17. *Long-term* effects from radiation exposure are often referred to as:

   _____.

18. In diagnostic radiology, we are most concerned about which radiation effect?

   _____

19. When radiation damage affects the reproductive cells of the irradiated person, this effect is the:

   _____.

20. An observable *short-term* effect of radiation exposure is called:

   _____.

21. Describe the LD 50/30.

   _____

22. What is the LD for human beings?

   _____

23. How much radiation does the skin have to receive for an erythema to develop?

_____

24. Which effect of radiation exposure is not predictable?

_____

25. Name at least four *long-term* somatic effects from radiation exposure.

1. _____

2. _____

3. _____

4. _____

26. The greatest percentage of *long-term* effects of radiation exposure will be seen in how many years?

_____

27. Which effect from radiation exposure will cause mutations in babies?

_____

28. Which body part should be protected with a lead shield to prevent mutations?

_____

29. Mutations caused by radiation exposure may be seen in a baby as:

1. _____

2. _____

3. _____

30. How much radiation is the average person living in the United States exposed to?

_____

31. Describe the ALARA principle.

_____

32. The greatest cause of unnecessary radiation to patients that can be controlled by limited operators is:

_____.

33. Name four ways in which patients can be protected from unnecessary radiation.

    1. _____

    2. _____

    3. _____

    4. _____

34. Gonad shields are used to reduce the likelihood of:

    _____.

35. The two categories of gonad shields are:

    1. _____

    2. _____

36. Gonad shields must be used when the primary x-ray beam is near the gonads. The dose will be significantly reduced with a shield when the radiation field is within:

    _____.

37. The greatest risks of occupational exposure to radiation occur when the operator is working in which two areas of radiography?

    1. _____

    2. _____

38. The three principal methods used to protect limited operators from unnecessary radiation exposure are:

    1. _____

    2. _____

    3. _____

39. Lead aprons and gloves must have a quality control check every:

    _____.

40. The lead equivalency of aprons and gloves must be:

    Aprons: _____

    Gloves: _____

41. OSL personal dosimeters have what advantages?

    1. _____

    2. _____

    3. _____

    4. _____

42. What is the purpose of the control badge that comes with the department's personal dosimeters?

    _____

43. Where should personal dosimeters be worn?

    _____

44. The upper limit of occupational exposure, as determined by the National Council on Radiation Protection and Measurements (NCRP), is called the:

    _____.

45. The lifetime risk of occupational exposure is referred to as the:

    _____.

46. What is the maximum *effective dose* that an occupational worker can receive in 1 year?

    _____

47. What is the formula for determining the *cumulative effective dose?*

    _____

48. What is the cumulative *effective dose* for a 42-year-old occupational worker?

    _____

49. NCRP studies confirm that a pregnant female exposed to radiation in excess of _____ to the uterus is a cause for concern for the fetus.

50. The greatest risk to a fetus exists during which portion of pregnancy?

    _____

51. The NCRP-recommended monthly *equivalent dose* limit to the embryo or fetus for a pregnant worker is:

    _____.

52. The NCRP-recommended "9-month" *equivalent dose* limit to the embryo or fetus for a pregnant worker is:

_____.

53. When a pregnant worker wears a second personal dosimeter, where is it worn?

_____

54. Describe ARS.

_____

55. Describe LET.

_____

56. What is the effect of oxygen in tissues?

_____

57. Describe why effective communication helps to reduce a dose to the patient.

_____

58. Why are children more vulnerable to radiation than adults?

_____

12 Introduction to Anatomy, Positioning, and Pathology

EXERCISE 1

Answer the following questions by selecting the best choice.

1. The study of diseases that cause abnormal changes in the structure or function of body tissues and organs is called:
   A. anatomy.
   B. physiology.
   C. pathology.
   D. inflammation.

2. How many bones are there in the skeletal system?
   A. 206
   B. 412
   C. 103
   D. 260

3. Bone tissue that has a "honeycomb," or trabecular, structure is called:
   A. cartilage.
   B. marrow.
   C. cancellous tissue.
   D. cortex.

4. All of the following are examples of long bones, *except*:
   A. femur.
   B. humerus.
   C. tibia.
   D. vertebrae.

5. When a limb is moved away from the central part of the body, this motion is called:
   A. extension.
   B. aversion.
   C. adduction.
   D. abduction.

6. A position in which the patient is lying face up is called:
   A. supine.
   B. anatomic.
   C. prone.
   D. lateral decubitus.

7. When the patient is prone or facing the image receptor (IR), the projection will be:
   A. anteroposterior (AP).
   B. posteroanterior (PA).
   C. lateral.
   D. oblique.

8. A disease that is relatively severe and that is characterized by a sudden onset and a short duration is described as:
   A. acute.
   B. chronic.
   C. exogenous.
   D. anomalous.

9. Which of the following are examples of short bones?
   1. Carpal bones
   2. Tarsal bones
   3. Vertebrae
   A. 1 and 2 only
   B. 1 and 3 only
   C. 2 and 3 only
   D. 1, 2, and 3

10. Which one of the following conditions is NOT classified as a neoplasm?
    A. Carcinoma
    B. Sarcoma
    C. Nosocomial disorder
    D. Lipoma

11. A rounded process that forms part of a joint is called a:
    A. crest.
    B. condyle.
    C. cortex.
    D. styloid.

12. A hole in bone that provides a passage for nerves and blood vessels is called a:
    A. foramen.
    B. styloid.
    C. fissure.
    D. sinus.

13. What term is used to describe a straightened joint?
    A. Abduction
    B. Adduction
    C. Extension
    D. Flexion

14. What does the term *cephalad* mean?
    A. Toward the head
    B. Away from the head
    C. The front part of the body
    D. The back part of the body

15. Which plane divides the body into equal right and left halves?
    A. Midcoronal
    B. Midsagittal
    C. Transverse
    D. Axial

16. In radiography, what three items must be precisely aligned?
    A. The x-ray tube, the IR, and the central ray (CR)
    B. The CR, the IR, and the collimator field light
    C. The CR, the body part, and the collimator field light
    D. The x-ray tube, the IR, and the body part

17. What term is used to describe the patient's comments about their perception of the condition?
    A. Symptoms
    B. Signs
    C. Syndromes
    D. Lesions

18. Diseases that occur as the result of treatment by health professionals are termed:
    A. iatrogenic.
    B. idiopathic.
    C. endogenous.
    D. nosocomial.

19. Which disease classification refers to those diseases acquired within the hospital?
    A. Iatrogenic
    B. Idiopathic
    C. Endogenous
    D. Nosocomial

20. Which of the following is the proper medical term for swelling?
    A. Degeneration
    B. Regeneration
    C. Atrophy
    D. Edema

21. Refer to the diagram. What is the patient position?

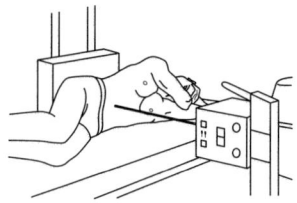

Fig. 12.1 Positioning.

    A. Recumbent left lateral
    B. Recumbent right lateral
    C. Right lateral decubitus
    D. Left lateral decubitus

22. Refer to the image in Question 21. What is the x-ray projection?
    A. AP
    B. PA
    C. Lateral
    D. Tangential

23. Which part of an obese patient's body poses the greatest challenge in imaging?
    A. Skull
    B. Trunk
    C. Limbs
    D. Pelvis

24. Which of the following disease processes causes tissues to waste away?
    A. Idiopathic
    B. Inflammation
    C. Atrophy
    D. Metastasis

25. Name the body plane that divides the body into equal front and back portions.
    A. Horizontal
    B. Transverse
    C. Coronal
    D. Sagittal

Match the following radiographic positioning terms with the correct descriptors.

1. _____ Caudad

A. Movement of the hand toward the lateral side of the wrist.

2. _____ Proximal

B. Outside or referring to the walls of a cavity

3. _____ Lateral

C. Away from the head

4. _____ Plantar

D. Near center of the body or a body part, deep.

5. _____ Visceral

E. To the side, or away from the center

6. _____ Radial deviation

F. Toward the head

7. _____ Internal

G. Pertaining to organs

8. _____ Parietal

H. Away from the source or point of origin

9. _____ Distal

I. Referring to the sole of the foot

10. _____ Cephalad

J. Lower or lower in position

11. _____ Inferior

K. Toward the source or point of origin

Label the fractures in the following figure.

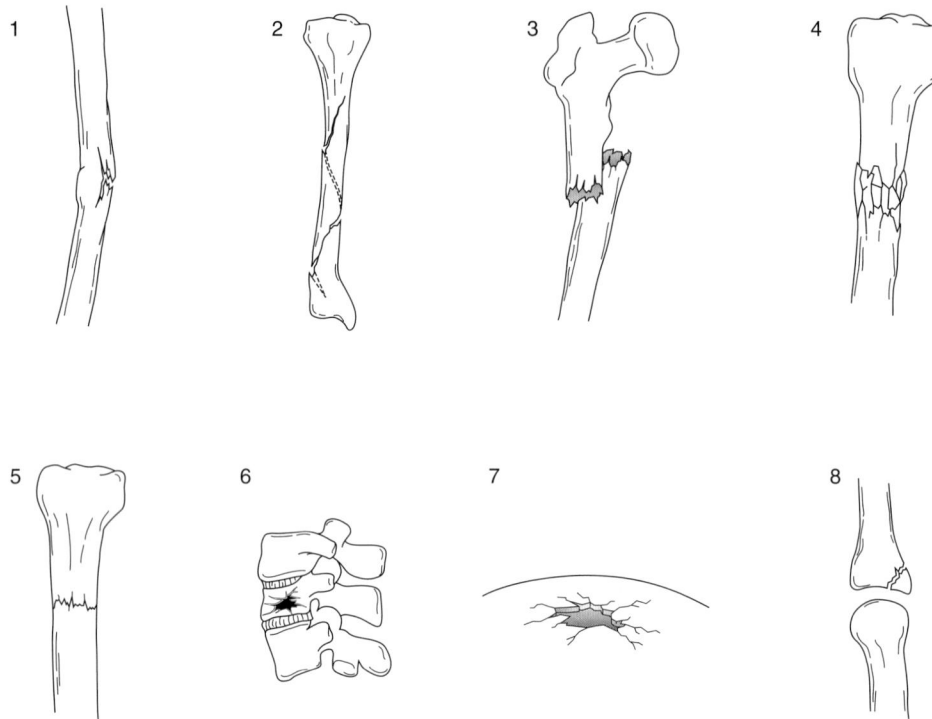

Fig. 12.2 Fractures.

1. _____

2. _____

3. _____

4. _____

5. _____

6. _____

7. _____

8. _____

Answer the following questions.

1. Describe the x-ray projection *tangential*.

   _____

2. Why does imaging part of the trunk in an obese patient pose a great challenge?

   _____

3. Name and describe the three commonly used planes of the body.

   1. _____

   2. _____

   3. _____

4. Describe the term *tuberosity*.

   _____

5. Describe the function of the skeletal system.

   _____

   _____

6. What is the hard, outer portion of most bones called? What is the inner, honeycomb portion called?

   _____

   _____

7. Describe the *midcoronal* plane.

   _____

8. Define the following terms used to describe joint motion:

   Abduction: _____

   Adduction: _____

   Extension: _____

   Flexion: _____

   Pronate: _____

   Supinate: _____

9. Name the joint that is proximal to the hands and distal to the shoulders.

_____

10. What is the radiographic term for a body position in which the patient is lying on the left side?

_____

11. What is the name, and its abbreviation, for the projection in which the CR enters the anterior surface and exits the posterior surface of the body?

_____

12. When the patient is lying on the left side and the CR is vertical, what is the name of the projection?

_____

13. What phase of respiration does the patient hold for chest radiography? For abdominal radiography?

_____

14. For a PA oblique projection of the chest, two oblique positions can be done. Name the two positions.

_____

15. Describe the *axial* projection.

_____

16. When the x-ray tube is angled for axial projections, how is the source-image receptor distance (SID) adjusted?

_____

17. Explain the differences between (1) acute and chronic conditions and between (2) benign and malignant conditions.

_____

_____

18. For oblique projections, how is it determined which side marker, right or left, to use?

_____

19. Which vertebra is located at each of the following landmarks?

    1. Thyroid cartilage: _____

    2. Vertebra prominens: _____

    3. Jugular notch: _____

4. Inferior angles of the scapulae: _____

5. Superior aspect of iliac crests: _____

6. Level of the anterior superior iliac spine: _____

20. (True/False). Electronic markers should never be used in place of lead markers.

21. (True/False). Markers are placed outside the radiation field.

22. (True/False). For AP and PA projections that include both sides of the body, a right marker should be used.

23. (True/False). For lateral projections of the head and truck, the side closest to the IR is marked.

24. (True/False). For decubitus positions of the chest and abdomen, the marker is placed on the side down on the table.

_____

CHALLENGE EXERCISE

This exercise does not have to be completed at the same time as the other exercises in this workbook chapter. The exercise is designed to assess retention of the essential information contained in the corresponding textbook chapter. It is recommended that you complete this exercise when you begin to study for the state limited licensure examination. This will help determine what you know and which information should be further reviewed.

1. Define *anterior* as it relates to radiographic positioning. _____

_____

2. Define *posterior* as it relates to radiographic positioning. _____

_____

3. Define *cephalad* as it relates to radiographic positioning. _____

_____

4. Define *caudad* as it relates to radiographic positioning. _____

_____

5. Define *superior* as it relates to radiographic positioning. _____

_____

6. Define *inferior* as it relates to radiographic positioning. _____

_____

7. Define *internal* as it relates to radiographic positioning. _____

_____

8. Define *external* as it relates to radiographic positioning. _____

_____

9. Define *medial* as it relates to radiographic positioning. _____

10. Define *lateral* as it relates to radiographic positioning. _____

_____

11. Define *proximal* as it relates to radiographic positioning. _____

_____

12. Define *distal* as it relates to radiographic positioning. _____

_____

13. Define *supine* as it relates to radiographic positioning. _____

_____

14. Define *prone* as it relates to radiographic positioning. _____

_____

15. Define *recumbent* as it relates to radiographic positioning. _____

_____

16. Define *upright* as it relates to radiographic positioning. _____

_____

17. Define *decubitus position* as it relates to radiographic positioning. _____

_____

18. Define *lateral position* as it relates to radiographic positioning. _____

_____

19. Define *oblique position* as it relates to radiographic positioning. _____

_____

20. Name the radiographic projection that is described as "the CR enters the anterior surface and exits the posterior surface of the body or anatomic structure."

_____

21. Name the radiographic projection that is described as "the CR enters the posterior surface and exits the anterior surface of the body or anatomic structure."

_____

22. Name the radiographic projection that is described as "that in which the sagittal plane of the body or body part is parallel to the IR."

_____

23. Name the radiographic projection that is described as "that in which the body is rotated so that the CR travels through the body on an oblique plane rather than following an anatomic plane."

_____

24. Name the radiographic projection that is described as "a radiograph taken with a longitudinal angulation of the CR of 10 degrees or more."

_____

25. Name the radiographic projection that is described as "produced by directing the CR to 'skim' the profile of the subject."

_____

26. Describe the *coronal* plane.

_____

27. Describe the *midsagittal* plane.

_____

28. How is the SID adjusted when the x-ray tube is angled for an axial projection?

_____

Chapter **12** **Introduction to Anatomy, Positioning, and Pathology**

29. Where is the side marker placed for decubitus projections?

_____

30. For AP and PA projections of the head and trunk, which side marker is used?

_____

31. Define *acute* and *chronic* conditions.

Acute: _____

Chronic: _____

13 Upper Limb and Shoulder Girdle

EXERCISE 1

Answer the following questions by selecting the best choice.

1. The small, long bones of the digits are called:
   A. metacarpals.
   B. carpals.
   C. phalanges.
   D. epicondyles.

2. The long, narrow bone located anterior to the upper portion of the rib cage and commonly known as the collarbone is the:
   A. humerus.
   B. clavicle.
   C. scapula.
   D. sternum.

3. How many degrees is the coronal plane of the hand rotated for a PA oblique projection?
   A. 15 degrees
   B. 30 degrees
   C. 45 degrees
   D. 45 to 50 degrees

4. The head of the radius articulates with the rounded process of the distal humerus that is called the:
   A. lateral epicondyle.
   B. olecranon process.
   C. trochlea.
   D. capitulum.

5. Why is a stair-step sponge used for a PA oblique projection of the hand, when the fingers are of interest?
   A. Improves patient comfort
   B. Closer proximity of the digits to the image receptor (IR)
   C. Improves visualization of the interphalangeal (IP) joints
   D. More precise degree of obliquity

6. Which aspect of the hand is in contact with the IR for a lateral projection?
   A. Medial
   B. Lateral
   C. Anteromedial
   D. Anterolateral

7. The PA projection of the wrist in ulnar deviation is ordered in cases of suspected:
   A. Colles fracture.
   B. osteoarthritis.
   C. scaphoid fracture.
   D. posterior dislocation.

8. Where is the central ray (CR) directed for finger projections?
   A. Proximal phalanx
   B. Metacarpophalangeal (MCP) joint
   C. Distal IP joint
   D. Proximal IP joint

9. All of the following are important positioning points when performing a lateral projection of the elbow, *except*:
   A. flex the elbow 90 degrees.
   B. place the central ray perpendicular to the region of the lateral epicondyle.
   C. place the coronal plane of the humeral epicondyles perpendicular to the IR.
   D. Stand the patient at the end of the table and lean in.

10. AP projections centered 1 inch inferior to the coracoid process, and with the humerus in both internal and external rotation, will provide an image of the:
    A. scapula.
    B. acromioclavicular joints.
    C. clavicle.
    D. shoulder girdle.

11. When performing a lateral projection of the left scapula with the patient in a PA oblique position, the body would be placed in what position?
    A. RPO
    B. LAO
    C. RAO
    D. LPO

12. Bilateral projections of the shoulders, with and without weights, are used to demonstrate what pathology?
    A. Acromioclavicular separation
    B. Glenohumeral dislocation
    C. Calcific tendinitis or bursitis
    D. Rotator cuff tears

13. An AP axial projection of the shoulder region in which the central ray is directed 30 degrees cephalad is taken to demonstrate:
    A. a fracture of the proximal humerus.
    B. the clavicle.
    C. the glenohumeral articulation.
    D. the acromioclavicular articulations.

14. For an acute shoulder injury, which of the projections below may be ordered by the physician?
    1. AP
    2. Transthoracic lateral
    3. PA oblique (scapular Y)
    A. 1 and 2
    B. 1 and 3
    C. 2 and 3
    D. 1, 2, and 3

15. The most common type of chronic degenerative joint disease that causes hypertrophy of the bone is:
    A. osteomyelitis.
    B. osteochondroma.
    C. osteoarthritis.
    D. osteoma.

16. All of the following accessory devices should be in the x-ray room when performing upper limb radiographs, *except*:
    A. a ruler.
    B. a stair-step sponge.
    C. sandbags.
    D. a 45-degree-angle sponge.

17. The IR, along with the wrist and hand, is placed at what angle for PA projection (Stecher method) of the wrist?
    A. 10 degrees
    B. 15 degrees
    C. 20 degrees
    D. 15 to 20 degrees

18. What is the primary structure demonstrated on a PA axial (Stecher method) projection of the wrist?
    A. Ulna styloid process
    B. Radial styloid process
    C. Scaphoid in lateral position
    D. Scaphoid with minimal foreshortening

19. For a PA oblique projection of the thumb, the hand is placed in what position?
    A. Prone (palmer surface on IR)
    B. Supine (back of hand on IR)
    C. 30-degree lateral oblique
    D. 45-degree medial oblique

20. The CR is directed perpendicular to which body part for projections of the thumb?
    A. 1st MCP joint
    B. Proximal IP joint
    C. Distal IP joint
    D. Body of the proximal phalanx

21. The scaphoid bone is located:
    A. above (posterior) the 1st MCP joint.
    B. behind (anterior) the 1st MCP joint.
    C. directly above (distal) the radial styloid process.
    D. directly above (distal) the ulnar styloid process.

22. The proximal aspect of the ulna has a large, bony process called the:
    A. coracoid.
    B. coronoid.
    C. olecranon.
    D. capitulum.

23. Oblique projections of the elbow will require the arm to be rotated how many degrees?
    A. 20
    B. 30
    C. 45
    D. 40 to 50

24. For a lateral projection of the humerus in the upright position, the elbow is flexed:
    A. 20 degrees.
    B. 25 degrees.
    C. 30 degrees.
    D. 45 degrees.

25. How is the hand positioned for an AP humerus when the patient is in the recumbent position?
    A. Supine
    B. Prone
    C. Natural position
    D. Internally rotated 45 degrees

26. Which prominent aspect of the humerus should be demonstrated in profile on an AP projection, external rotation?
    A. Lesser tubercle
    B. Greater tubercle
    C. Medial epicondyle
    D. Lateral epicondyle

27. Which projection of the shoulder requires the coronal plane of the body to be 35 to 45 degrees from the IR?
    A. AP
    B. AP oblique (Grashey method)
    C. Transthoracic lateral
    D. PA oblique (scapular Y)

28. How far is the top of the IR above the top of the shoulder for a PA oblique (scapular Y) projection?
    A. 1 inch
    B. 1.5 inches
    C. 2 inches
    D. 1.5 to 2 inches

29. What primary structure will be seen on an AP oblique (Grashey method) of the shoulder that tells you the projection was positioned properly?
    A. Glenohumeral joint with open joint space
    B. Glenohumeral joint, posterior aspect
    C. Greater tubercle in profile
    D. Lessor tubercle in profile

30. The AP or PA axial projections of the clavicle require a CR angulation of:
    A. 25 degrees.
    B. 30 degrees.
    C. 15 to 30 degrees.
    D. 30 to 45 degrees.

EXERCISE 2

Label the following illustrations.

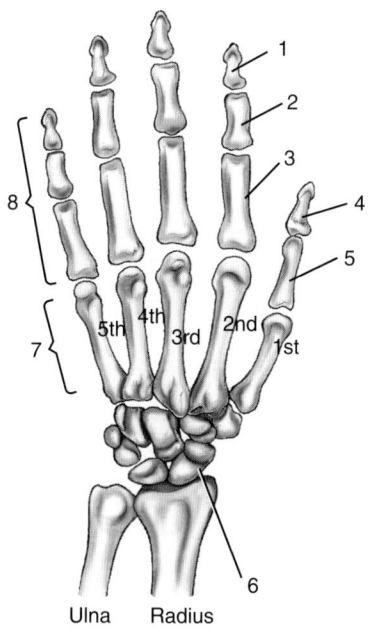

Fig. 13.1 Posterior aspect of the left hand and wrist.

1. _____
2. _____
3. _____
4. _____
5. _____
6. _____
7. _____
8. _____

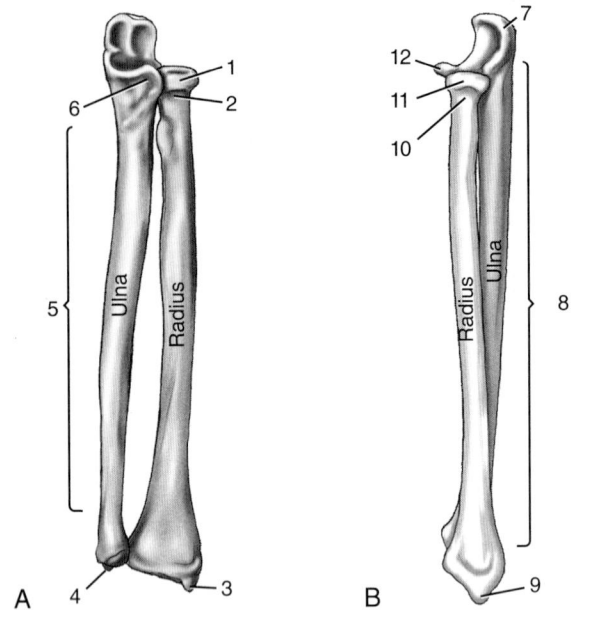

Fig. 13.2 Forearm. (A) Anterior aspect. (B) Lateral aspect.

1. _____
2. _____
3. _____
4. _____
5. _____
6. _____
7. _____
8. _____
9. _____
10. _____
11. _____
12. _____

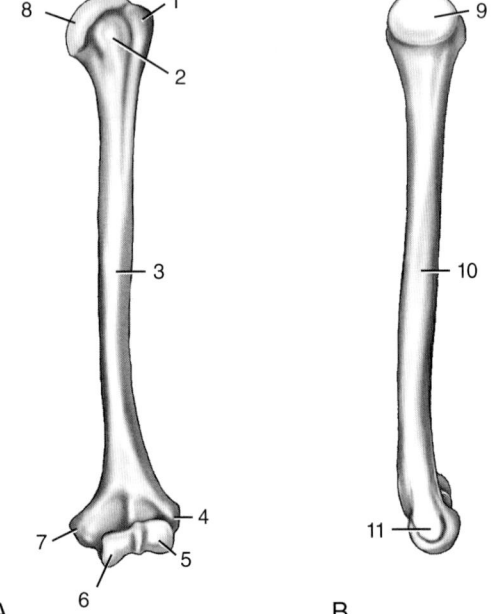

Fig. 13.3 Humerus. (A) Anterior aspect. (B) Medial aspect.

1. _____
2. _____
3. _____
4. _____
5. _____
6. _____
7. _____
8. _____
9. _____
10. _____
11. _____

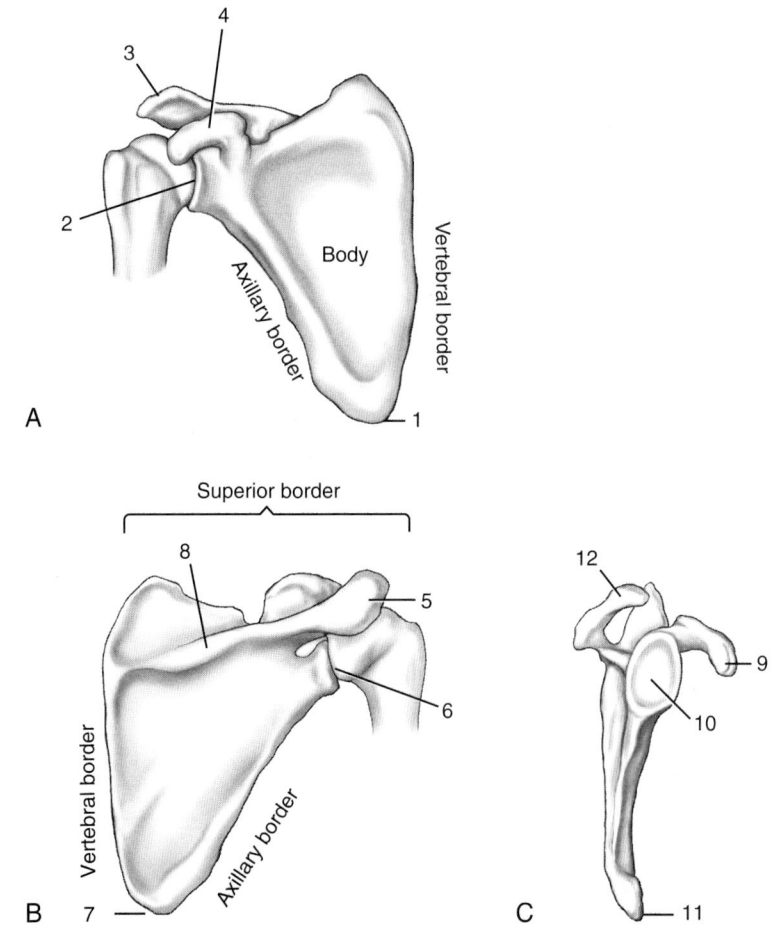

Fig. 13.4 Scapula. (A) Anterior aspect. (B) Posterior aspect. (C) Lateral aspect.

1. _____   7. _____

2. _____   8. _____

3. _____   9. _____

4. _____   10. _____

5. _____   11. _____

6. _____   12. _____

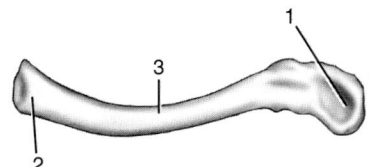

Fig. 13.5 Anterior aspect of the clavicle.

1. _____

2. _____

3. _____

125

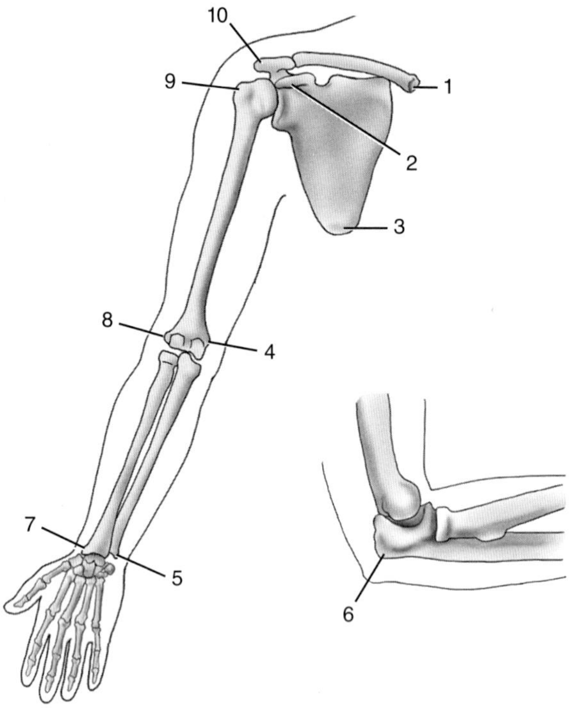

Fig. 13.6 Palpable bony landmarks of the upper limb.

1. _____

2. _____

3. _____

4. _____

5. _____

6. _____

7. _____

8. _____

9. _____

10. _____

EXERCISE 3

Answer the following questions.

1. Name (1) the middle bone of the third digit and (2) the most frequently fractured carpal bone.

   1. _____

   2. _____

2. Is the ulna bone medial or lateral to the radius?

   _____

3. Name the two articular processes of the distal humerus.

   1. _____

   2. _____

4. What are the two projections of the elbow that can be done if the arm is not able to be extended?

   1. _____

   2. _____

5. For the AP projection of the humerus in the recumbent position, how is the hand placed?

   _____

126

Chapter **13 Upper Limb and Shoulder Girdle**

6. Describe the differences in positioning for a PA wrist projection and a PA hand projection.

_____

_____

_____

_____

7. Name two special projections used specifically to demonstrate the scaphoid.

   1. _____

   2. _____

8. What are the three shoulder projections that can be done if a patient has an acute shoulder injury?

   1. _____

   2. _____

   3. _____

9. What two projections are commonly performed for a radiographic examination of the clavicle?

   1. _____

   2. _____

10. How is the arm and hand positioned for an AP projection of the shoulder?

_____

_____

_____

_____

11. How are the epicondyles positioned for a lateral projection of the humerus?

_____

12. How many degrees is the coronal plane of the chest rotated for a PA oblique (scapular Y) projection of the

    shoulder? _____

13. Which breathing technique is used for the transthoracic lateral projection of the shoulder?

_____

14. Where is the CR directed for a PA oblique (Grashey method) projection of the shoulder?

_____

15. Describe the position of the arm for an AP projection of the scapula.

_____

16. Describe the projections required for demonstration of the acromioclavicular (A-C) joints.

_____

_____

17. What is the position of the hand when a lateral projection of the elbow is positioned?

_____

EXERCISE 4

Label the following figures.

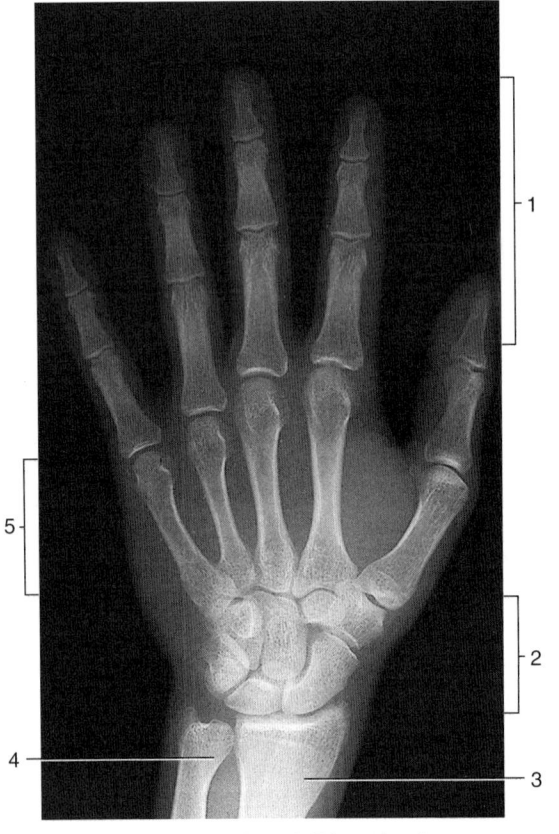

Fig. 13.7 Left hand. PA projection.

1. _____

2. _____

3. _____

4. _____

5. _____

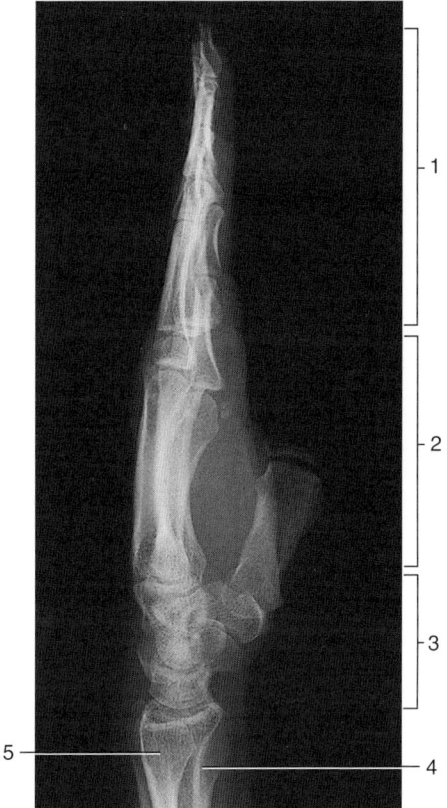

Fig. 13.8 Left hand. Lateral projection.

1. _____

2. _____

3. _____

4. _____

5. _____

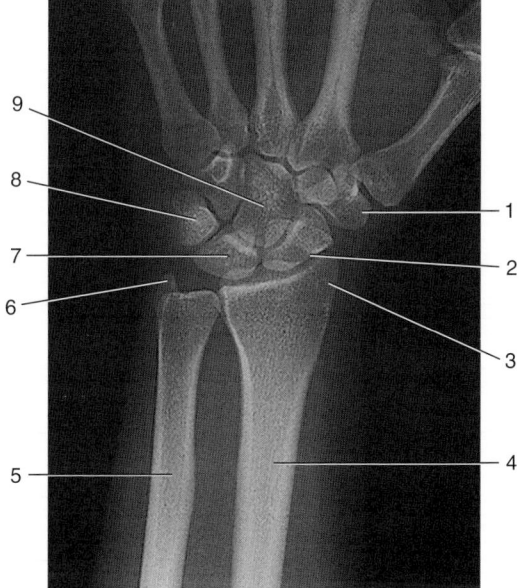

Fig. 13.9 Left wrist. PA radiograph.

1. _____

2. _____

3. _____

4. _____

5. _____

6. _____

7. _____

8. _____

9. _____

Chapter **13 Upper Limb and Shoulder Girdle**

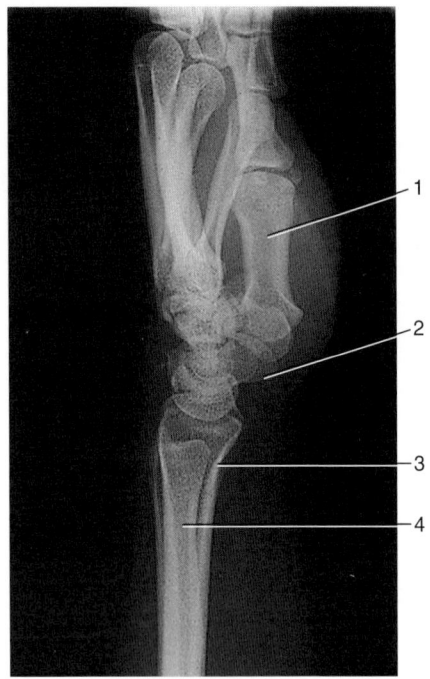

Fig. 13.10 Left wrist. Lateral projection.

1. _____

2. _____

3. _____

4. _____

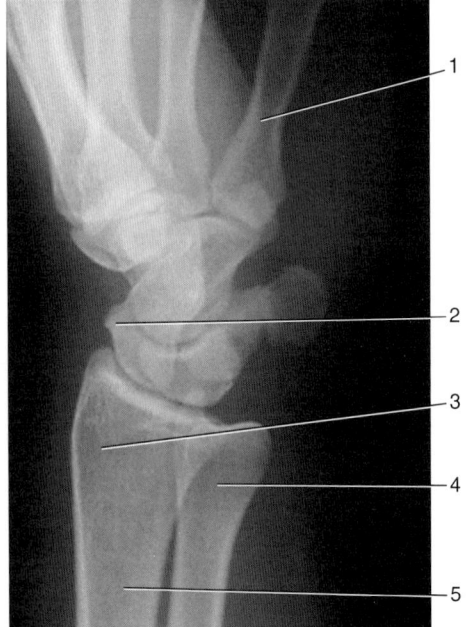

Fig. 13.11 Left wrist. AP oblique projection.

1. _____

2. _____

3. _____

4. _____

5. _____

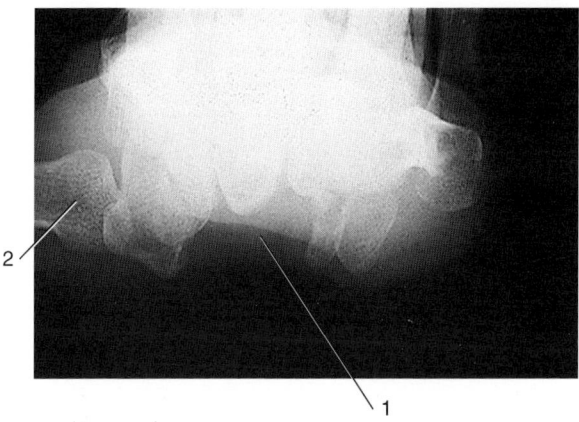

Fig. 13.12 Carpal canal. Tangential (Gaynor-Hart) projection.

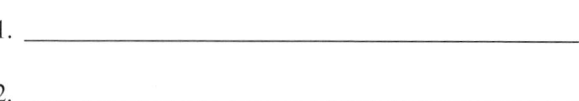

1. _____

2. _____

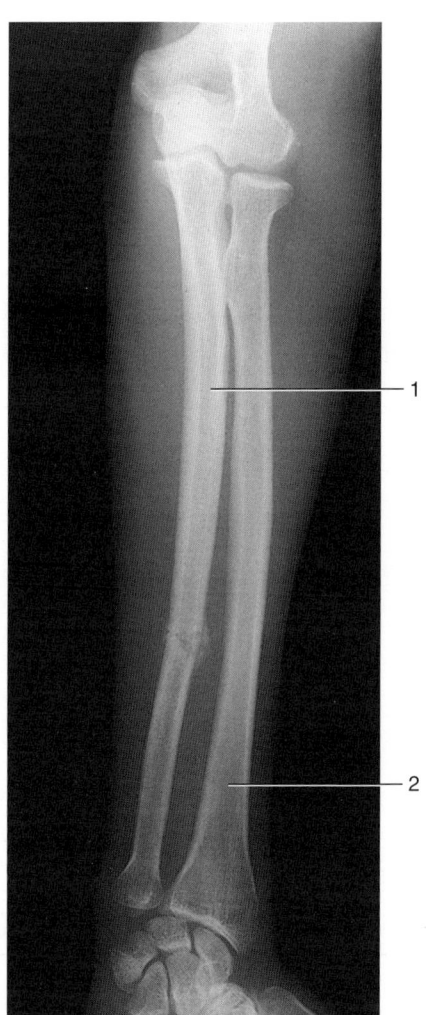

Fig. 13.13 Left forearm. AP projection with fracture.

1. _____

2. _____

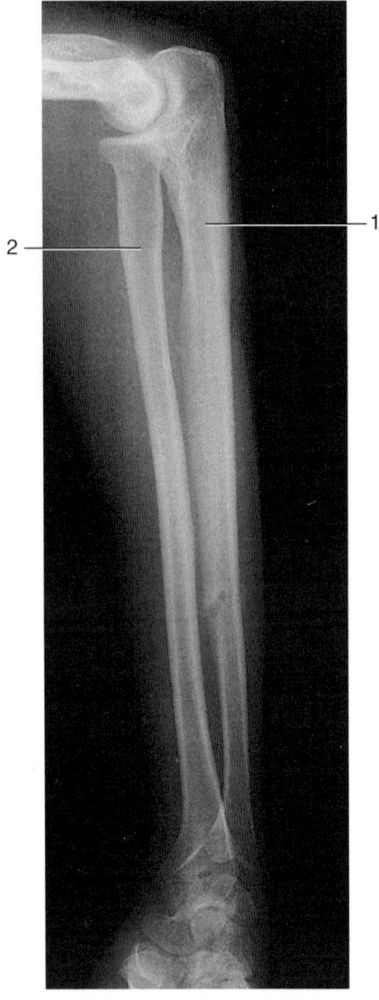

Fig. 13.14 Left forearm. Lateral projection with fracture.

1. _____

2. _____

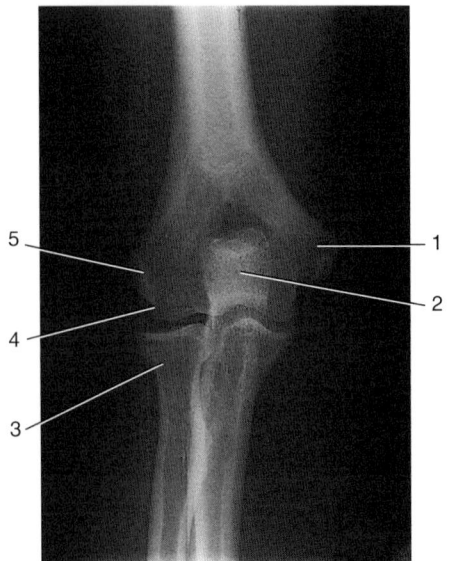

Fig. 13.15 Right elbow. AP projection.

1. _____

2. _____

3. _____

4. _____

5. _____

Chapter **13 Upper Limb and Shoulder Girdle**

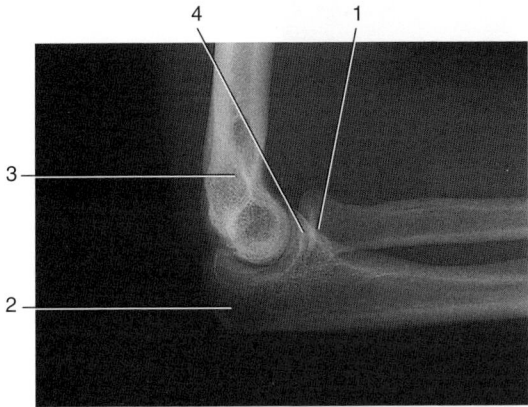

Fig. 13.16 Right elbow. Lateral projection.

1. _____

2. _____

3. _____

4. _____

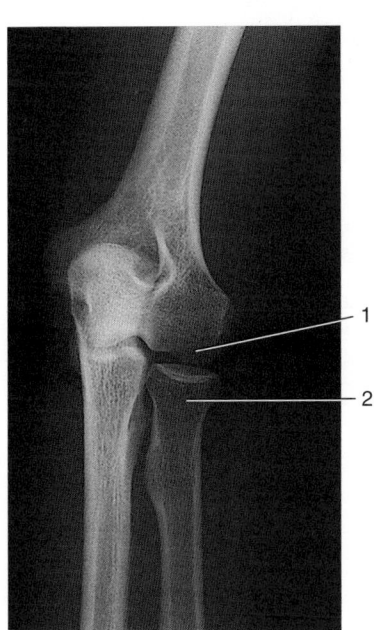

Fig. 13.17 Left elbow. AP oblique projection.

1. _____

2. _____

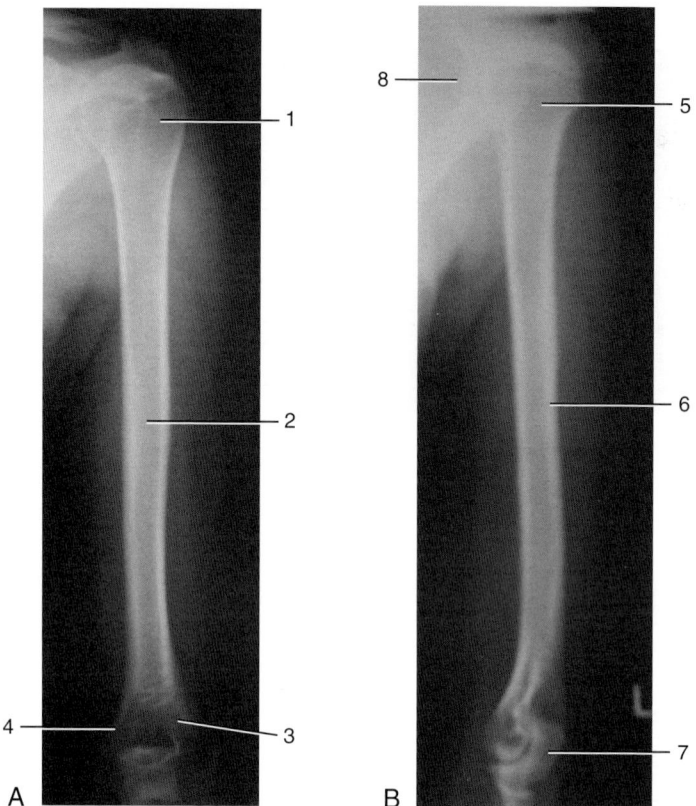

Fig. 13.18 Left humerus. (A) AP projection. (B) Lateral projection.

1. _____

2. _____

3. _____

4. _____

5. _____

6. _____

7. _____

8. _____

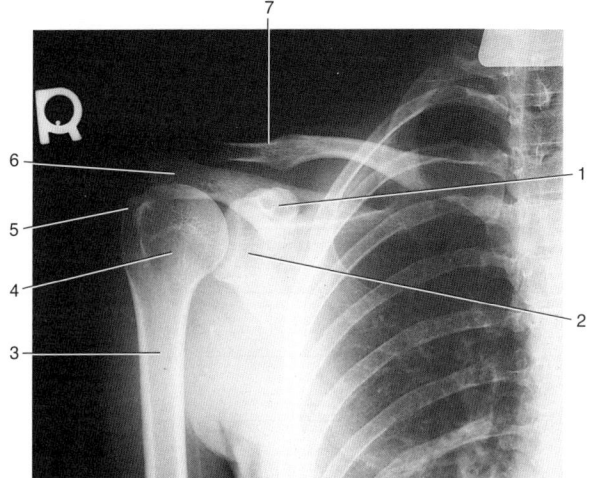

Fig. 13.19 Right shoulder. AP projection, external arm rotation.

1. _____
2. _____
3. _____
4. _____
5. _____
6. _____
7. _____

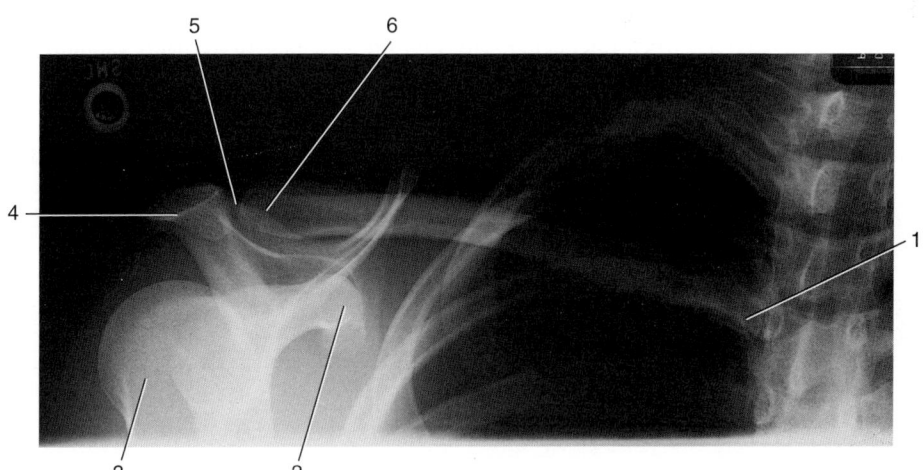

Fig. 13.20 Right clavicle. PA projection.

1. _____
2. _____
3. _____
4. _____
5. _____
6. _____

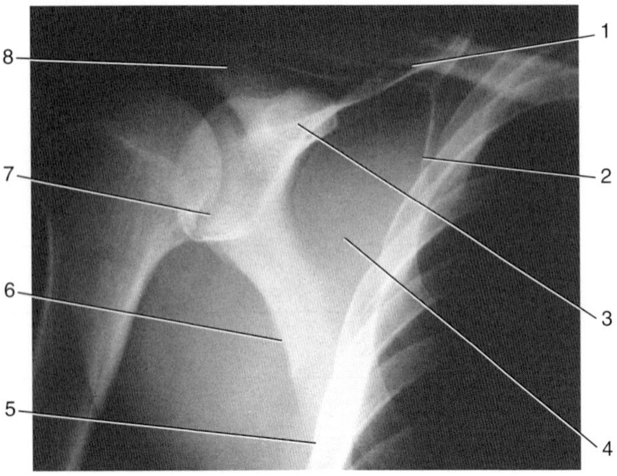

Fig. 13.21 Right scapula. AP projection.

1. _____

2. _____

3. _____

4. _____

5. _____

6. _____

7. _____

8. _____

CHALLENGE EXERCISE

This exercise does not have to be completed at the same time as the other exercises in this workbook chapter. The exercise is designed to assess retention of the essential information contained in the corresponding textbook chapter. It is recommended that you complete this exercise when you begin to study for the state limited licensure examination. This will help determine what you know and which information should be further reviewed.

1. What is the minimum source-image receptor distance used for nearly all radiographic images of the upper limb?

   _____

2. Describe how the hand is positioned for the PA projection. _____

   _____

3. What is the CR centering point for the PA projection of the hand?

   _____

4. What is the amount of lateral rotation needed to achieve a PA oblique projection of the hand?

   _____

   _____

5. Describe the positioning details for the PA oblique projection of the fourth (ring) finger.

   _____

   _____

6. Why is the PA projection *not* the routine projection for the thumb? _____

_____

7. Describe the positioning details for the PA projection of the wrist. _____

_____

8. What is the CR centering point for the PA projection of the wrist?

_____

9. Describe the positioning details for the lateral projection of the wrist. _____

_____

10. Describe the positioning details for the AP projection of the forearm. _____

_____

11. Describe the positioning details for the AP projection of the elbow. _____

_____

12. What is the degree of flexion needed for the lateral projection of the elbow? _____

_____

13. Describe the positioning details for the AP projection of the humerus.

_____

_____

14. When performing an AP projection of the shoulder, what is the orientation of the coronal plane of the humeral epicondyles to achieve external rotation of the humerus?

_____

_____

15. When performing an AP projection of the shoulder, what is the orientation of the coronal plane of the humeral epicondyles to achieve internal rotation of the humerus?

_____

_____

16. What are the amount and direction of central ray angulation for an AP axial projection of the clavicle?

_____

17. Why is it necessary to attach weights to the patient's wrists when performing radiography of the A-C joints?

_____

_____

14 Lower Limb and Pelvis

LIMITED-SCOPE STUDENTS

Exercises 1 and 2 in this section are for students studying for the *Extremity Procedures Module* in the ARRT Limited-Scope examination. **Podiatry** student exercises are later in this chapter's exercises.

EXERCISE 1, LIMITED-SCOPE

Answer the following questions by selecting the best choice.

1. The bones of the midfoot are called the:
   A. phalanges.
   B. tarsals.
   C. metatarsals.
   D. sesamoid bones.

2. Small, flat, oval bones in the region of the first metatarsophalangeal joint are called:
   A. phalanges.
   B. tarsals.
   C. metatarsals.
   D. sesamoid bones.

3. The sesamoid bone that is anterior to the distal femur and is commonly known as the *kneecap* is the:
   A. fibula.
   B. tibia.
   C. patella.
   D. fabella.

4. Which of the following bones are in the hindfoot portion of the foot?
   1. Cuneiforms
   2. Calcaneus
   3. Talus
   A. 1 and 2 only
   B. 1 and 3 only
   C. 2 and 3 only
   D. 1, 2, and 3

5. What tarsal bone is commonly referred to as the "heel bone"?
   A. Talus
   B. Cuneiforms
   C. Navicular
   D. Calcaneus

6. When performing an anteroposterior (AP) axial projection of the foot, the central ray is directed:
   A. 10 degrees toward the toes.
   B. 10 degrees toward the heel.
   C. 15 degrees toward the heel.
   D. perpendicular to the image receptor (IR).

7. When the leg is extended, the ankle is dorsiflexed 90 degrees between the foot and leg, the leg is rotated medially approximately 15 to 20 degrees, and the CR is perpendicular between the malleoli, the resulting image will demonstrate:
   A. an axial projection of the calcaneus.
   B. a medial oblique projection of the tarsals and metatarsals.
   C. the ankle mortise.
   D. the cuboid and the third cuneiform.

8. When the leg is extended in the supine position, the foot is maximally dorsiflexed, and the central ray is directed 40 degrees cephalad through the sole of the foot entering near the third metatarsal base, the resulting image will demonstrate:
   A. an axial projection of the calcaneus.
   B. a medial oblique projection of the tarsals and metatarsals.
   C. the cuboid and the third cuneiform.
   D. distal portions of the tibia and fibula.

9. Which of the following projections requires a central ray that is angled 5 to 7 degrees cephalad?
   A. An AP projection of the ankle
   B. A lateral projection of the knee
   C. An AP projection of the foot
   D. An axial projection of the calcaneus

10. When the patient is prone, the knee is flexed 75 to 80 degrees between the femur and the lower leg, and the CR is 15 to 20 degrees cephalad through the patella, the resulting radiograph will demonstrate all of the following, *except*:
    A. a tangential projection of the patella.
    B. the patella in profile.
    C. the patellofemoral joint.
    D. the tibial plateaus

11. When there is suspicion of a fracture of the patella, flexion of the knee joint for the lateral projection should be limited to:
    A. 5 to 7 degrees.
    B. 10 degrees.
    C. 20 to 30 degrees.
    D. 30 to 45 degrees.

12. When an AP projection of the proximal femur is performed, the IR should be placed so that the:
    A. superior margin is at the level of the greater trochanter.
    B. superior margin is at the level of the iliac crest.
    C. superior margin is at the level of the anterior superior iliac spine.
    D. center is aligned to the midfemur.

13. How are the toes identified?
    A. The toes are numbered 1 to 5 beginning on the medial side.
    B. The toes are numbered 1 to 5 beginning on the lateral side.
    C. The toes are referred to as digits without identifying numbers.
    D. The toes have individual names.

14. Which of the following bones are located in the lower leg?
    A. Tibia and femur
    B. Fibula and femur
    C. Tibia and fibula
    D. Tibula and fibia

15. A systemic disorder that increases the uric acid content of the blood and may cause a joint condition that commonly affects the feet (particularly the joints of the great toe) is called:
    A. osteoarthritis.
    B. gout.
    C. rheumatoid arthritis.
    D. osteoporosis.

16. _____ may cause degeneration of any of the joints of the lower limb but is most common in the knee and the hip.
    A. Osteoarthritis
    B. Osteomyelitis
    C. Osteogenic sarcoma
    D. Osteoporosis

17. A normal variation in which an additional small sesamoid bone is located posterior to the knee is termed
    A. patella.
    B. fabella.
    C. meniscus.
    D. mortise.

18. Which bone of the lower leg is on the medial side?
    A. Tibia
    B. Fibula
    C. Femur
    D. Ulna

19. Where is the intercondylar fossa located?
    A. On the proximal, anterior aspect of the femur
    B. On the distal, anterior aspect of the femur
    C. On the distal, posterior aspect of the femur
    D. On the proximal, posterior aspect of the tibia

20. What name is given to the articular surface of the proximal, superior aspect of the tibia?
    A. Intercondylar fossa
    B. Intercondylar eminence
    C. Tibial spine
    D. Tibial plateau

21. What is the name given to the distal end of the fibula?
    A. Talus
    B. Medial malleolus
    C. Lateral malleolus
    D. Astragalus

22. Which of the following are the bones that articulate to form the ankle mortise?
    A. Talus, tibia, and fibula
    B. Tibia, fibula, and calcaneus
    C. Talus and tibia
    D. Calcaneus and tibia

23. Which bone does the distal tibia articulate with directly?
    A. cuboid
    B. talus
    C. navicular
    D. calcaneus

24. The distal aspect of the femur has two large round prominences called the
    A. heads
    B. trochanters
    C. malleoli
    D. condyles

25. On what bone is the prominent landmark, greater trochanter, located?
    A. calcaneus
    B. fibula
    C. femur
    D. tibia

26. Where does the CR enter the patient for the AP axial projection of the foot?
    A. At the third metatarsophalangeal (MTP) joint
    B. At the first MTP joint
    C. At the base of the third metatarsal
    D. At the head of the third metatarsal

27. Which surface of the foot should be in contact with the IR for the lateral projection of the foot?
    A. Lateral
    B. Medial
    C. Dorsal
    D. Plantar

28. How much is the plantar surface of the foot rotated medially from the IR for the AP oblique projection of the foot?
    A. 45 degrees
    B. 30 degrees
    C. 10 degrees
    D. 25 degrees

29. What is the proper CR angle and direction for the axial projection of the calcaneus when the ankle is dorsiflexed so that the plantar surface of the foot is perpendicular to the IR?
    A. 10 degrees cephalad
    B. 40 degrees cephalad
    C. 10 degrees caudad
    D. 40 degrees caudad

30. Where should the CR enter the patient for the AP projection of the ankle joint?
    A. Perpendicular to a point midway between the malleoli
    B. Perpendicular to the base of the third metatarsal
    C. Angled 10 degrees cephalic to a point midway between the malleoli
    D. Angled 10 degrees cephalic to the base of the third metatarsal

31. Which of the following is true regarding the lateral projection of the foot?
    A. The ankle does not have a specific position when performing the lateral projection of the foot.
    B. The ankle should be dorsiflexed so that the long axis of the foot forms a 45-degree angle with the tibia.
    C. The ankle should be extended so that the plantar surface of the foot forms a 45-degree angle with the IR.
    D. The ankle should be dorsiflexed so that the long axis of the foot is perpendicular to the tibia.

32. Which foot projection and position demonstrate the metatarsals without superimposition?
    A. AP projection with plantar surface of foot in contact with IR
    B. AP oblique projection in 30-degree lateral rotation
    C. AP oblique projection in 30-degree medial rotation
    D. Lateral projection with MTP joints perpendicular to IR

33. What device may help provide an even brightness on a radiograph of an AP axial projection of the foot?
    A. Lead shield
    B. Wedge compensating filter
    C. Wedge positioning sponge
    D. Sandbag

34. Which of the following must be included on an AP projection of the lower leg?
    1. Entire tibia and fibula
    2. Knee joint
    3. Ankle joint
    A. 1 and 2 only
    B. 1 and 3 only
    C. 2 and 3 only
    D. 1, 2, and 3

35. Where should the CR enter the patient for the AP projection of the knee?
    A. ½ inch below the apex of the patella
    B. ½ inch below the base of the patella
    C. 1 inch distal to the medial epicondyle of the femur
    D. 1 inch proximal to the medial epicondyle of the femur

36. Which of the following radiographic methods are used to demonstrate the intercondylar fossa?
    1. Holmblad method
    2. Camp-Coventry method
    3. Settegast method
    A. 1 and 2 only
    B. 1 and 3 only
    C. 2 and 3 only
    D. 1, 2, and 3

37. Which of the following radiographic methods is used to demonstrate the patella and the patellofemoral joint space?
    A. Holmblad method
    B. Camp-Coventry method
    C. Settegast method
    D. Grashey method

38. What is the position of the CR for an AP knee when the part measures less than 19 cm?
    A. 0 degrees
    B. 3-5 degrees caudad
    C. 3-5 degrees cephalad
    D. 5-7 degrees cephalad

39. How many degrees is the leg rotated for an AP oblique-mortise position?
    A. 15-20 degrees medially
    B. 30 degrees laterally
    C. 30 degrees medially
    D. 45 degrees medially

40. What is the CR angle for the PA axial projection, Holmblad method, of the intercondylar fossa (tunnel)?
    A. 0 degrees
    B. 40 degrees
    C. 50 degrees
    D. 40–50 degrees depending upon position of the leg

41. Which of the following are true regarding the correct position for an AP projection of the lower leg?
    1. The leg should be extended and resting on the IR.
    2. The ankle should be dorsiflexed so that the foot forms a 90-degree angle with the lower leg.
    3. The sagittal plane of the leg should be placed parallel to the IR.
    A. 1 and 2 only
    B. 1 and 3 only
    C. 2 and 3 only
    D. 1, 2, and 3

42. An infection of the bone, leading to bony destruction in the acute phase, is called:
    A. gout
    B. bone hypertrophy
    C. osteoarthritis
    D. osteomyelitis

EXERCISE 2, LIMITED-SCOPE

Answer the following questions.

1. How many phalanges are there in the great toe? The second toe?

   _____

2. Is the fibula medial or lateral to the tibia?

   _____

3. Name the two bones that form the knee joint.

   1. _____

   2. _____

4. Which bone of the lower leg is located on the lateral side?

   _____

5. The palpable portion at the distal end of the tibia is called the

   _____

6. Describe the position of the leg for an AP oblique projection (mortise joint) of the ankle.

_____

_____

_____

7. Name the two projections of the knee that will demonstrate the intercondylar fossa (tunnel) of the femur.

    1. _____

    2. _____

8. When the ankle is flexed and raises the foot, the movement is termed:

_____

9. Which is the largest and heaviest bone in the body?

_____

10. What is the name of the hinge joint between the metatarsals and the proximal phalanges?

_____

11. The largest of the tarsal bones is the:

_____

12. What is the location of the two small sesamoid bones in the lower limb?

_____

13. The palpable boney landmark on the proximal lateral side of the femur is the?

_____

14. The inferior pointed part of the patella is called the:

_____

15. Which tarsal bone articulates with the distal tibia?

_____

16. The large lateral prominences on the distal femur which serve as boney landmarks are called:

_____

17. Where does the CR enter the patient for the AP projection of the first toe?

_____

18. Which surface of the ankle is placed in contact with the IR for the lateral projection of the ankle?

_____

19. On a lateral projection of the knee, what anatomy is used to determine if the knee joint is properly positioned?

_____

20. Where is the CR directed for an AP axial foot?

_____

21. Where is the CR directed for a lateral calcaneus projection?

_____

22. Where is the CR directed for an AP projection of the knee?

_____

23. How much is the plantar surface of the foot rotated medially for an AP oblique projection?

_____

24. What is the degree of angulation and the CR position for an AP knee that measures over 24 cm?

_____

25. How many degrees is the leg flexed for a lateral projection of the knee?

_____

Exercises 1 and 2 in this section are for completion by students studying for the *Podiatric Procedures Module* in the ARRT Limited-Scope examination. These questions all relate to the *foot, calcaneus, sesamoid bones and ankle* only. All positioning and projection questions are written from the perspective that they are all performed on the floor-based Podiatry x-ray machine, and with the patient standing.

EXERCISE 1 - PODIATRY

1. The bones of the midfoot are called the:
   A. phalanges.
   B. tarsals.
   C. metatarsals.
   D. sesamoid bones.

2. Unintentional inversion or eversion of the foot caused by stepping on something will cause a:
   A. stress fracture
   B. fracture of the malleoli
   C. sprained ankle
   D. dislocation of the ankle

3. Which of the following bones are in the hindfoot portion of the foot?
   1. Cuneiforms
   2. Calcaneus
   3. Talus
   A. 1 and 2 only
   B. 1 and 3 only
   C. 2 and 3 only
   D. 1, 2, and 3

4. What tarsal bone is commonly referred to as the "heel bone"?
   A. Talus
   B. Cuneiforms
   C. Navicular
   D. Calcaneus

5. How are the toes and metatarsals identified?
   A. The toes are numbered 1 to 5 beginning on the medial side.
   B. The toes are numbered 1 to 5 beginning on the lateral side.
   C. The toes are referred to as digits without identifying numbers.
   D. The toes have individual names.

6. Which of the following bones are located in the lower leg?
   A. Tibia and femur
   B. Fibula and femur
   C. Tibia and fibula
   D. Tibula and fibia

7. Which bone of the lower leg is on the medial side?
   A. Tibia
   B. Fibula
   C. Femur
   D. Ulna

8. Which of the following are the bones that articulate to form the ankle mortise?
   A. Talus, tibia, and fibula
   B. Tibia, fibula, and calcaneus
   C. Talus and tibia
   D. Calcaneus and tibia

9. Which bone does the distal tibia articulate with directly?
   A. cuboid
   B. talus
   C. navicular
   D. calcaneus

10. Which of the following would be seen on the medial side of the foot?
    1. cuneiform
    2. cuboid
    3. navicular
    A. 1 and 2
    B. 1 and 3
    C. 2 and 3
    D. 1, 2, and 3

11. Where is the "ball" of the foot located?
    A. On the plantar surface directly below the MTP joints
    B. On the plantar surface directly below the IP joints
    C. On the plantar surface directly below the navicular bone
    D. On the plantar surface directly below the phalanges

12. All of the following articulate with the talus, *except*:
    A. cuboid
    B. tibia
    C. navicular
    D. medial malleolus

13. When the ankle joint flexes to raise the foot, the motion is called:
    A. eversion
    B. inversion
    C. dorsiflexion
    D. plantar flexion

14. When the plantar surface of the foot is flexed inward, the movement is called:
    A. abduction
    B. dorsiflexion
    C. eversion
    D. inversion

15. Small, flat, oval bones in the region of the first metatarsophalangeal joint are called:
    A. phalanges.
    B. tarsals.
    C. metatarsals.
    D. sesamoid bones.

16. The hinge joint between the proximal phalanges and the metatarsals is called the _____ joint:
    A. tarsocuniform (TC)
    B. interphalangeal (IP)
    C. metatarsophalangeal (MTP)
    D. metatarsocuniform (MC)

17. When performing a dorso-plantar (DP) projection of the foot, the central ray is directed:
    A. 10 degrees toward the toes.
    B. 10 degrees cephalad.
    C. 10 to 15 degrees toward the heel.
    D. perpendicular to the image receptor (IR).

18. When the leg is extended, the ankle is dorsiflexed 90 degrees between the foot and leg, the leg is rotated medially approximately 15 to 20 degrees, and the CR is perpendicular between the malleoli, the resulting image will demonstrate:
    A. an axial projection of the calcaneus.
    B. a medial oblique projection of the tarsals and metatarsals.
    C. the ankle mortise.
    D. the cuboid and the third cuneiform

19. Where does the CR enter the patient for the AP axial projection of the foot?
    A. At the third metatarsophalangeal (MTP) joint
    B. At the first MTP joint
    C. At the base of the third metatarsal
    D. At the head of the third metatarsal

20. Which surface of the foot should be in contact with the IR for the lateral projection of the foot?
    A. Lateral
    B. Medial
    C. Dorsal
    D. Plantar

21. How much is the leg and plantar surface of the foot rotated medially from the IR for the AP oblique projection of the foot?
    A. 45 degrees
    B. 30 degrees
    C. 10 degrees
    D. 25 degrees

22. What is the CR angle and direction for the axial calcaneal (Harris-Beath method) projection of the calcaneus?
    A. 10 degrees cephalad
    B. 20 degrees cephalad
    C. 25 degrees anteriorly
    D. 35 to 45 degrees anteriorly

23. Where should the CR enter the patient for the AP projection of the ankle joint?
    A. Perpendicular to a point midway between the malleoli
    B. Perpendicular to the base of the third metatarsal
    C. Angled 10 degrees cephalic to a point midway between the malleoli
    D. Angled 10 degrees cephalic to the base of the third metatarsal

24. Which foot projection and position demonstrate the metatarsals without superimposition?
    A. AP projection with plantar surface of foot in contact with IR
    B. AP oblique projection in 45-degree lateral rotation
    C. AP oblique projection in 45-degree medial rotation
    D. Lateral projection with MTP joints perpendicular to IR

25. What device may help provide an even brightness on a radiograph of an DP axial projection of the foot?
    A. Lead shield
    B. Wedge compensating filter
    C. Wedge positioning sponge
    D. Sandbag

26. How many degrees is the leg rotated for an AP oblique-mortise position of the ankle?
    A. 15-20 degrees medially
    B. 15-20 degrees laterally
    C. 30 degrees medially
    D. 45 degrees medially

27. For the AP oblique projection of the foot in medial rotation, where is the CR directed?
    A. navicular bone
    B. 3rd metatarsal head
    C. 1st metatarsal base
    D. 3rd metatarsal base

146

28. Where is the CR directed for the lateral projection of the foot?
    A. talus
    B. navicular bone
    C. cuniform-cuboid joint
    D. base of the 5th metatarsal

29. What are the primary structures seen on the AP oblique projection of the foot, medial rotation?
    A. metatarsals and some tarsals
    B. all the tarsal bones
    C. talus and calcaneus
    D. ankle joint, talus and calcaneus

30. For the lateral projection of the ankle, the CR enters the:
    A. medial malleolus
    B. lateral malleolus
    C. anterior talus
    D. anterior calcaneus

31. The AP oblique projections of the ankle require the foot to be angled:
    A. 30 degrees
    B. 45 degrees
    C. 10 to 15 degrees
    D. 15 to 20 degrees

32. The primary structures seen on the lateral projection of the ankle are the:
    A. tibiotalar, subtalar and base of the 5th metatarsal
    B. talus and calcaneus and base of the 5th metatarsal
    C. medial and intermediate cuniforms
    D. medial and intermediate cuniforms and talus

33. How is the ball of the foot placed into position for the sesamoid axial (Lewis method) projection?
    A. toes are pulled up with a strap
    B. foot placed in an angulation device
    C. perpendicular to the IR
    D. parallel to the IR

34. All of the following are tarsal bones, *except*:
    A. cuboid
    B. navicular
    C. sesamoids
    D. talus

EXERCISE 2 - PODIATRY

1. What are the three basic parts of the foot?

2. How many phalanges are on the first toe?

3. When the foot flexes so it is raised, the motion is called:

4. Where is the CR directed for the sesamoid axial projection (Lewis method) of the sesamoids?

5. Which two projections done in Podiatry practice would benefit from the use of a compensating filter?

6. The standard degree of rotation of the foot for the AP oblique, medial and lateral rotations, is:

_____

7. For which projection is the patient instructed to "flex the knees slightly" and into the "ski-jump" position?

_____

8. Which ankle projection requires the leg and foot to be internally rotated 15 to 20 degrees?

_____

9. The AP oblique projection of the ankle with the foot in a 45-degree internal rotation will demonstrate which joint?

_____

10. The superior aspect of the calcaneus is best demonstrated using which projection?

_____

11. The hinge joint located between the metatarsals and the phalanges is called the:

_____

12. Which two bones make up the hindfoot?

_____

13. When the foot is rolled into medial and lateral flexion, the two terms are called:

_____

14. For the AP oblique projections of the foot in medial and lateral rotations the foot is angled 45 degrees from the IR as the standard. As an alternate the foot is commonly rotated how many degrees?

_____

15. The AP oblique projection of the foot will primarily demonstrate the:

_____

Both limited-scope and Podiatry students will complete Exercises 3 and 4 in this section. **Podiatry** students will only complete the anatomy and radiographic Figures that relate to the *toe, foot, ankle, and calcaneus.*

EXERCISE 3

Label the following illustrations.

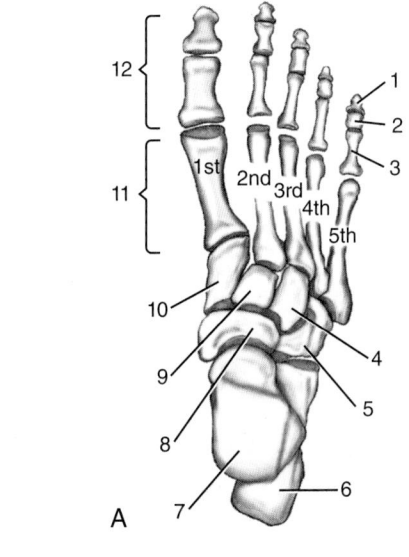

Fig. 14.1 Foot. **A**, Anterior (dorsal) aspect. **B**, Medial aspect.

1. _____

2. _____

3. _____

4. _____

5. _____

6. _____

7. _____

8. _____

9. _____

10. _____

11. _____

12. _____

13. _____

14. _____

15. _____

16. _____

17. _____

18. _____

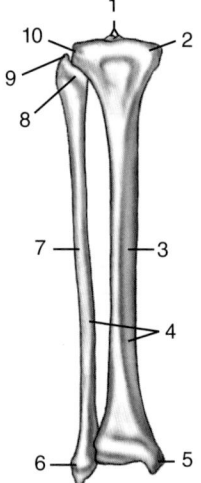

Fig. 14.2 Anterior aspect of the tibia and fibula.

1. _____
2. _____
3. _____
4. _____
5. _____
6. _____
7. _____
8. _____
9. _____
10. _____

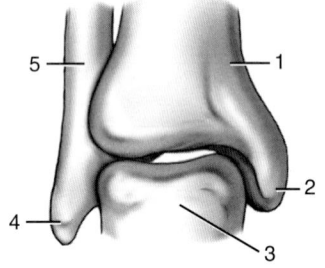

Fig. 14.3 Anterior aspect of the ankle joint.

1. _____
2. _____
3. _____
4. _____
5. _____

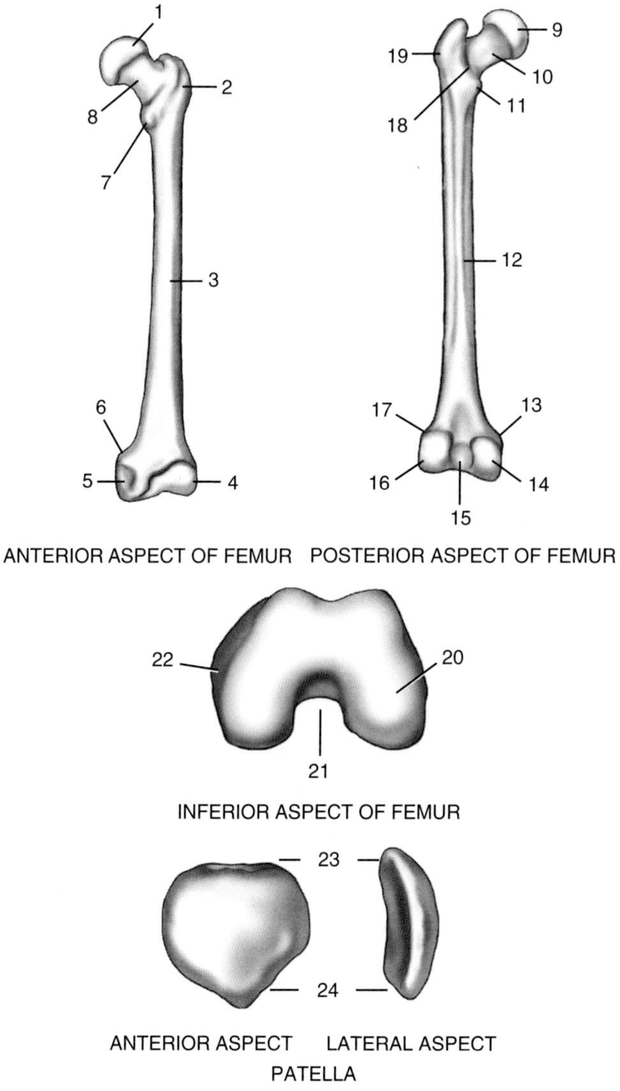
1
2
8
7
3
6
5
4
9
19
10
18
11
12
17
13
16
14
15
ANTERIOR ASPECT OF FEMUR
POSTERIOR ASPECT OF FEMUR
22
20
21
INFERIOR ASPECT OF FEMUR
23
24
ANTERIOR ASPECT
LATERAL ASPECT
PATELLA

Fig. 14.4 Femur and patella.

1. ____________________
2. ____________________
3. ____________________
4. ____________________
5. ____________________
6. ____________________
7. ____________________
8. ____________________
9. ____________________
10. ____________________
11. ____________________
12. ____________________
13. ____________________
14. ____________________
15. ____________________
16. ____________________
17. ____________________
18. ____________________
19. ____________________
20. ____________________
21. ____________________
22. ____________________
23. ____________________
24. ____________________

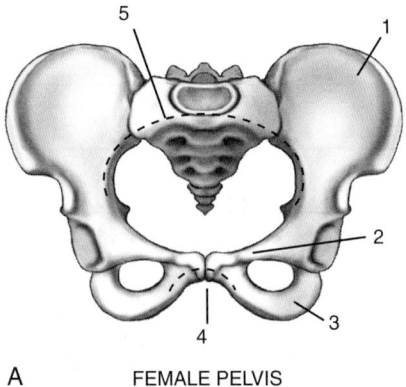

5

1

A   FEMALE PELVIS

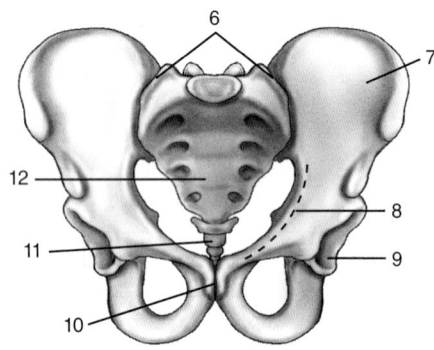

6

7

12

8

11

9

10

B   MALE PELVIS

Fig. 14.5 Pelvis. (A) Female. (B) Male.

1. _____

2. _____

3. _____

4. _____

5. _____

6. _____

7. _____

8. _____

9. _____

10. _____

11. _____

12. _____

EXERCISE 4

Label the following figures.

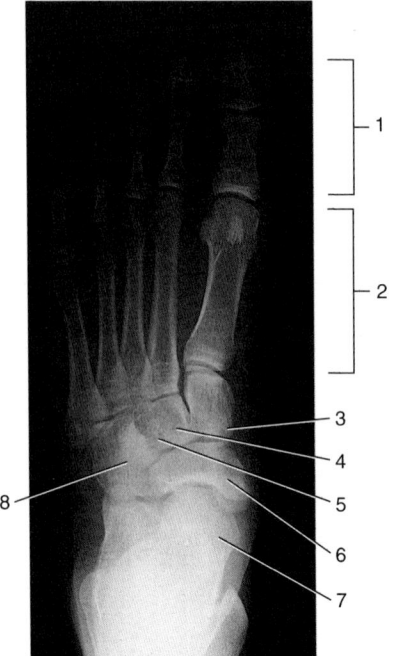

1

2

3

4

8

5

6

7

Fig. 14.6 Foot. AP projection.

1. _____

2. _____

3. _____

4. _____

5. _____

6. _____

7. _____

8. _____

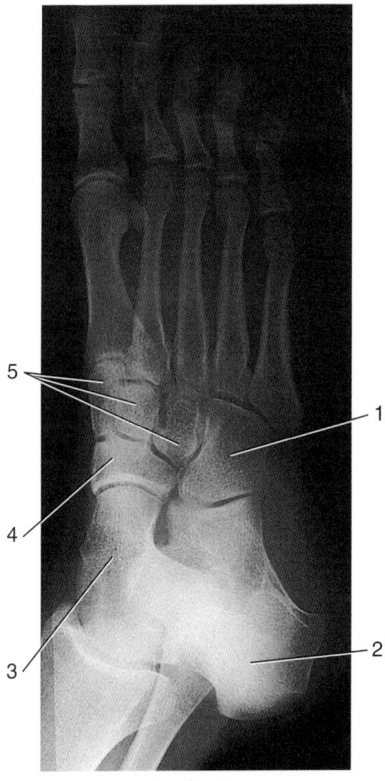

Fig. 14.7 Foot. AP oblique projection.

1. _____

2. _____

3. _____

4. _____

5. _____

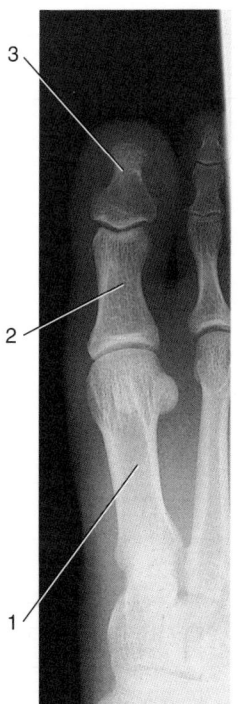

Fig. 14.8 Toes. AP projection.

1. _____

2. _____

3. _____

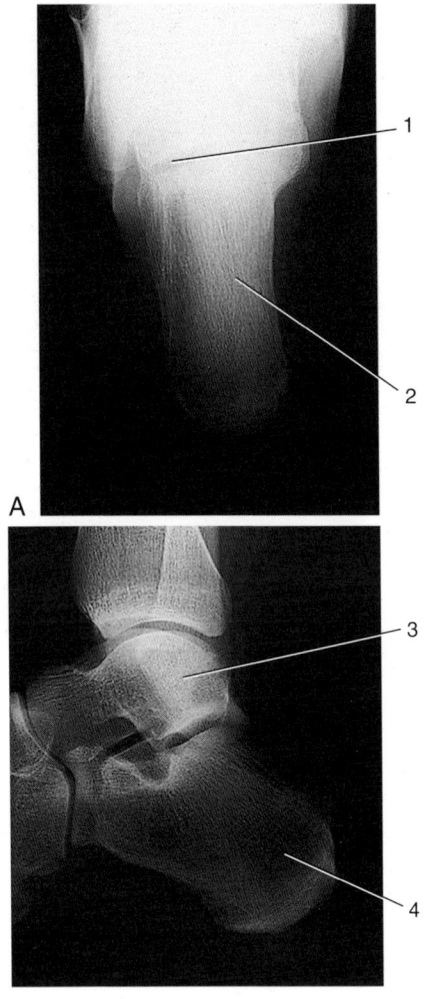

A

B

Fig. 14.9 Calcaneus. (A) Axial projection. (B) Lateral projection.

1. _____
2. _____
3. _____
4. _____

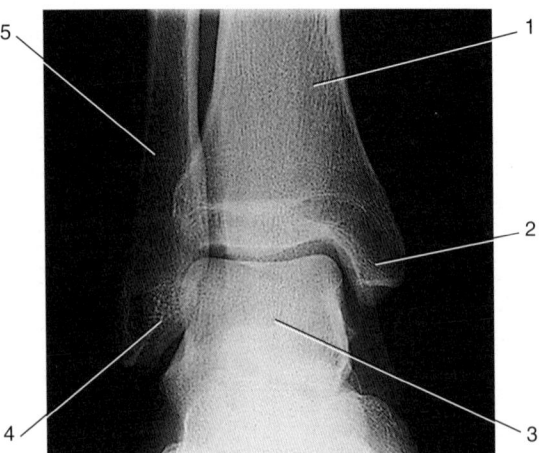

Fig. 14.10 Ankle. AP projection.

1. _____
2. _____
3. _____
4. _____
5. _____

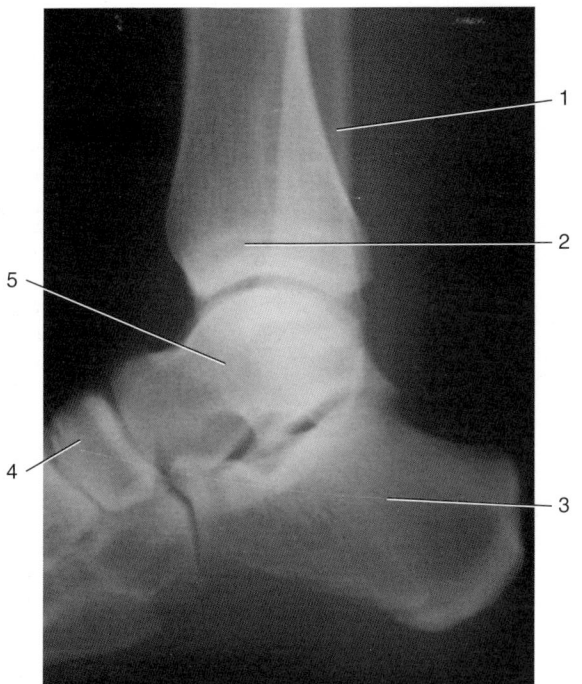

Fig. 14.11 Ankle. Lateral projection.

1. _____

2. _____

3. _____

4. _____

5. _____

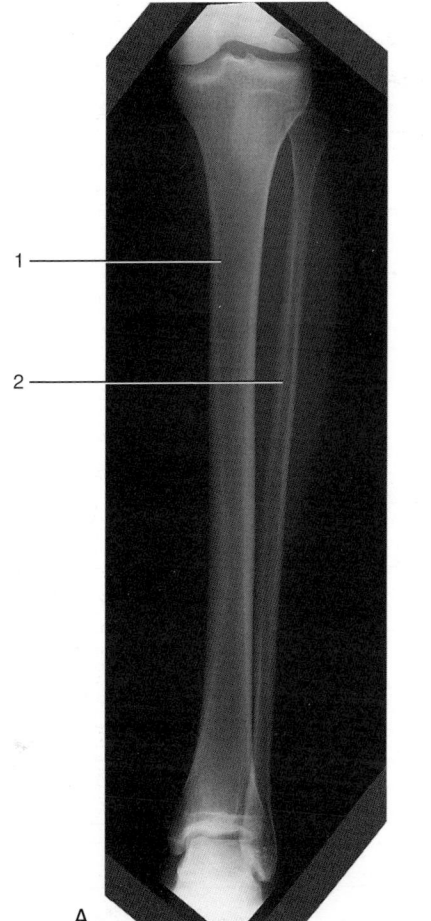

A

Fig. 14.12A Lower leg. (A) AP projection.

1. _____

2. _____

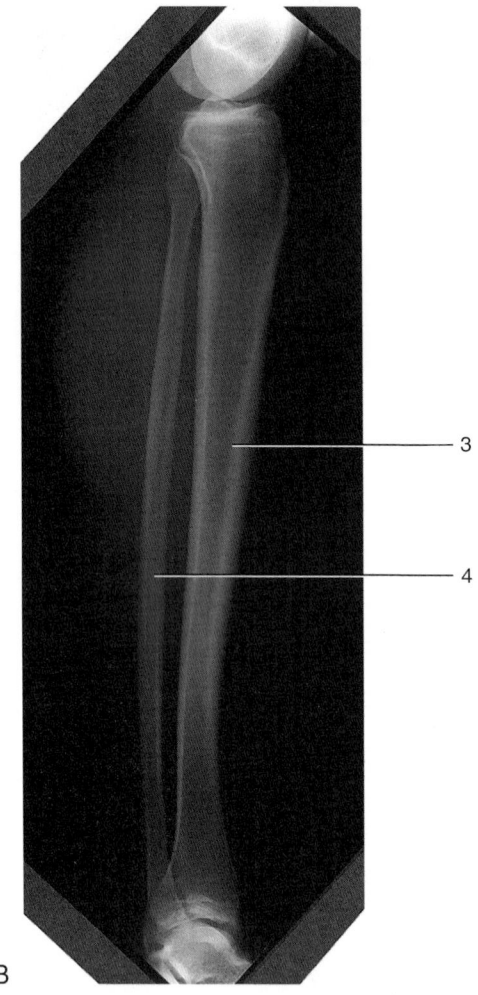

B

Fig. 14.12B Lower leg. (B) Lateral projection.

3. _____

4. _____

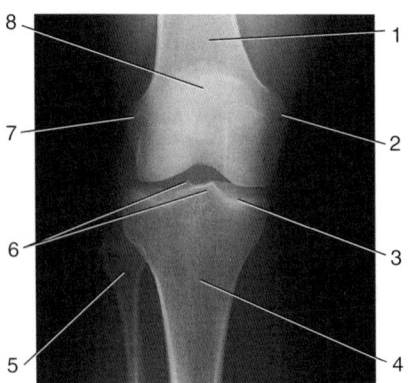

Fig. 14.13 Knee. AP projection.

1. _____

2. _____

3. _____

4. _____

5. _____

6. _____

7. _____

8. _____

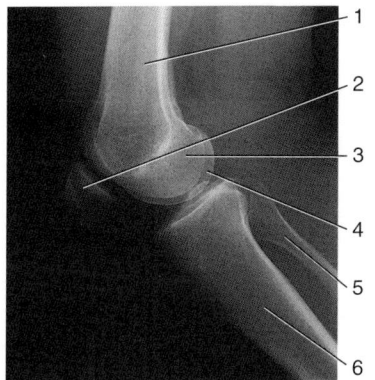

Fig. 14.14 Knee. Lateral projection.

1. _____
2. _____
3. _____
4. _____
5. _____
6. _____

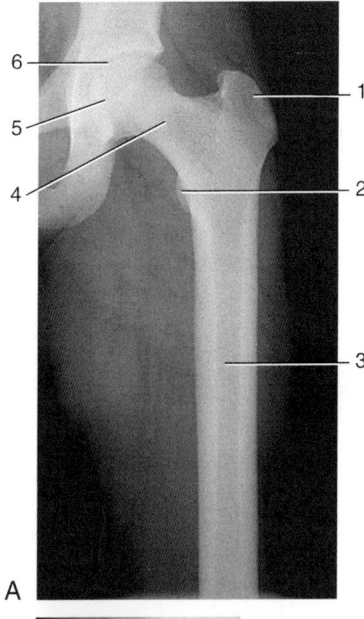

A

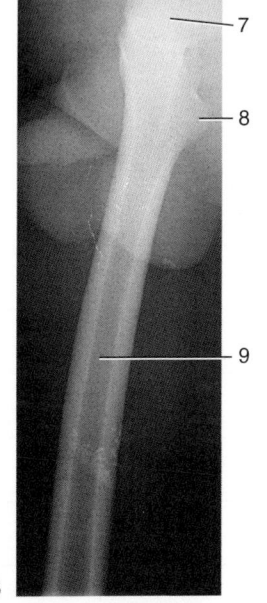

B

Fig. 14.15 Femur. (A) AP projection. (B) Lateral projection.

1. _____
2. _____
3. _____
4. _____
5. _____
6. _____
7. _____
8. _____
9. _____

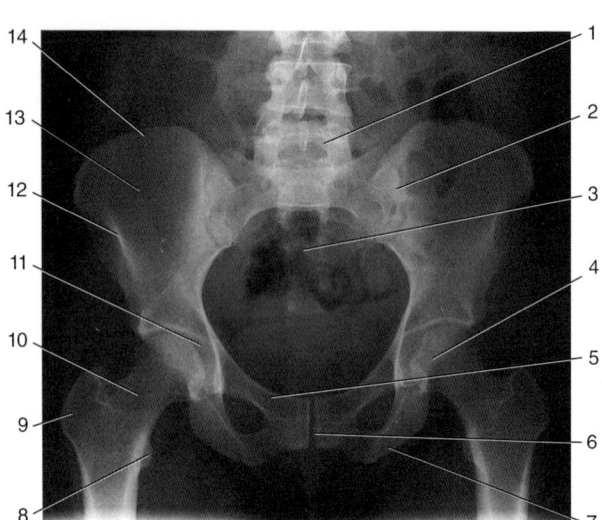

Fig. 14.16 Pelvis. AP projection.

1. _____
2. _____
3. _____
4. _____
5. _____
6. _____
7. _____
8. _____
9. _____
10. _____
11. _____
12. _____
13. _____
14. _____

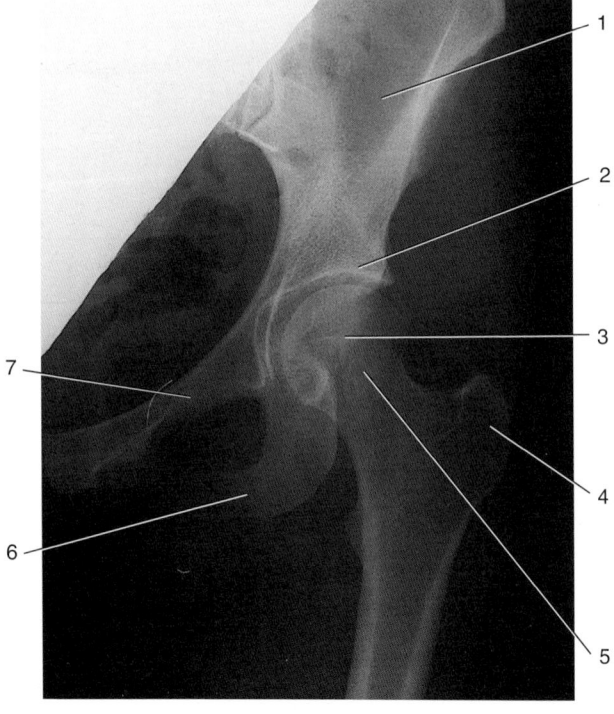

Fig. 14.17 Hip. AP projection.

1. _____
2. _____
3. _____
4. _____
5. _____
6. _____
7. _____

CHALLENGE EXERCISE

This exercise does not have to be completed at the same time as the other exercises in this workbook chapter. The exercise is designed to assess retention of the essential information contained in the corresponding textbook chapter. It is recommended that you complete this exercise when you begin to study for the state limited licensure examination. This will help determine what you know and which information should be further reviewed.

1. What is the minimum source-image receptor distance (SID) used for nearly all radiography of the lower limb?

   _____

2. Describe how the foot is positioned for the AP axial projection._____

   _____

3. Describe the central ray placement for the AP axial projection of the foot._____

   _____

4. What is the amount of medial rotation needed to achieve an AP oblique projection of the foot?_____

   _____

5. What are the amount and direction of central ray angulation for an axial (plantodorsal) projection of the calcaneus?

   _____

6. Describe the positioning details for the AP projection of the ankle._____

   _____

7. Describe the central ray placement for the AP projection of the ankle._____

   _____

8. Describe the positioning details for the lateral projection of the ankle._____

   _____

9. Describe the central ray placement for the lateral projection of the ankle._____

   _____

10. What are the amount and direction of leg rotation needed for an AP oblique projection of the ankle to demonstrate the distal tibiofibular joint?

    _____

11. What are the amount and direction of leg rotation needed for an AP oblique projection of the ankle to demonstrate the mortise joint?

_____

12. Describe the positioning details for the AP projection of the knee._____

_____

13. Describe the central ray placement for the AP projection of the knee, for all 3 sizes of patients._____

_____

14. Describe the positioning details for the lateral projection of the knee._____

_____

15. Describe the central ray placement and angle for the lateral projection of the knee._____

_____

16. Where is the superior margin of the IR or collimated field placed for an AP projection of the proximal femur?

_____

_____

17. Where is the inferior margin of the IR or collimated field placed for a lateral projection of the distal femur?

_____

_____

18. What are the amount and direction of leg rotation needed for an AP projection of the pelvis?

_____

19. What are the amount and direction of leg rotation needed for an AP projection of the hip?

_____

20. What is the amount of femur abduction needed for a lateral projection (frog-leg position) of the hip?

_____

15 Spine

EXERCISE 1

Answer the following questions by selecting the best choice.

1. The region of the spine that consists of five vertebrae and has a lordotic curve is the:
   A. cervical spine.
   B. thoracic spine.
   C. lumbar spine.
   D. sacrum.

2. What is the name of the most distal (or caudal) portion of the spine?
   A. Lumbar
   B. Thoracic
   C. Coccyx
   D. Sacrum

3. The cylindrical anterior portion of a typical vertebra is called the:
   A. body.
   B. lamina.
   C. pedicle.
   D. articular process.

4. The number of vertebrae in the normal cervical spine is:
   A. 4.
   B. 5.
   C. 7.
   D. 12.

5. The axis is another name for which vertebra?
   A. C1
   B. C2
   C. T1
   D. L5

6. The toothlike projection on the axis, around which the atlas rotates, is called the:
   A. spinous process.
   B. facet.
   C. articular process.
   D. dens or odontoid process.

7. When an anteroposterior (AP) projection of the cervical spine is performed, the central ray is directed:
   A. perpendicular to the image receptor (IR).
   B. 15 degrees caudad.
   C. 15 degrees cephalad.
   D. 25 degrees cephalad.

8. When the midsagittal plane of the body is parallel to the IR and the central ray is directed perpendicular to C4, the resulting image will be a(n):
   A. AP projection of the lower cervical spine.
   B. lateral projection of the cervical spine.
   C. anterior oblique projection of the cervical spine.
   D. AP projection of the upper cervical spine (open mouth).

9. A shallow breathing technique is used to advantage when taking a lateral projection of the:
   A. cervical spine.
   B. thoracic spine.
   C. lumbar spine.
   D. sacrum.

10. For which of the following projections is it most important to consider the anode heel effect when positioning the patient?
    A. AP projection of the lower cervical spine
    B. AP projection of the thoracic spine
    C. Lateral projection of the thoracic spine
    D. AP projection of the lumbar spine

11. A supine position with the central ray directed 10 degrees caudad 1 inch inferior to the anterior superior iliac spine is used to demonstrate an:
    A. AP axial projection of the lumbosacral joint.
    B. AP axial projection of the sacrum.
    C. AP axial projection of the coccyx.
    D. AP projection of the pelvis.

12. All of the following patient positions can be used for spine radiography, except:
    A. upright.
    B. supine.
    C. prone.
    D. decubitus.

13. Patient breathing instructions for all projections of the lumbar spine should include:
    1. suspend breathing on inspiration.
    2. suspend breathing on expiration.
    3. shallow breathing.
    A. 1 only
    B. 2 only
    C. 3 only
    D. 1, 2, and 3

161

14. The CR for a lateral projection of the lumbar spine is centered:
    1. perpendicular to the IR through L4.
    2. perpendicular to the IR through L3.
    3. in the midaxillary line.
    A. 1 and 2
    B. 1 and 3
    C. 2 and 3
    D. 1, 2, and 3

15. The projection commonly called the *swimmer's technique* will demonstrate which region of the spine?
    A. Cervical region
    B. Cervicothoracic region
    C. Thoracic region
    D. Lumbar region

16. The positioning steps for the AP projection of the upper cervical spine *open-mouth technique* include which of the following?
    1. Align the midsagittal plane perpendicular to the IR.
    2. Align the occlusal plane and base of the skull parallel to the horizontal plane.
    3. Use close collimation.
    A. 1 and 2
    B. 1 and 3
    C. 2 and 3
    D. 1, 2, and 3

17. Which palpable landmark would be used when positioning for an AP projection of the lumbar spine?
    A. Iliac crest
    B. Jugular notch
    C. Xiphoid process
    D. Lower costal margin

18. When the posterior portions of the neural arch fail to close during early embryonic development, the condition is known as:
    A. spina bifida.
    B. meningomyelocele.
    C. herniated nucleus pulposus.
    D. stenosis.

19. Which region of the spine is the most common site of pathologic compression fractures of vertebral bodies due to osteoporosis in elderly females?
    A. Cervical region
    B. Thoracic region
    C. Lumbar region
    D. Sacral region

20. The opening in each vertebra that serves as the passage for the spinal cord is called the
    A. vertebral foramen.
    B. intervertebral foramen.
    C. vertebral arch.
    D. body.

21. The blocklike, anterior portion of a typical vertebra is called the
    A. pedicle.
    B. lamina.
    C. body.
    D. articular process.

22. What structures serve as cushions in the anterior portion of the vertebral column?
    A. Longitudinal ligaments
    B. Facets
    C. Articular processes
    D. Intervertebral disks

23. Which of the following is another name for C2?
    A. Atlas
    B. Axis
    C. Vertebra prominens
    D. Dens

24. What is the CR angle and direction for the AP axial projection of the sacrum?
    A. 10 degrees cephalad
    B. 10 degrees caudad
    C. 15 degrees cephalad
    D. 15 degrees caudad

25. Which projection of the lumbar spine demonstrates open intervertebral foramina?
    A. AP
    B. PA
    C. Lateral
    D. AP oblique

26. What positioning maneuver is used to improve patient comfort and reduce the lordotic curve of the lumbar spine when positioning a recumbent patient for an AP projection of the lumbar spine?
    A. Raising the patient's arms above the head
    B. Crossing the patient's arms across the chest
    C. Flexing the knees and using a support under them
    D. Having the patient distribute weight equally on both feet

27. Where does the CR enter the patient for the AP projection of the lumbar spine?
    A. At the level of the iliac crest, centered to the midsagittal plane
    B. At the level of the xiphoid process of the sternum, centered to the midcoronal plane
    C. At a level 1.5 inches above the iliac crest, centered to the midcoronal plane
    D. The CR entrance point depends on the size of the IR

28. Which of the following helps position the entire thoracic spine parallel to the IR when the patient is in a lateral recumbent position?
    A. Radiolucent support under the head and neck
    B. Radiolucent support under the shoulders and hips
    C. Radiolucent support under the waist and/or hips
    D. Radiolucent support between the knees

29. Which structures are seen on the lateral projection of the thoracic spine?
    A. C7 through L1
    B. T3 through T12
    C. C5 through T7
    D. C6 through L2

30. Where does the CR enter the patient for the AP projection of the thoracic spine?
    A. Perpendicular to T10
    B. Perpendicular to T5
    C. Perpendicular to T7
    D. Perpendicular to C7

31. The toothlike projection from the superior surface of the body of the axis is called the
    A. spinous process.
    B. anterior tubercle.
    C. dens or odontoid process.
    D. superior articular process.

32. Which portion of the spine is made up of five vertebrae and has a lordotic curve?
    A. Cervical
    B. Thoracic
    C. Lumbar
    D. Sacrum

33. What projection of the cervical spine should precede flexion and extension positions?
    A. AP projection, open-mouth position of the upper cervical spine
    B. Lateral projection of the cervical spine
    C. AP axial projection of the cervical spine
    D. Lateral projection of the skull

34. What is the CR angle and direction for the AP oblique projections of the cervical spine?
    A. 45 degrees cephalic
    B. 45 degrees caudal
    C. 15 degrees cephalic
    D. 15 degrees caudal

35. What is the minimum SID for standing full-spine projections?
    A. 40 inches
    B. 48 inches
    C. 60 inches
    D. 72 inches

36. Where is the top of the IR margin placed for standing full-spine projections?
    A. At C4
    B. At the ear
    C. Bottom of the ear
    D. Top of the ear

37. All of the following should be in the x-ray room when standing full-spine x-rays are taken, *except*:
    A. positioning sponges.
    B. compensating filters.
    C. lead waist apron.
    D. shadow shields.

EXERCISE 2

Answer the following questions.

1. List the sections of the spine and state the number of vertebrae or vertebral segments in each.

_____

_____

_____

_____

_____

163

2. Which spinal segments have a kyphotic curve? Which have a lordotic curve?

_____

_____

_____

3. How do the atlas and axis differ from the other cervical vertebrae?

_____

_____

_____

4. How many vertebrae comprise the thoracic spine?

_____

5. An AP projection of the upper cervical spine (open-mouth technique) is unsatisfactory because the patient's upper teeth are superimposed over the atlas and the dens. How should you adjust the position for a satisfactory radiograph?

_____

_____

_____

6. On which projection of the spine is the "Scottie dog" configuration demonstrated?

_____

7. An order for radiographic examination of the cervical spine includes a request for lateral flexion and extension positions. The patient was in a car accident this morning. What precautions are needed? Why?

_____

_____

_____

_____

8. An AP projection of the thoracic spine appears to be quite dark in the region of T1 to T4 and a bit too light in the region of T7 to T12. List possible causes and suggest solutions.

_____

_____

_____

_____

9. How would you instruct a female patient to prepare for a lumbar spine examination?

_____

_____

_____

10. What is the rationale for using a 72-inch SID for the lateral projection of the cervical spine?

_____

11. What type of spinal fracture is common among older females with osteoporosis?

_____

12. What anatomic structures are best demonstrated by the AP oblique projections of the cervical spine?

_____

13. What device is used to improve visualization of the spinous processes of the thoracic spine on the lateral projection?

_____

14. An abnormal lateral curvature of the spine is called

_____

15. State where the CR is positioned for a lateral projection of the sacrum?

_____

16. To protect a patient's sensitive tissues—thyroid, breasts and gonads—during standing full-spine x-rays, which projection should be used?

_____

Label the following figures.

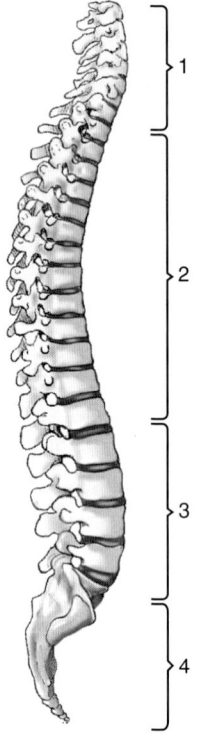

Fig. 15.1 Lateral aspect of the spine.

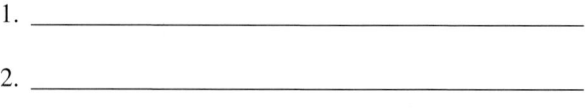

1. _____

2. _____

3. _____

4. _____

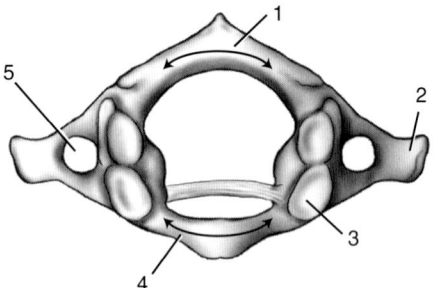

Fig. 15.2 Superior aspect of the atlas (C1).

1. _____

2. _____

3. _____

4. _____

5. _____

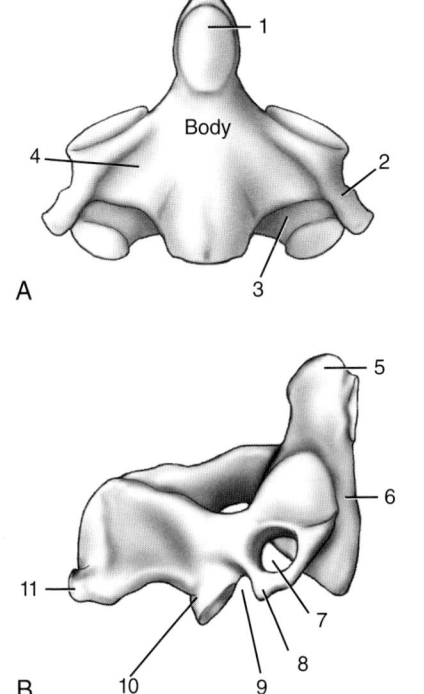

Body

A

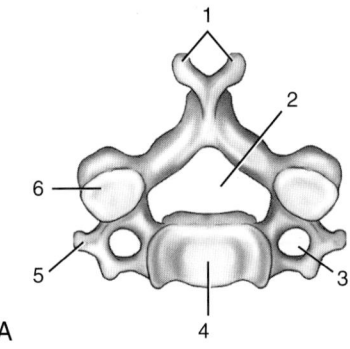

B

Fig. 15.3 Atlas. (A) Anterior aspect. (B) Lateral aspect.

1. _____
2. _____
3. _____
4. _____
5. _____
6. _____
7. _____
8. _____
9. _____
10. _____
11. _____

A

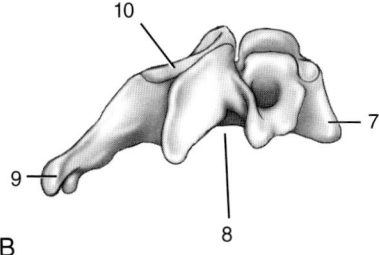

B

Fig. 15.4 Typical cervical vertebra. (A) Superior aspect.
(B) Lateral aspect.

1. _____
2. _____
3. _____
4. _____
5. _____
6. _____
7. _____
8. _____
9. _____
10. _____

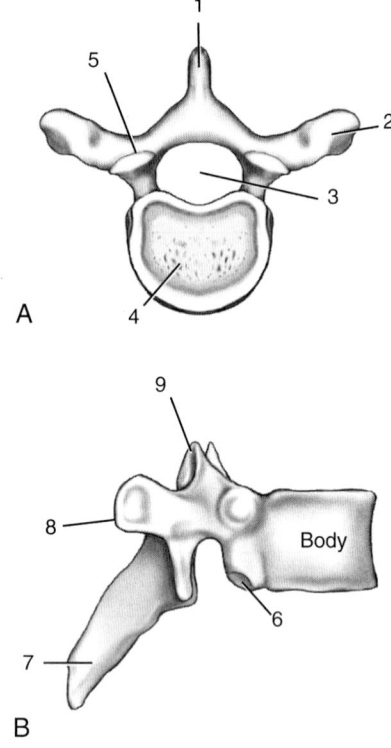

A

B

Fig. 15.5 Thoracic vertebra. (A) Superior aspect. (B) Lateral aspect.

1. _____
2. _____
3. _____
4. _____
5. _____
6. _____
7. _____
8. _____
9. _____

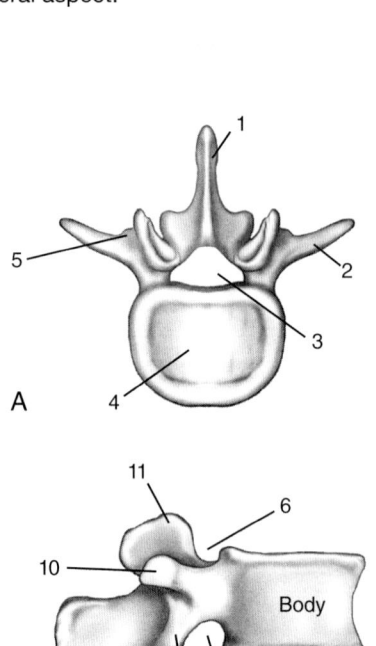

A

B

Fig. 15.6 Lumbar vertebra. (A) Anterior aspect. (B) Lateral aspect.

1. _____
2. _____
3. _____
4. _____
5. _____
6. _____
7. _____
8. _____
9. _____
10. _____
11. _____

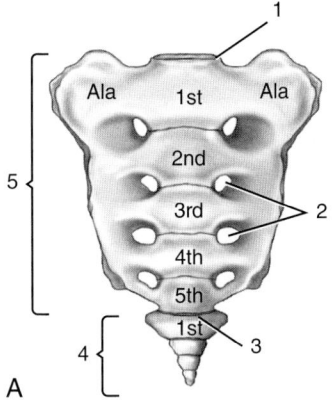

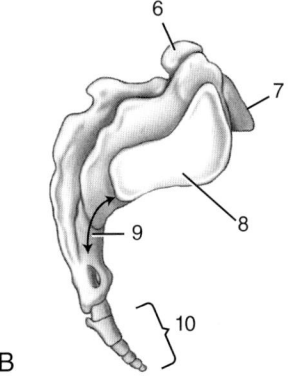

Fig. 15.7 Sacrum and coccyx. (A) Anterior aspect. (B) Lateral aspect.

1. _____
2. _____
3. _____
4. _____
5. _____
6. _____
7. _____
8. _____
9. _____
10. _____

Label the following images.

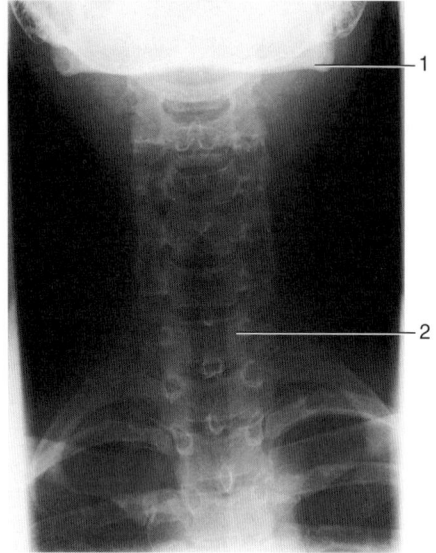

Fig. 15.8 Cervical spine (lower). AP projection.

1. _____

2. _____

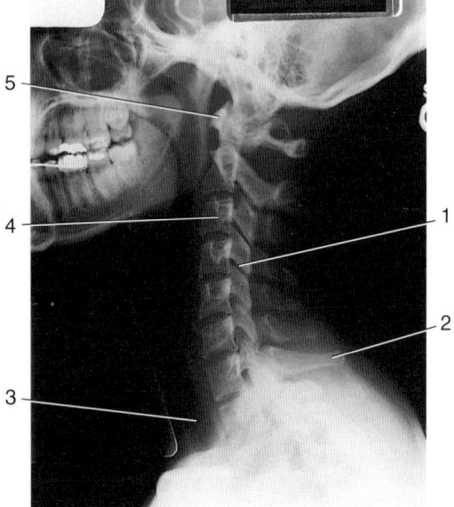

Fig. 15.9 Cervical spine. Lateral projection.

1. _____

2. _____

3. _____

4. _____

5. _____

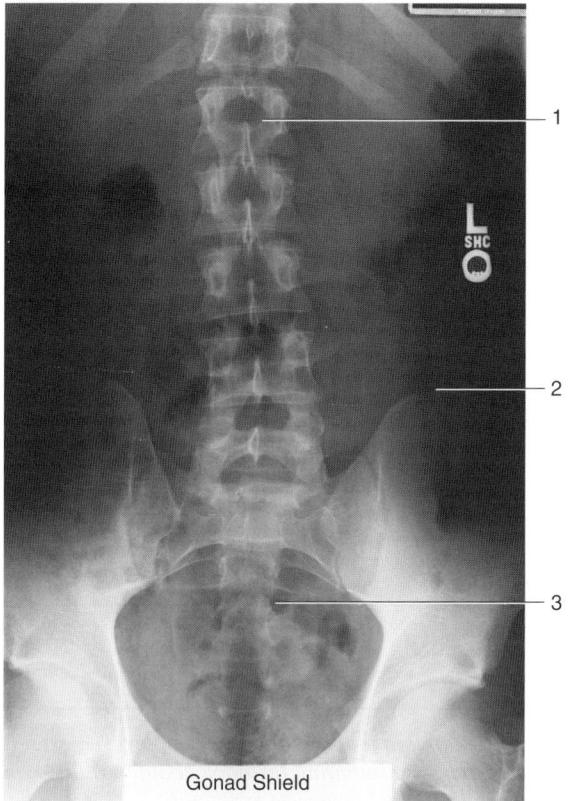

Fig. 15.10 Lumbar spine. AP projection, patient recumbent with knees flexed.

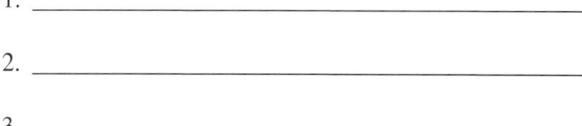

Gonad Shield

1. _____

2. _____

3. _____

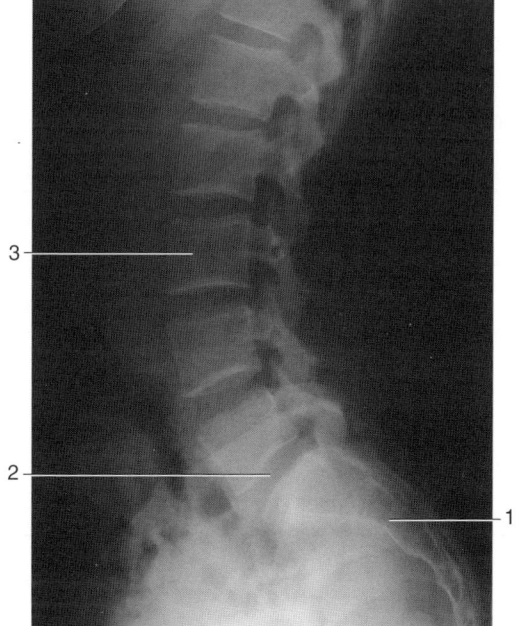

Fig. 15.11 Lumbar spine. Lateral projection.

1. _____

2. _____

3. _____

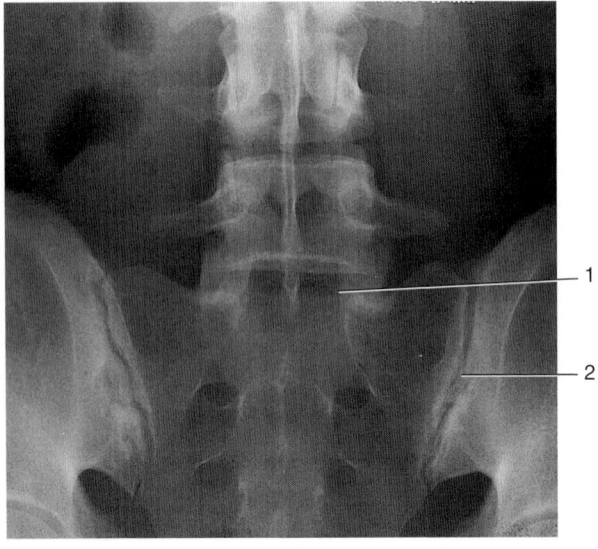

Fig. 15.12 Lumbosacral junction and sacroiliac joints. AP axial projection.

1. _____

2. _____

CHALLENGE EXERCISE

This exercise does not have to be completed at the same time as the other exercises in this workbook chapter. The exercise is designed to assess retention of the essential information contained in the corresponding textbook chapter. It is recommended that you complete this exercise when you begin to study for the state limited licensure examination. This will help determine what you know and which information should be further reviewed.

1. Describe the positioning details for the AP axial projection of the lower cervical spine.

   _____

   _____

2. Describe the central ray angle and placement for the AP axial projection of the lower cervical spine.

   _____

3. Describe the positioning details for the AP projection of the upper cervical spine.

   _____

   _____

4. Describe the central ray angle and placement for the AP projection of the upper cervical spine.

   _____

5. Describe the positioning details for the lateral projection of the cervical spine.

   _____

   _____

6. Describe the central ray angle and placement for the lateral projection of the cervical spine.

_____

7. What is the source-image receptor distance (SID) range used for the lateral projection of the cervical spine?

_____

8. Describe the positioning details for the AP axial oblique projection of the cervical spine.

_____

_____

9. Describe the central ray angle and placement for the AP axial oblique projection of the cervical spine. _____

_____

10. What is the common name for the lateral projection of the cervicothoracic region? (Hint: You do this in the water.)

_____

11. Describe how the "breathing technique" is performed for the lateral projection of the thoracic spine.

_____

_____

12. Describe the positioning details for the AP projection of the lumbar spine.

_____

_____

13. Describe the central ray angle and placement for the AP projection of the lumbar spine.

_____

14. Describe the positioning details for the lateral projection of the lumbar spine.

_____

_____

15. Describe the central ray angle and placement for the lateral projection of the lumbar spine.

_____

16. Describe the positioning details for the AP oblique projection of the lumbar spine.

_____

_____

17. Describe the central ray angle and placement for the AP oblique projection of the lumbar spine.

_____

18. What is the purpose of the lateral projection of the L5 to S1 lumbosacral junction?

_____

_____

19. Describe the positioning details for the AP oblique projection of the sacroiliac joint.

_____

_____

20. Describe the central ray angle and placement for the AP oblique projection of the sacroiliac joint.

_____

21. Describe the positioning details for the AP axial projection of the sacrum.

_____

_____

22. Describe the central ray angle and placement for the AP axial projection of the sacrum.

_____

23. Describe the central ray angle and placement for the AP axial projection of the coccyx.

_____

24. Describe the positioning details for the lateral projection of the sacrum.

_____

_____

25. Describe the central ray angle and placement for the lateral projection of the sacrum.

_____

16 Bony Thorax, Chest, and Abdomen

EXERCISE 1

Answer the following questions by selecting the best choice.

1. Which of the following terms does *not* refer to a portion of the sternum?
   A. Body
   B. Jugular notch
   C. Mediastinum
   D. Xiphoid process

2. The lower five pairs of ribs are called:
   A. true ribs.
   B. false ribs.
   C. floating ribs.
   D. cervical ribs.

3. All of the following organs are found within the mediastinum, *except:*
   A. heart.
   B. lungs.
   C. trachea.
   D. ascending aorta.

4. The inferior lateral "corners" of the lungs are called the:
   A. hila.
   B. inferior lobes.
   C. cardiophrenic angles.
   D. costophrenic angles.

5. Which of the following make up the bony thorax?
   A. 12 pairs of ribs
   B. 12 ribs, 12 thoracic vertebrae, and the sternum
   C. 12 pairs of ribs, 12 thoracic vertebrae, and the sternum
   D. 12 pairs of ribs, 7 thoracic vertebrae, the sternum, and clavicles

6. How many lobes are in the right lung?
   A. Three
   B. Four
   C. Two
   D. One

7. What body habitus term is applied to a person of normal size?
   A. Asthenic
   B. Sthenic
   C. Hypersthenic
   D. Hyposthenic

8. Which of the following describes the importance of using an upright position for chest radiography?
      1. Demonstrates air-fluid levels.
      2. Allows maximum lung expansion.
      3. Minimizes magnification of the heart.
   A. 1 and 2 only
   B. 1 and 3 only
   C. 2 and 3 only
   D. 1, 2, and 3

9. What is the purpose of rotating the patient's shoulders anteriorly for the posteroanterior (PA) projection of the chest?
   A. Rotates the scapulae out of the lungs.
   B. Reduces magnification of the heart shadow.
   C. Makes the position more comfortable for the patient.
   D. Places the coronal plane parallel to the upright grid cabinet.

10. The essential factor for the demonstration of air-fluid levels in radiography is:
   A. the decubitus position.
   B. the semiupright position.
   C. a horizontal x-ray beam.
   D. a perpendicular x-ray beam.

11. Which of the following is true regarding persons with a hypersthenic body habitus?
   A. Average body build
   B. Organs are located higher and more horizontally
   C. Tall and slender body build
   D. Organs are longer and narrower in shape

12. Where is the jugular notch located?
   A. At the end of the body of the sternum
   B. At the end of the xiphoid process
   C. At the top of the sternum
   D. At the bottom of the manubrium

13. When a posteroanterior (PA) projection of the chest is performed, the correct source-image receptor distance (SID) is:
   A. 40 inches.
   B. 48 inches.
   C. 60 inches.
   D. 72 inches.

175

14. Why are lateral projections of the chest taken with the left side against the image receptor (IR)?
    A. Magnification of the cardiac silhouette is minimized with the left side nearer the IR.
    B. It is conventional to have a routine standard, and the left has been established as the standard.
    C. Lung pathology is more common on the left side.
    D. The right hilum provides high-contrast details that may be confusing.

15. Which of the following techniques is desirable for chest radiography?
    A. High kVp, high milliamperes (mA), and short exposure time
    B. Low kVp and 72-inch SID
    C. Low kVp, high milliampere-seconds (mAs)
    D. High kVp, 72-inch SID, and low mA

16. What structure separates the thoracic cavity from the abdominal cavity?
    A. The aortic arch
    B. The parietal membrane
    C. The visceral membrane
    D. The diaphragm

17. All of the following are true for demonstrating air-fluid levels in radiography, *except*:
    A. the decubitus position.
    B. the upright position.
    C. a horizontal x-ray beam.
    D. a 40-inch SID

18. Breathing instructions for a PA projection of the chest should include:
    A. suspend breathing on the first deep inspiration.
    B. suspend breathing on the second deep inspiration.
    C. suspend breathing on the first expiration.
    D. suspend breathing on the second expiration.

19. The presence of air in the pleural cavity is called:
    A. pneumothorax.
    B. emphysema.
    C. pneumonia.
    D. pleural effusion.

20. Why is a grid used for chest radiography?
    A. To increase the exposure time
    B. To reduce fog from scatter radiation
    C. To enhance image contrast
    D. To enhance spatial resolution

21. Evidence of full inspiration on a chest radiograph is seen when how many ribs can be counted superior to the diaphragm?
    A. 8 ribs
    B. 10 ribs
    C. 8 to 10 ribs
    D. 12 ribs

22. Which body habitus is characterized as very slender?
    A. Sthenic
    B. Asthenic
    C. Hypersthenic
    D. Hyposthenic

23. Where does the CR enter the patient for the upright, PA projection of the chest?
    A. Midsagittal plane at the level of T7
    B. Midcoronal plane at the level of T7
    C. Midsagittal plane at the level of the iliac crests
    D. Midcoronal plane at the level of the iliac crests

24. Which body position is recommended for maximum lung expansion in chest radiography?
    A. Supine
    B. Prone
    C. Upright
    D. Decubitus

25. When a patient is unable to stand for an upright PA projection of the chest, which of the following projections should be substituted?
    A. Anteroposterior (AP) projection (usually supine)
    B. PA projection (prone position)
    C. AP projection (lateral decubitus position)
    D. PA projection (lateral decubitus position)

26. The xiphoid process is the _____ of the sternum.
    A. proximal portion
    B. distal tip
    C. middle portion
    D. longest portion

27. In chest radiography, which body habitus is best imaged by placing the 35 × 43-cm IR crosswise in the upright grid cabinet?
    A. Sthenic
    B. Asthenic
    C. Hyposthenic
    D. Hypersthenic

28. The structures seen on an AP axial projection (lordotic position) of the chest are the:
    A. mediastinum and trachea.
    B. mediastinum including the aortic arch.
    C. apices of both lungs and mediastinum.
    D. apices of both lungs free of superimposition by the clavicles.

29. The definition of pneumonia is:
    A. an inflammation of the lung caused by a bacterial or viral infection.
    B. a type of chronic obstructive pulmonary disease.
    C. a collapse of the lung, usually caused by trauma.
    D. chronic lung disease caused by the inhalation of irritating dust.

30. How high should the down side of the chest be elevated for a decubitus position x-ray?
    A. 2 to 3 inches
    B. 2 to 4 inches
    C. 2 inches for females and 4 inches for males
    D. 4 inches for all adults

31. For an AP chest projection, where is the CR centered?
    A. 1 in. below the jugular notch
    B. 3 in. below the jugular notch
    C. Centered to the manubrium
    D. Centered on the xiphoid process

EXERCISE 2

Answer the following questions.

1. The indentation on the top of the sternum that is used as a positioning landmark is the:

    _____

2. What is the name of the upper portion of both lungs?

    _____

3. Name the three main structures located within the mediastinum.

    1. _____

    2. _____

    3. _____

4. Name three characteristics of the asthenic body habitus.

    1. _____

    2. _____

    3. _____

5. What is the proper placement of the arms for the upright, lateral projection of the chest?

    _____

6. What is the definition of *emphysema*?

    _____

7. What is the recommended SID for x-ray projections of the chest?_____

    _____

8. State three reasons why it is important to use the upright position for chest radiography.

   1. _____

   2. _____

   3. _____

9. What are the three primary structures seen on a PA projection of the chest?

   1. _____

   2. _____

   3. _____

10. Why are lateral projections of the chest taken with the patient's left side against the IR?

    _____

11. Which body habitus is characterized by a massive stocky build?_____

    _____

12. What primary movement is performed on the patient to move the scapulae out of the way of the lungs for a PA projection?

    _____

13. How far is the IR placed above C7 for a PA chest?

    _____

14. What is the purpose of using a 72-inch SID for chest radiography?

    _____

15. What is the definition of atelectasis?

    _____

16. When air-fluid levels need to be evaluated on a chest x-ray, how is the x-ray tube positioned?

    _____

17. Which projection is performed to demonstrate the apices of the lungs?

    _____

Label the following figures.

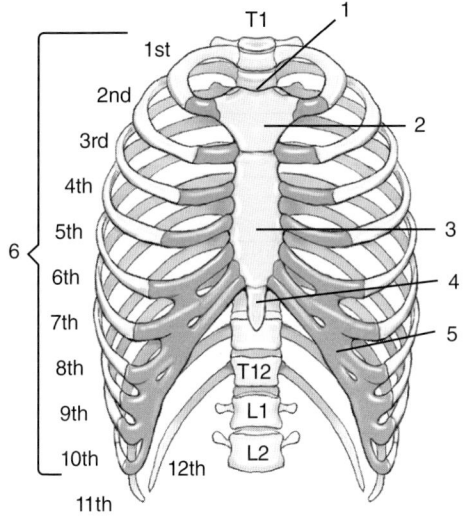

Fig. 16.1 Bony thorax.

1. _____

2. _____

3. _____

4. _____

5. _____

6. _____

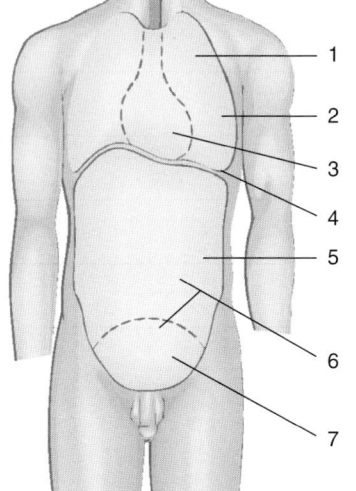

Fig. 16.2 Body cavities, anterior aspect.

1. _____

2. _____

3. _____

4. _____

5. _____

6. _____

7. _____

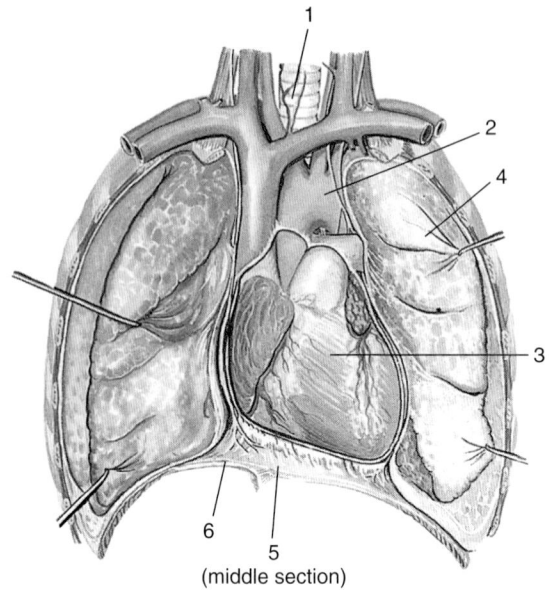

Fig. 16.3 Thoracic cavity.

1. _____

2. _____

3. _____

4. _____

5. _____

6. _____

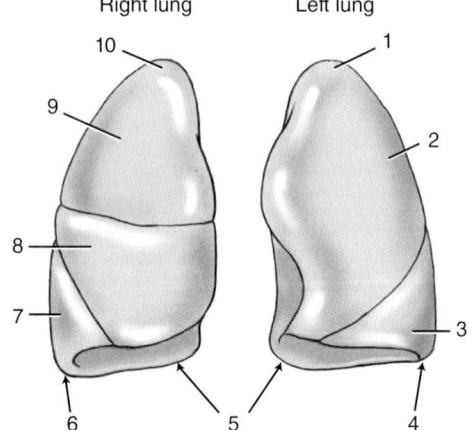

Right lung   Left lung

Fig. 16.4 Anterior aspect of lungs.

1. _____

2. _____

3. _____

4. _____

5. _____

6. _____

7. _____

8. _____

9. _____

10. _____

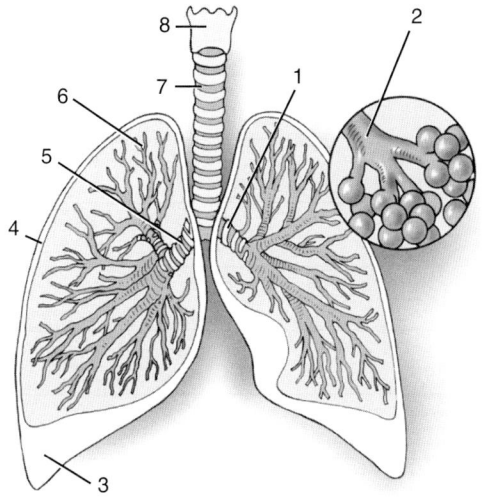

Fig. 16.5 Organs of the respiratory system in the thoracic cavity.

1. _____
2. _____
3. _____
4. _____
5. _____
6. _____
7. _____
8. _____

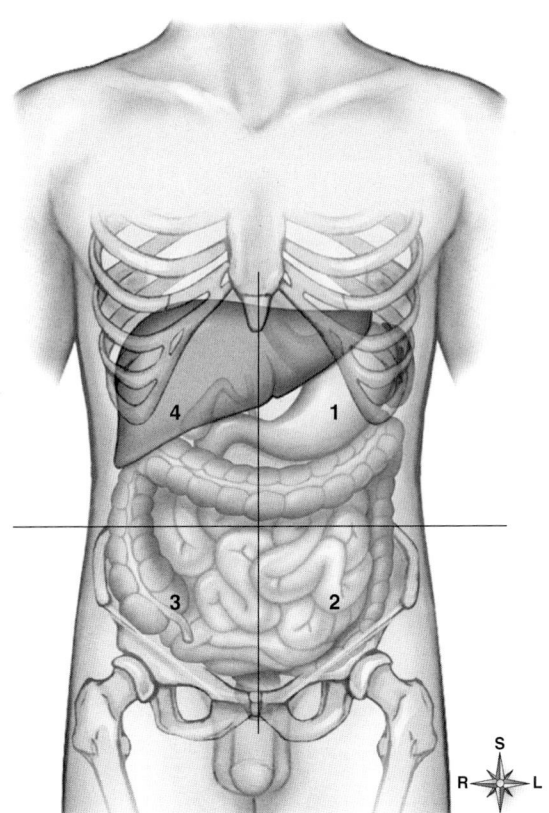

Fig. 16.6 Abdominopelvic cavity divided into quadrants.

1. _____
2. _____
3. _____
4. _____

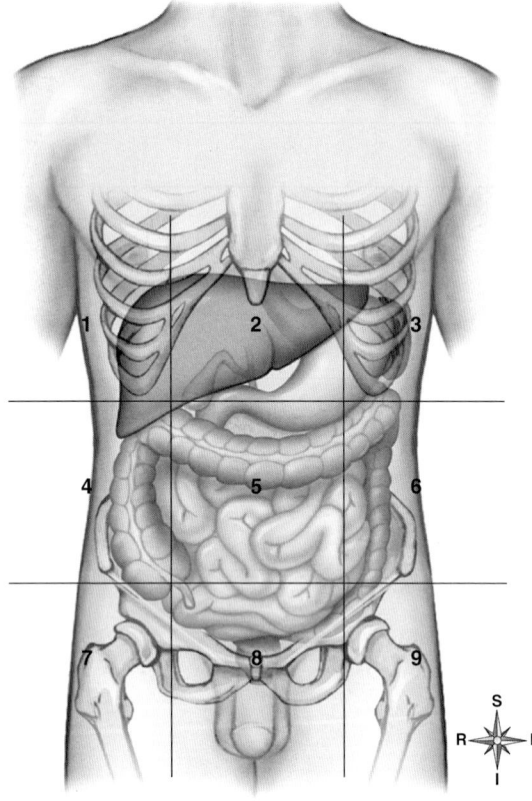

Fig. 16.7 Nine abdominal regions.

1. _____

2. _____

3. _____

4. _____

5. _____

6. _____

7. _____

8. _____

9. _____

Label the following figures.

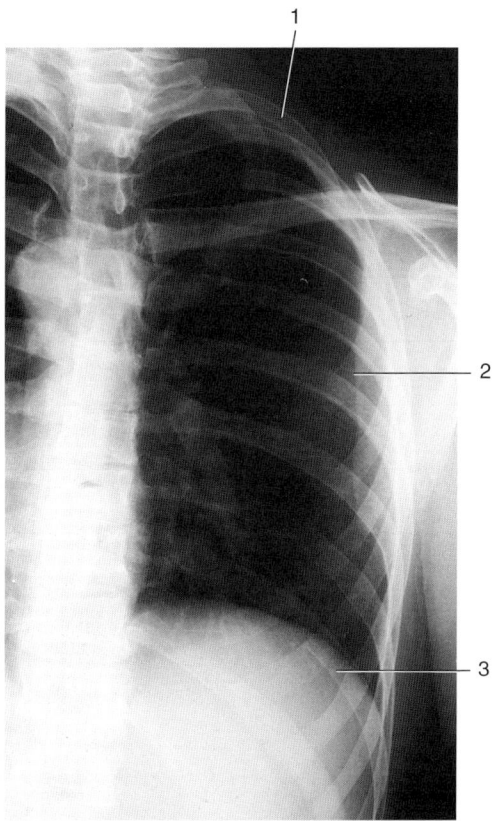

Fig. 16.8 Upper posterior chest. AP projection.

1. _____

2. _____

3. _____

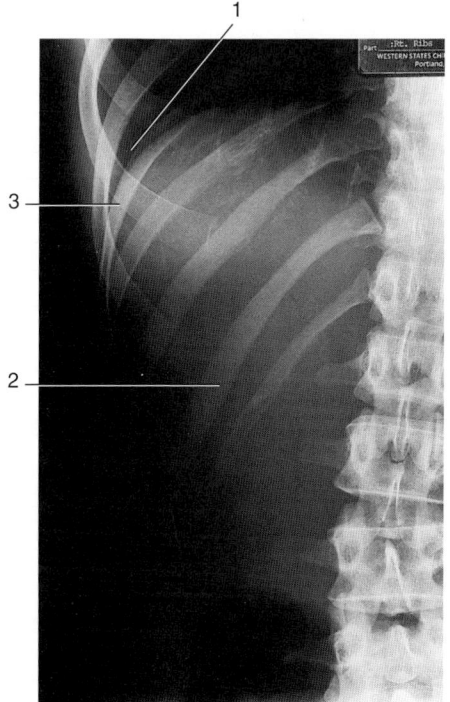

Fig. 16.9 Lower posterior ribs. AP projection.

1. _____

2. _____

3. _____

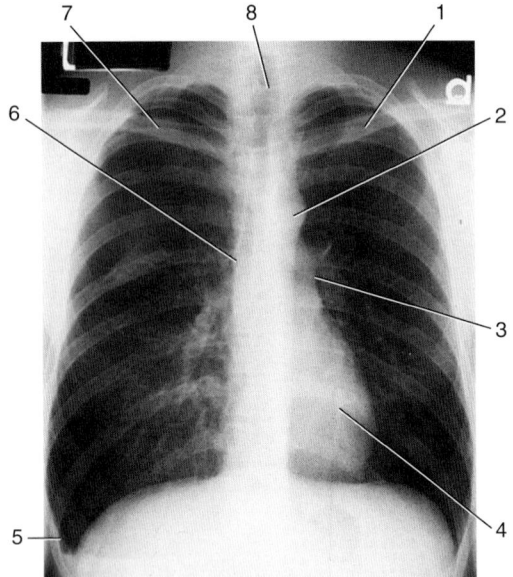

Fig. 16.10 Chest. PA projection.

1. _____

2. _____

3. _____

4. _____

5. _____

6. _____

7. _____

8. _____

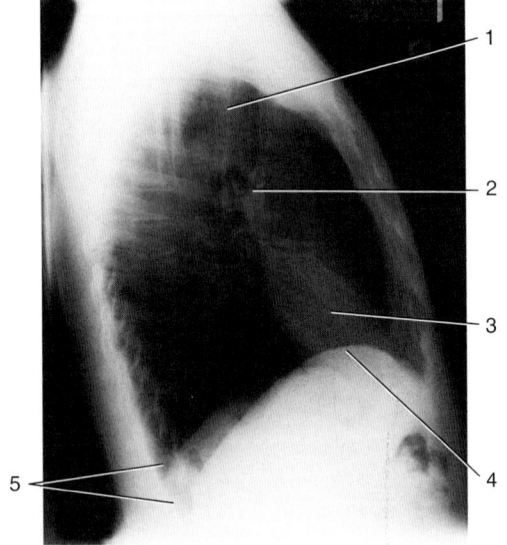

Fig. 16.11 Chest. Lateral projection.

1. _____

2. _____

3. _____

4. _____

5. _____

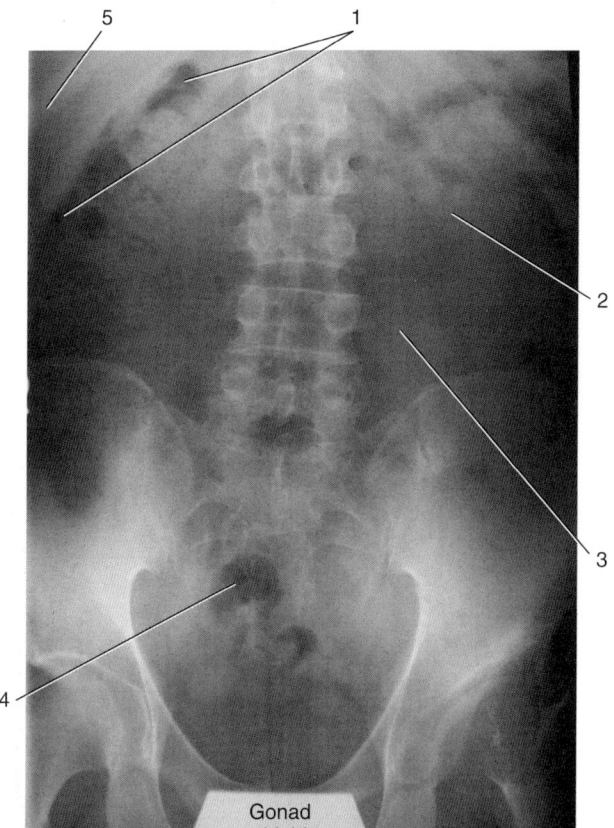

Gonad
shield

Fig. 16.12 Abdomen. AP projection, patient recumbent.

1. _____

2. _____

3. _____

4. _____

5. _____

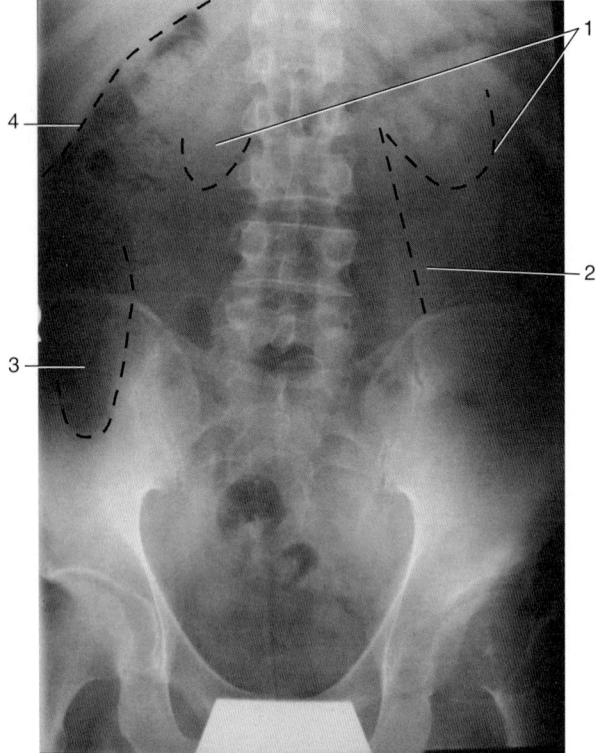

Fig. 16.13 AP abdomen radiograph showing kidney shadows, liver margin, and psoas muscles.

1. _____

2. _____

3. _____

4. _____

CHALLENGE EXERCISE

This exercise does not have to be completed at the same time as the other exercises in this workbook chapter. The exercise is designed to assess retention of the essential information contained in the corresponding textbook chapter. It is recommended that you complete this exercise when you begin to study for the state limited licensure examination. This will help determine what you know and which information should be further reviewed.

1. Describe the movement of the diaphragm during inspiration.

   _____

2. Describe the movement of the diaphragm during expiration.

   _____

3. What is the recommended SID for routine radiography of the chest?

   _____

4. Describe the positioning details for the PA projection of the chest.

   _____

   _____

5. Describe the central ray placement for the PA projection of the chest.

_____

6. Describe the patient's breathing instructions for the PA projection of the chest.

_____

7. Describe the positioning details for the lateral projection of the chest.

_____

_____

8. Describe the central ray placement for the lateral projection of the chest.

_____

9. Describe the positioning details for the AP projection (lateral decubitus position) of the chest

_____

_____

10. Describe positioning details to position for an AP axial chest (lordotic position).

_____

_____

17 Skull, Facial Bones, and Paranasal Sinuses

EXERCISE 1

Answer the following questions by selecting the best choice.

1. Which of the following bones are NOT parts of the cranium?
   A. Parietal
   B. Frontal
   C. Maxillary
   D. Temporal

2. The bony prominence on the frontal bone between the eyebrows is called the:
   A. acanthion.
   B. glabella.
   C. gonion.
   D. nasion.

3. Which of the following is the positioning landmark located at the junction of the nose and upper lip?
   A. Acanthion
   B. Glabella
   C. Gonion
   D. Nasion

4. All of the following bones contain paranasal sinuses, *except* the:
   A. frontal bone.
   B. ethmoid bone.
   C. temporal bone.
   D. maxilla.

5. When a posteroanterior (PA) projection of the skull is performed, the central ray (CR) is directed:
   A. perpendicular to the image receptor (IR).
   B. 15 degrees cephalad.
   C. 15 degrees caudad.
   D. 30 degrees cephalad.

6. A projection of the skull in which the sagittal plane is parallel to the IR and the interpupillary line is perpendicular to the IR is a(n):
   A. PA projection.
   B. AP axial projection (Towne method).
   C. Waters projection.
   D. lateral projection.

7. How many bones are there in the skull?
   A. 14
   B. 18
   C. 22
   D. 31

8. When the patient is supine, the sagittal plane of the skull is perpendicular to the IR, the orbitomeatal line is perpendicular to the IR, and the CR is angled 30 degrees caudad, the resulting radiograph will demonstrate the:
   A. frontal bones.
   B. temporal bones.
   C. posterior parietal bones and occipital bone.
   D. maxillary sinuses.

9. Which of the following bones are categorized as cranial bones?
   1. Maxilla
   2. Ethmoid
   3. Parietal
   A. 1 and 2 only
   B. 1 and 3 only
   C. 2 and 3 only
   D. 1, 2, and 3

10. When the right and left halves of the skull do not appear symmetric on a PA or an AP projection, this is a sign that:
    A. the neck is extended too much.
    B. the neck is flexed too much.
    C. the sagittal plane is not perpendicular to the IR.
    D. the central ray is not centered to the IR.

11. A blowout fracture involves the:
    A. floor of the orbit.
    B. occipital bone.
    C. mandible.
    D. nasal bones.

12. The projection that will demonstrate all of the paranasal sinuses is:
    A. the lateral projection.
    B. the parietoacanthial projection.
    C. the PA axial projection.
    D. all of the above.

13. Which of the following cranial bones are paired (right and left)?
    1. Frontal
    2. Parietal
    3. Temporal
    A. 1 only
    B. 1 and 2 only
    C. 2 and 3 only
    D. 1, 2, and 3

14. What is the term for the articulations between the cranial bones?
    A. Glabellae
    B. Sutures
    C. Acanthions
    D. Foramina

15. Which projection best demonstrates the maxillary sinuses?
    A. Parietoacanthial (Waters method)
    B. SMV
    C. PA axial (Caldwell method)
    D. AP axial (Towne method)

16. In which bone can the foramen magnum be found?
    A. Frontal
    B. Temporal
    C. Ethmoid
    D. Occipital

17. Which structure houses the pituitary gland?
    A. EAM
    B. Foramen magnum
    C. Sella turcica
    D. Crista galli

18. The EAM is located in the _____ bone.
    A. temporal
    B. ethmoid
    C. occipital
    D. frontal

19. Which of the following bones contain paranasal sinuses?
    1. Frontal
    2. Ethmoid
    3. Temporal
    A. 1 and 2 only
    B. 1 and 3 only
    C. 2 and 3 only
    D. 1, 2, and 3

20. There are several imaginary lines used to position the skull. Which imaginary line connects the outer corner of the eye to the EAM?
    A. The infraorbitomeatal line
    B. The orbitomeatal line
    C. The acanthiomeatal line
    D. The mentomeatal line

21. When taking a PA axial projection (Caldwell method) of the skull, the CR is directed:
    A. 15 degrees cephalad.
    B. 15 degrees caudad.
    C. 30 degrees cephalad.
    D. 30 degrees caudad.

22. Which projection of the cranium demonstrates the petrous ridges within the orbits?
    A. AP axial (Towne method)
    B. PA
    C. PA axial (Caldwell method)
    D. SMV

23. What is the position of the OML for the PA axial projection (Caldwell method) of the cranium?
    A. Perpendicular to IR
    B. Parallel with IR
    C. Perpendicular to CR
    D. 37 degrees from IR

24. Which cranial projection best demonstrates the occipital bone?
    A. PA
    B. PA axial (Caldwell method)
    C. AP axial (Towne method)
    D. Lateral

25. Which of the following demonstrates the structures of the cranial base?
    A. Lateral
    B. PA axial
    C. SMV
    D. PA

26. A lateral projection of the face using a tabletop IR (nongrid) is used to demonstrate the:
    A. mandible.
    B. zygoma.
    C. orbits.
    D. nasal bones.

27. Which projection of the facial bones requires the CR to exit the acanthion?
    A. AP axial (Towne method)
    B. PA axial (Caldwell method)
    C. Lateral
    D. Parietoacanthial (Waters method)

28. What is the purpose of performing sinus radiography with the patient in the upright position?
    A. To demonstrate air-fluid levels
    B. For ease of patient positioning
    C. To prevent superimposition of the cranial structures on the paranasal sinuses
    D. Sinus radiography does not have to be performed with the patient upright

29. Which paranasal sinuses are best demonstrated on the PA axial projection (Caldwell method)?
    1. Maxillary
    2. Frontal
    3. Ethmoid
    A. 1 and 2 only
    B. 1 and 3 only
    C. 2 and 3 only
    D. 1, 2, and 3

30. Which of the following projections demonstrates the sphenoid sinus?
    A. Parietoacanthial (Waters method)
    B. Lateral
    C. AP axial (Towne method)
    D. PA axial (Caldwell method)

31. What is the name of the articulation between the parietal bones?
    A. Squamosal suture
    B. Lambdoidal suture
    C. Coronal suture
    D. Sagittal suture

32. When the patient is prone, the sagittal plane of the skull is perpendicular to the IR, the OML is perpendicular to the IR, and the CR is angled 15 degrees caudad, the resulting radiograph will demonstrate the:
    A. frontal bones.
    B. temporal bones.
    C. posterior parietal bones and occipital bone.
    D. maxillary sinuses.

EXERCISE 2

Answer the following questions.

1. Name the eight bones that make up the cranium.

_____

_____

_____

_____

_____

_____

_____

_____

2. Which cranial bones contain the auditory canals?

_____

3. What is the medical term for the bony sockets that house the eyes?

_____

4. Which cranial bone is most anterior?

_____

5. Name the projection that demonstrates the cranial base.

_____

6. What is the name of the articulation between the frontal bone and the parietal bones?

_____

7. Name two projections that demonstrate the maxillary sinuses.

   1. _____

   2. _____

8. How does the procedure for a lateral projection of the nasal bones differ from that for a lateral projection of the facial bones?

_____

_____

_____

9. What is the *foramen magnum*?

_____

10. If the petrous portion is projected over the floor of the maxillary sinuses on the parietoacanthial (Waters method) projection, how should the position be modified to clearly demonstrate this area?

_____

_____

11. What common positioning landmark is located on the anterior, lower margin of the mandible?

_____

12. Name three types of pathologic conditions that may be diagnosed by radiography of the cranium.

   1. _____

   2. _____

   3. _____

13. Air-filled cavities located in some bones of the face and cranium are called:

_____

14. The depression on the anterior surface of the skull between the orbits is called the:

_____

15. Which radiographic baseline is used to position the PA axial projection (Caldwell method) of the cranium?

_____

16. Which projections of the cranium best demonstrate the frontal bone?

_____

17. The patient is positioned supine with the midsagittal plane (MSP) and OML perpendicular to the IR. The CR is angled 30 degrees caudal and enters the MSP at approximately 2.5 inches superior to the glabella. What projection is imaged on the radiograph?

_____

18. What cranial structures are best demonstrated by the SMV projection?

_____

19. Which facial bones are demonstrated on the PA axial projection (Caldwell method)?

_____

20. Which paranasal sinuses are demonstrated by the parietoacanthial projection (Waters method)?

_____

21. Which paranasal sinuses are demonstrated by the SMV projection?

_____

22. Which facial bone(s) is (are) most frequently fractured?

_____

Label the following illustrations.

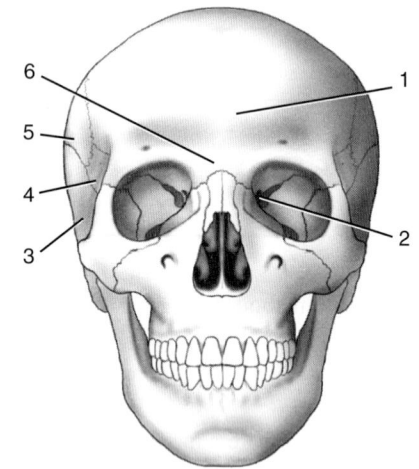

A

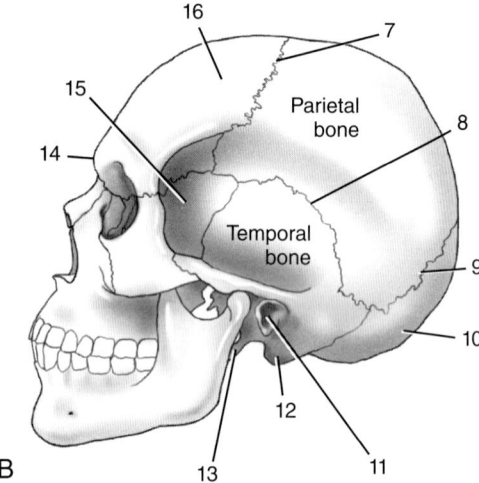

B

Fig. 17.1 Cranium. (A) Anterior aspect. (B) Lateral aspect.

1. _____

2. _____

3. _____

4. _____

5. _____

6. _____

7. _____

8. _____

9. _____

10. _____

11. _____

12. _____

13. _____

14. _____

15. _____

16. _____

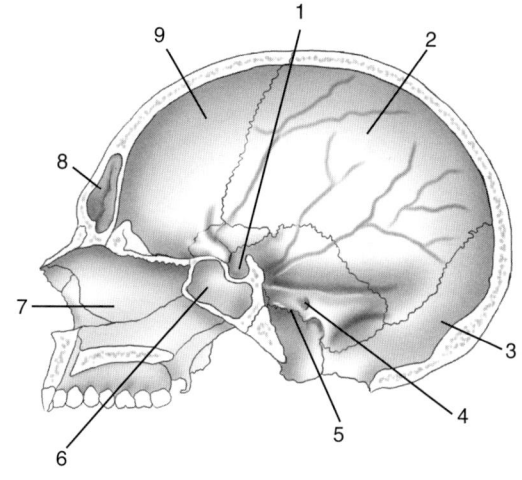

Fig. 17.1 cont'd (C) Lateral aspect of interior cranium.

C

1. _____

2. _____

3. _____

4. _____

5. _____

6. _____

7. _____

8. _____

9. _____

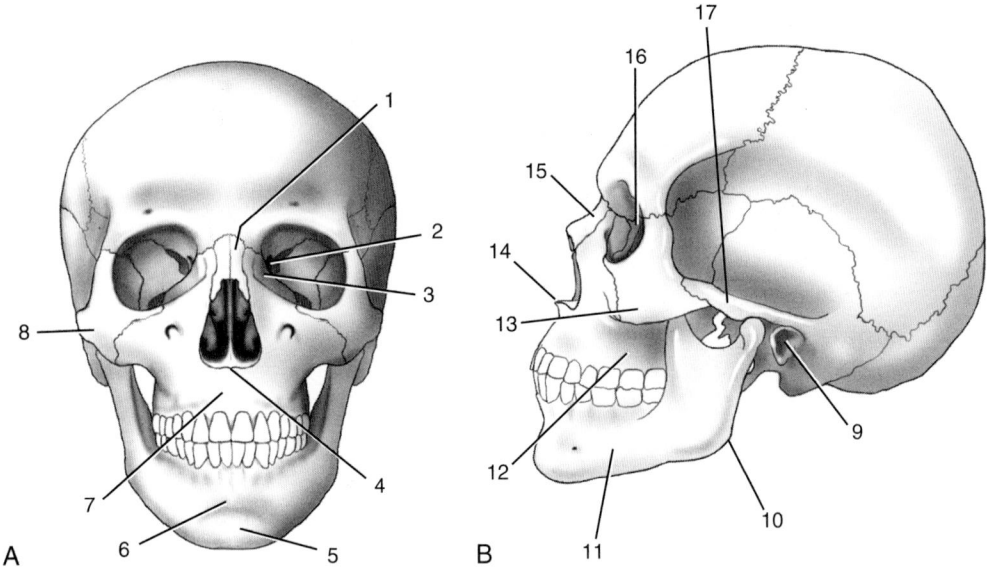

Fig. 17.2 Facial bones. (A) Anterior aspect. (B) Lateral aspect.

1. _____

2. _____

3. _____

4. _____

5. _____

6. _____

7. _____

8. _____

9. _____

10. _____

11. _____

12. _____

13. _____

14. _____

15. _____

16. _____

17. _____

Chapter **17 Skull, Facial Bones, and Paranasal Sinuses**

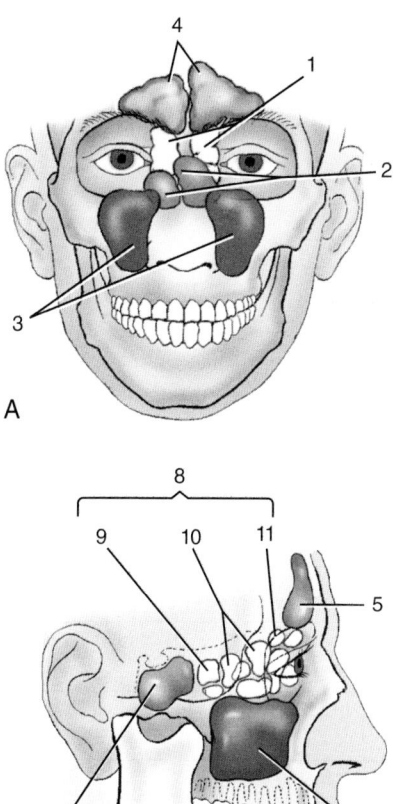

A

B

Fig. 17.3 Paranasal sinuses. (A) Anterior aspect. (B) Lateral aspect.

1. _____

2. _____

3. _____

4. _____

5. _____

6. _____

7. _____

8. _____

9. _____

10. _____

11. _____

Label the following figures.

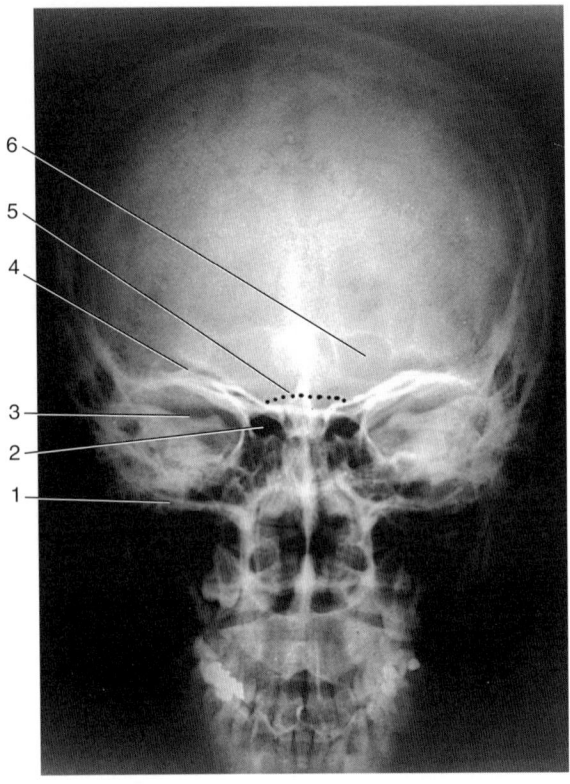

Fig. 17.4 Cranium. PA projection.

1. _____

2. _____

3. _____

4. _____

5. _____

6. _____

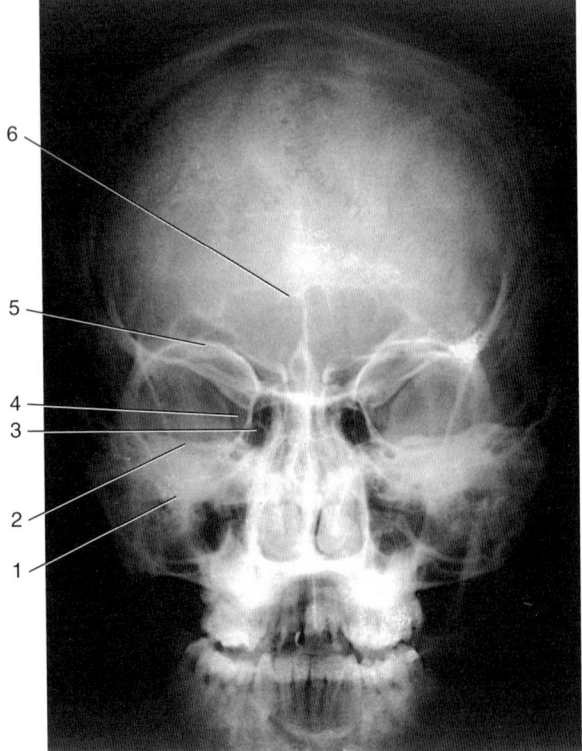

Fig. 17.5 Cranium. PA axial projection.

1. _____

2. _____

3. _____

4. _____

5. _____

6. _____

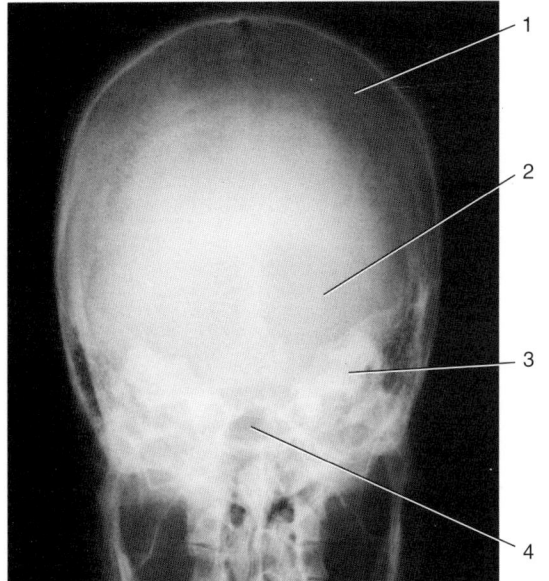

Fig. 17.6 Cranium. AP axial projection (Towne method).

1. _____

2. _____

3. _____

4. _____

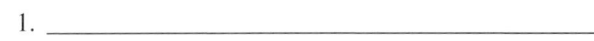
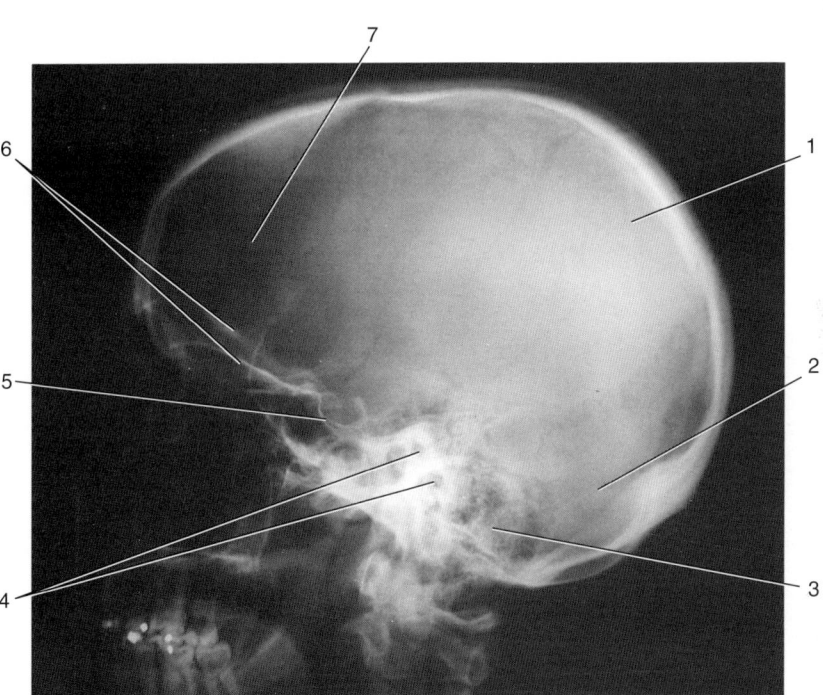

Fig. 17.7 Cranium. Lateral projection.

1. _____   5. _____

2. _____   6. _____

3. _____   7. _____

4. _____

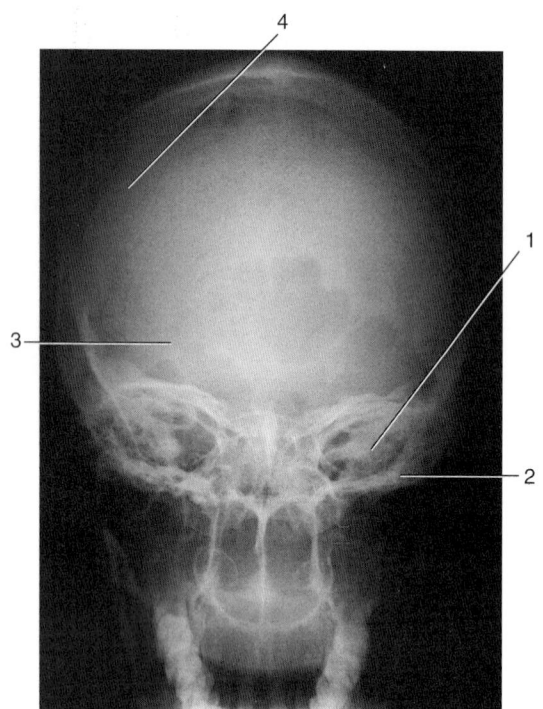

Fig. 17.8 Cranium. AP projection.

1. _____

2. _____

3. _____

4. _____

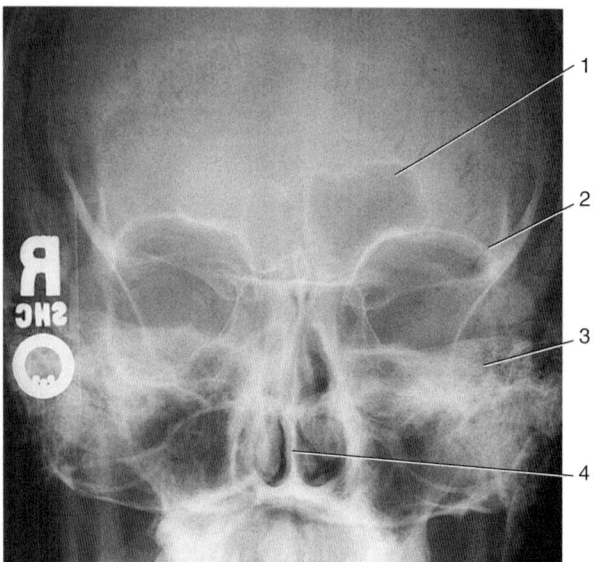

Fig. 17.9 Facial bones. PA axial projection (Caldwell method).

1. _____

2. _____

3. _____

4. _____

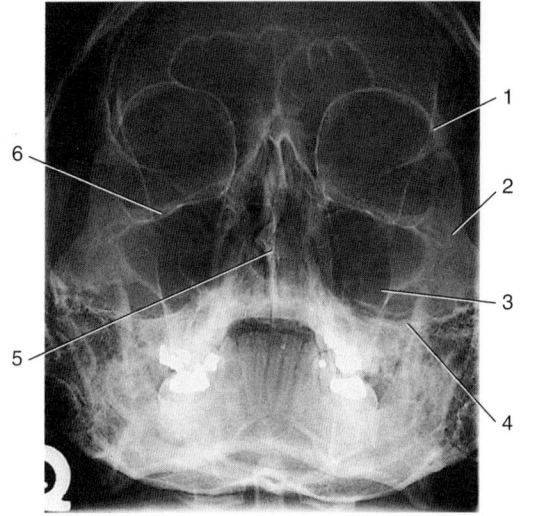

Fig. 17.10 Facial bones. Parietoacanthial projection (Waters method).

1. _____
2. _____
3. _____
4. _____
5. _____
6. _____

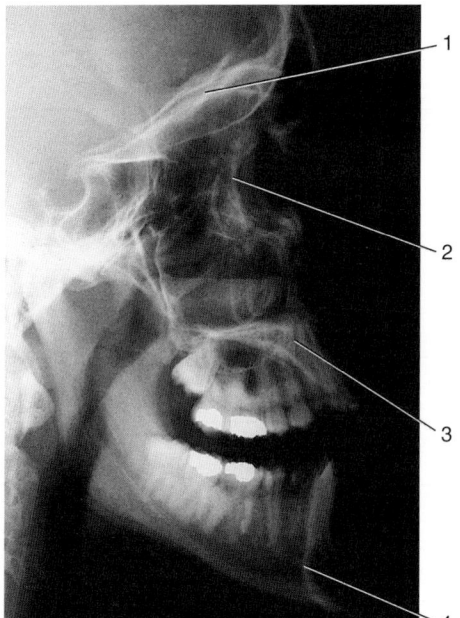

Fig. 17.11 Facial bones. Lateral projection.

1. _____
2. _____
3. _____
4. _____

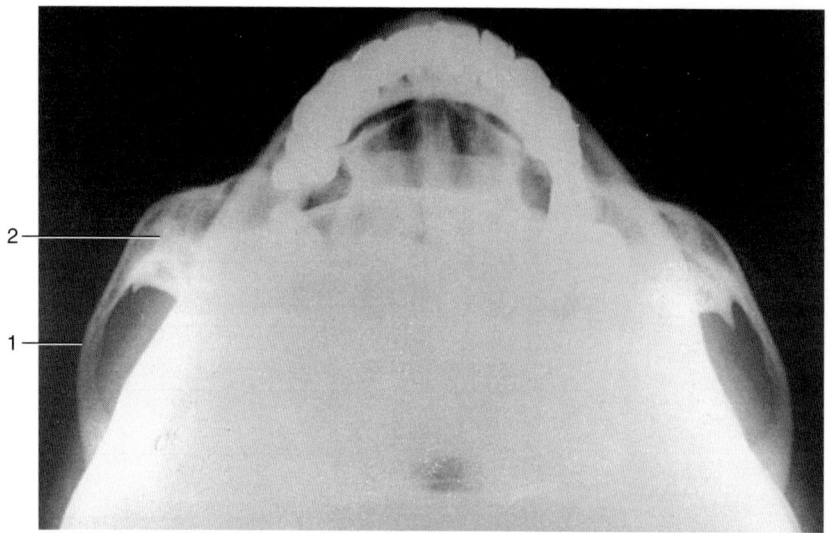

Fig. 17.12 Zygomatic arches. Verticosubmental projection.

1. _____

2. _____

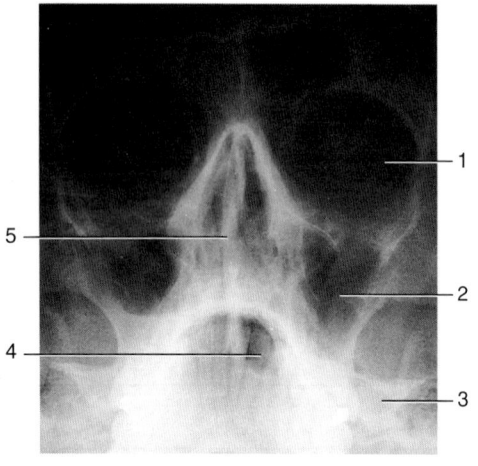

Fig. 17.13 Paranasal sinuses. Parietoacanthial projection (Waters method).

1. _____

2. _____

3. _____

4. _____

5. _____

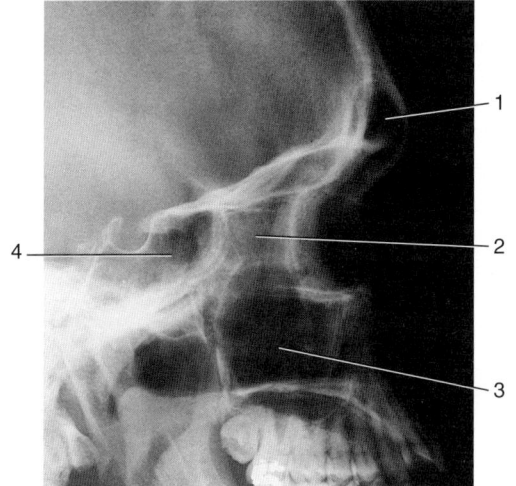

Fig. 17.14 Paranasal sinuses. Lateral projection.

1. _____
2. _____
3. _____
4. _____

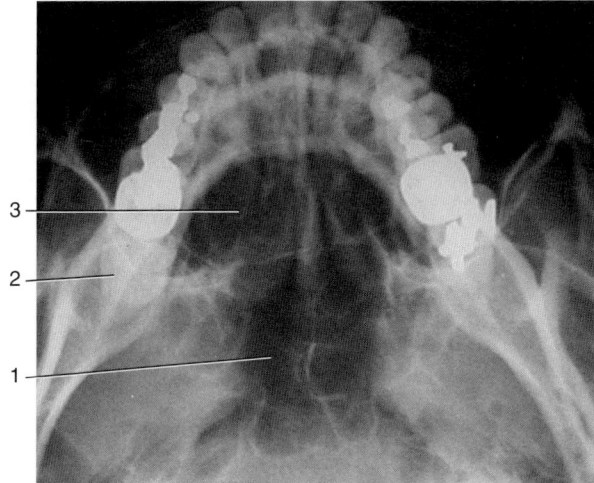

Fig. 17.15 Paranasal sinuses. Submentovertical projection.

1. _____
2. _____
3. _____

This exercise does not have to be completed at the same time as the other exercises in this workbook chapter. The exercise is designed to assess retention of the essential information contained in the corresponding textbook chapter. It is recommended that you complete this exercise when you begin to study for the state limited licensure examination. This will help determine what you know and which information should be further reviewed.

1. Describe the skull positioning landmark called the *glabella*.

   _____

2. Describe the skull positioning landmark called the *nasion*.

   _____

3. Describe the skull positioning landmark called the *acanthion*.

   _____

4. Describe the skull positioning landmark called the *mental protuberance*.

   _____

5. Describe the skull positioning landmark called the *gonion*.

   _____

6. Describe the positioning details for the PA axial projection of the skull.

   _____

7. Describe the central ray placement for the PA axial projection of the skull.

   _____

8. Describe the positioning details for the AP axial projection of the skull.

   _____

9. Describe the central ray placement for the AP axial projection of the skull.

   _____

10. What positioning and central ray adjustments are needed for the AP axial projection of the skull if the patient is unable to flex the neck sufficiently to get the orbitomeatal line perpendicular to the IR?

    _____

    _____

11. Describe the positioning details for the lateral projection of the skull.

_____

_____

12. Describe the central ray placement for the lateral projection of the skull.

_____

13. Describe the positioning details for the parietoacanthial projection of the facial bones and sinuses.

_____

_____

14. Describe the central ray placement for the parietoacanthial projection of the facial bones and sinuses.

_____

15. Describe the central ray placement for the lateral projection of the facial bones.

_____

16. Why do all sinus radiographs need to be performed upright?

_____

_____

17. Describe the positioning details for the PA axial projection of the sinuses.

_____

_____

18 Radiography of Pediatric and Geriatric Patients

EXERCISE 1

Answer the following questions.

1. The term that refers to the care of older adults is_____.

2. The term that refers to the care of infants and children is_____.

3. List three things you might do to calm an infant.

   1. _____

   2. _____

   3. _____

4. (True/False) More information is communicated nonverbally than with words.

5. When a toddler is refusing to cooperate, what are two things you can do that might change the child's attitude?

   1. _____

   2. _____

6. Explain what is meant by a "valid choice."

   _____

   _____

7. (True/False) When a child is to have a radiographic examination, a parent should never be allowed in the x-ray room.

8. (True/False) School-age children can think logically about anything that can be touched or seen.

9. Exaggerated modesty is a typical characteristic of what age group?

   _____

EXERCISE 2

1. (True/False) Mechanical immobilization is preferable to having someone hold a child during an x-ray exposure.

2. (True/False) When a child must be held during an x-ray exposure, x-ray personnel should hold the child.

3. The principal objective when immobilizing an infant or child for radiography is_____

_____

4. List three ways in which the anatomy of children differs from that of adults.

   1. _____

   2. _____

   3. _____

EXERCISE 3

1. Bilateral studies of the _____ and the _____ are seldom required for adults, but are usually performed for children.

2. (True/False) Chest radiography of small children does not require the use of a grid.

3. An adult knee measuring 13 cm requires an exposure of 5 milliampere-seconds (mAs) and 70 peak kilovoltage (kVp) at 40 inches source-image receptor distance with no grid. Suggest a set of exposure factors that will produce a satisfactory radiograph for a 9-year-old patient whose knee measures 8 cm.

_____

_____

4. (*Circle the correct word.*) When making radiographs of small children, it is usually advantageous to use a (high/low) mA setting.

5. Why might a physician order frontal chest radiographs of a child to be taken on both inspiration and expiration?

_____

6. An incomplete fracture in which the periosteum ruptures and the cortex separates on one side of the bone, but the

   other side remains intact, is called a _____ fracture.

7. A common anatomic area for radiography to determine bone age is the_____.

8. Nonaccidental trauma is another term for _____.

Chapter **18** **Radiography of Pediatric and Geriatric Patients**

9. List five signs in a child that should raise suspicion of nonaccidental trauma.

1. _____

2. _____

3. _____

4. _____

5. _____

EXERCISE 4

Answer the following questions.

1. (*Circle the correct word.*) The number of persons in the United States who are at or above retirement age is (increasing/decreasing).

2. List three common characteristics of aging that may affect communication.

1. _____

2. _____

3. _____

3. List four strategies that will help to improve communication with patients who are hard of hearing.

1. _____

2. _____

3. _____

4. _____

4. A term that refers to a large group of disorders associated with brain damage or impaired cerebral function, particularly in the aged, is_____.

5. (*Circle the correct phrase.*) Patients with Alzheimer disease or other conditions that affect mental function are more likely to lose their memory of (recent events/the distant past).

6. Demineralization, osteopenia, and osteoporosis are all terms that refer to the condition of aging that is characterized by

_____

7. List three soft tissue changes that occur as a result of aging.

   1. _____

   2. _____

   3. _____

8. Open sores over bony prominences that occur when pressure on a limited area inhibits circulation are called

   _____.

9. (*Circle the correct words.*) When adjusting exposure factors to compensate for osteopenia in the elderly, it is best to (increase/decrease) the (mA/kVp).

10. A degenerative inflammatory disease of the colon that is common in the elderly and is characterized by constipation and/or diarrhea with abdominal cramping is called

    _____

11. A degenerative condition of the nervous system that attacks the elderly and is characterized by fine tremors, a peculiar gait, and a lack of facial expression is called

    _____.

CHALLENGE EXERCISE

This exercise does not have to be completed at the same time as the other exercises in this workbook chapter. The exercise is designed to assess retention of the essential information contained in the corresponding textbook chapter. It is recommended that you complete this exercise when you begin to study for the state limited licensure examination. This will help determine what you know and which information should be further reviewed.

1. *Geriatrics* is a term that refers to the care of_____.

2. Children's anatomy differs from that of adults in four principal ways: proportions of the head and body, ossification,

   spinal curvature, and_____.

3. Is it acceptable to take a chest radiograph of a small child without using a grid?_____

   _____

4. How does a greenstick fracture differ from other fractures?_____

   _____

5. A currently used term for physical child abuse or battered child syndrome is_____

   _____.

6. Lack of bone density in the aged people is referred to as *demineralization* or

   _____.

7. A characteristic of Parkinson disease that creates problems during radiography is

   _____.

8. What age group is most commonly affected by the condition known as *organic brain syndrome?*

   _____

9. Black eyes, bulging fontanels, or unexplained unconsciousness in an infant should raise suspicion of

   _____.

10. Decubitus ulcers most commonly occur in the elderly and the bedridden as a result of

   _____

   _____.

19 Image Evaluation

EXERCISE 1

Answer the following questions by selecting the best choice.

1. Image evaluation is the process that determines whether an image:
    1. is correctly identified and marked.
    2. has sufficient diagnostic quality.
    3. meets the minimum requirements of the imaging order.
    A. 1 and 2
    B. 1 and 3
    C. 2 and 3
    D. 1, 2, and 3

2. Which of the following conditions should be observed when viewing radiographs?
    1. View images in a brightly lit room.
    2. Maintain a clean monitor screen.
    3. Maintain a low light level in the viewing area.
    A. 1 and 2
    B. 1 and 3
    C. 2 and 3
    D. 1, 2, and 3

3. When radiographs are viewed, the correct image orientation is:
    1. the way the anatomy was positioned when the image receptor (IR) was exposed.
    2. in the anatomic position.
    3. with the patient's right side toward the viewer's right side.
    A. 1 and 2
    B. 1 and 3
    C. 2 and 3
    D. 1, 2, and 3

4. The term *esthetic quality* refers to the:
    A. visual appeal of the radiograph.
    B. position of the part on the IR.
    C. amount of detail in the image.
    D. amount of contrast in the image.

5. Images that lack esthetic quality may:
    1. show artifacts.
    2. show blurring of anatomy.
    3. display poor alignment of the body part.
    A. 1 and 2
    B. 1 and 3
    C. 2 and 3
    D. 1, 2, and 3

6. Which of the following would be a factor used to evaluate evidence of radiation safety practices?
    A. Contrast
    B. Brightness
    C. Collimation
    D. Patient positioning

7. (True/False) The decision to repeat a radiograph should be based only on radiation safety considerations.

8. (True/False) Keeping a log of repeated radiographs aids the limited operator in evaluating problems and progressing toward esthetic quality.

9. Troubleshooting an image includes:
    1. deciding whether the image should be repeated.
    2. determining the cause of any problems.
    3. discussing the image with the patient's physician.
    A. 1 and 2
    B. 1 and 3
    C. 2 and 3
    D. 1, 2, and 3

10. (True/False) Radiographs with markings added after exposure are not admissible in court.

11. (True/False) Errors in diagnosis can occur with incorrect position and exposure factors.

12. The factors that affect spatial resolution include which of the following?
    1. Object-image receptor distance (OID)
    2. Motion
    3. kVp
    A. 1 and 2
    B. 1 and 3
    C. 2 and 3
    D. 1, 2, and 3

13. Which of the following will decrease patient motion in the radiograph?
    A. Use of low-mA (milliampere) techniques
    B. Use of low-kVp (peak kilovoltage) techniques
    C. Providing clear patient instructions
    D. Use of long exposure time techniques

14. (True/False) The visual quality check for proper radiation exposure in digital radiography systems is to check the Exposure Indicator number.

213

15. Anatomic structures may be excluded in the image because of:
    1. inaccurate collimation.
    2. improper part centering.
    3. improper selection of mA or kVp.
    A. 1 and 2
    B. 1 and 3
    C. 2 and 3
    D. 1, 2, and 3

16. Radiographs of fingers, hands, toes, and feet are positioned on the viewing monitor with the:
    A. distal aspects pointing up.
    B. distal aspects pointing down.

17. A limited operator would be repeating radiographs unnecessarily if his or her repeat rate exceeded:
    A. 1%.
    B. 4%.
    C. 10%.
    D. 15%.

18. Most experienced limited operators have a repeat rate of about:
    A. 1%.
    B. 4%.
    C. 10%.
    D. 15%.

19. (True/False) Gonad shielding is required on patients under 55 when the gonads are within 5 cm of the radiation field, and the shield will not interfere with the purpose of the examination.

20. (True/False) Decubitus projections are often viewed horizontally, in the same position as they are taken.

EXERCISE 2

Answer the following questions.

1. What is the acronym that can help you remember how to accurately assess image quality?

   _____

2. What does each letter stand for in the acronym that answers Question 1?

   Letter   Definition

   _____   _____

   _____   _____

   _____   _____

   _____   _____

   _____   _____

   _____   _____

3. Describe the anatomic position.

_____

_____

_____

_____

_____

CHALLENGE EXERCISE

This exercise does not have to be completed at the same time as the other exercises in this workbook chapter. The exercise is designed to assess retention of the essential information contained in the corresponding textbook chapter. In addition, many other chapters will need to be consulted to fully answer many of these questions, because image evaluation requires comprehensive understanding of imaging principles and procedural details. It is recommended that you complete this exercise when you begin to study for the state limited licensure examination. This will help determine what you know and which information should be further reviewed.

1. Describe the appearance of a digital radiograph that has been overexposed.

_____

2. Describe the appearance of a digital radiograph that has been exposed with a kVp that was too low for the body part.

_____

3. What is the most common cause of poor spatial resolution in a digital radiograph?

_____

4. Describe the appearance of a radiograph in which the OID of the part was too great.

_____

5. How could you correct the appearance of the radiograph in Question 4 if the OID of the part could not be decreased?

_____

6. Does central ray angulation result primarily in size distortion or shape distortion?

_____

7. Describe the correct placement of radiographic markers.

_____

215

8. Describe the cause and appearance of *noise* on a radiograph.

_____

9. Because there is no direct link between exposure level and image brightness in digital radiographic systems, how do you determine whether a radiograph was taken with an appropriate exposure level?

_____

10. Describe radiation exposure conditions that will result in unsatisfactory digital images.

_____

_____

_____

20 Ethics, Legal Considerations, and Professionalism

Answer the following questions.

1. List at least four characteristics that distinguish a profession from a nonprofessional occupation.

   1. _____

   2. _____

   3. _____

   4. _____

2. (True/False) Limited radiography is considered to be a profession.

3. (True/False) Professional attitudes and behaviors are expected of limited x-ray machine operators.

4. Define the following terms and give an example of each.

   1. Morals: _____

   2. Values: _____

   3. Ethics: _____

5. An aspirational document that establishes a high standard of professional conduct and assists the members of the radiologic technology profession in practicing ethical principles is the

   _____.

6. Mandatory standards of minimally acceptable professional conduct for all registered radiologic technologists are contained in the document called the

   _____.

7. Write a brief phrase that characterizes the behavior prescribed in each principle of the code of ethics of the American Registry of Radiologic Technologists.

Principle 1: _____

Principle 2: _____

Principle 3: _____

Principle 4: _____

Principle 5: _____

Principle 6: _____

Principle 7: _____

Principle 8: _____

Principle 9: _____

Principle 10: _____

Principle 11: _____

8. (True/False) The confidentiality of conversations between patients and limited operators is not protected by "legal privilege."

9. (True/False) It is ethical to discuss your patients with your friends as long as you do not mention the patients' names.

10. List the four basic steps involved in solving ethical dilemmas using the process of ethical analysis.

1. _____

2. _____

3. _____

4. _____

EXERCISE 2

Answer the following questions.

1. (True/False) Most procedures commonly performed by limited operators require that the patient sign an informed consent document.

2. (True/False) Parents, grandparents, or adult siblings may sign an informed consent form for a minor.

3. (True/False) Informed consent may be revoked by the patient at any time after signing.

4. Explain briefly why it is essential to maintain all the credentials that are required for practice.

_____

_____

_____

5. Match the types of intentional misconduct with their legal definitions.

1. _____ Assault   A. Unjustifiable detention

2. _____ Battery   B. Unlawful touching

3. _____ False imprisonment   C. Written information that causes defamation of character

4. _____ Invasion of privacy   D. Disclosure of confidential information

5. _____ Libel   E. Omission of reasonable care

6. _____ Slander   F. The threat of touching in an injurious way

                                               G. Verbal dissemination of information that causes loss of reputation

6. Failure to use reasonable care or caution is termed _____.

7. What is the standard of care that is used to legally define negligence?

_____

8. The responsibility of healthcare providers for accountability in the area of patient confidentiality is legally prescribed in a federal law known by the acronym

_____.

9. An act of negligence in the context of a professional relationship is defined as professional negligence or

_____.

10. The employer is liable for employees' negligent acts that occur in the course of their work, according to the legal

doctrine of _____.

11. List three important steps you can take to reduce the likelihood of malpractice litigation.

1. _____

2. _____

3. _____

Chapter **20 Ethics, Legal Considerations, and Professionalism**

Answer the following questions.

1. Number the following list of human needs in order according to the hierarchy of needs, with 1 being the most basic level of needs and 6 being the highest level.

   _____ Love and acceptance   _____ Recreation

   _____ Nutrition and oxygen   _____ Self-actualization

   _____ Recognition   _____ Safety

2. List good practices that represent responsible self-care by limited operators.

   _____

   _____

   _____

   _____

   _____

3. List three positive actions for promoting teamwork and cooperation in the workplace.

   1. _____

   2. _____

   3. _____

4. Sensitivity to the needs of others that allows you to meet those needs constructively is called

   _____.

5. What is the best strategy for dealing with clinical situations in which you find it difficult to cope because the patient is vomiting, bleeding, or acting inappropriately?

   _____

6. List reasons why limited operators should pursue continuing education, even if it is not required for the renewal of credentials.

   _____

   _____

   _____

EXERCISE 4

Answer the following questions.

1. List three nonverbal behaviors that enhance communication.

    1. _____

    2. _____

    3. _____

2. Explain what is meant by validation of communication.

    _____

    _____

3. Write two questions other than those presented in the text that could be used to offer an adult patient a valid choice.

    1. _____

    2. _____

4. Match the following communication terms with the correct definitions.

    1. _____ Validation   A. Sensitivity to the needs of others

    2. _____ Aggression   B. Reaction to the distress of others

    3. _____ Empathy   C. Calm, firm expression of feelings or opinions

    4. _____ Assertion   D. Confirmation that a message is understood

    5. _____ Sympathy   E. Expression of angry or hostile feelings

                                  F. Disregard for the feelings of others

EXERCISE 5

Answer the following questions.

1. List signs or characteristics that might alert you to the fact that a patient is totally deaf.

    1. _____

    2. _____

    3. _____

    4. _____

2. List three ways in which the deaf may communicate.

   1. _____

   2. _____

   3. _____

3. (True/False) Patients who do not speak English are responsible for communicating effectively in a healthcare situation despite language barriers.

4. (True/False) When patients do not speak English, translation by a family member is preferable to translation by an interpreter who is not known by the patient.

5. (True/False) When using an interpreter, you should talk directly to the patient as if he or she could understand you.

6. List common social practices in the United States that might be different in other cultures.

   _____

   _____

   _____

7. An old superstition of Mediterranean origin that is occasionally seen among Hispanic patients is called the *evil eye*, or *mal ojo*. This is a belief that _____

   _____.

8. Check the cultural groups listed below in which direct eye contact is generally acceptable.

   _____ Many cultures in the United States

   _____ Most Asian cultures

   _____ Native American cultures

   _____ Hispanic culture

   _____ Russian culture

9. Aggressive demands for service and attention by patients' families are most commonly the results of _____

   _____.

10. List three things you can do to support the anxious relatives of an injured patient.

   1. _____

   2. _____

   3. _____

EXERCISE 6

Answer the following questions.

1. A legal document that contains a record of the care and treatment received by a patient is called a_____

_____.

2. Diagnostic images are owned by_____.

3. What should you do if a physician calls from across town and requests images that are in your files?

_____

_____

CHALLENGE EXERCISE

This exercise does not have to be completed at the same time as the other exercises in this workbook chapter. The exercise is designed to assess retention of the essential information contained in the corresponding textbook chapter. It is recommended that you complete this exercise when you begin to study for the state limited licensure examination. This will help determine what you know and which information should be further reviewed.

1. What constitutes a medical chart?

_____

_____

2. Who owns diagnostic images?

_____

3. Who bears responsibility for communication when a patient is unable to speak or understand English?

_____

4. *Negligence* is defined as the failure to use reasonable care or caution. How is this standard defined?

_____

5. The use of physical restraints without the patient's permission or a physician's order could be the basis for a legal

charge of _____.

6. Failure to maintain confidence in a clinical situation could result in a legal charge of _____

_____.

7. What is the ethical responsibility of a limited operator with respect to the diagnosis or interpretation of images?

   _____

8. A limited operator should not discriminate against any patient on the basis of sex, age, race, ethnicity, or diagnosis.

   Such discrimination is a violation of _____

9. When the solution to a problem is sought through a process that includes identification of the problem, development of alternate solutions, selecting the best solution, and defending the selection, this process is called

   _____.

10. The aspirational document that establishes ethical standards for those involved in medical imaging is

   _____.

21 Safety and Infection Control

EXERCISE 1

Answer the following questions.

1. In the list below, check the three elements that must be present in order for a fire to burn.

   _____ Open flames

   _____ Fuel

   _____ Smoke

   _____ Oxygen

   _____ Electricity

   _____ Heat

2. (True/False) In case of an electrical fire, you should use a class A fire extinguisher or a water supply to put out the fire.

3. (True/False) Oxygen does not burn.

4. List three important fire safety precautions that should be observed when oxygen is in use.

   1. _____

   2. _____

   3. _____

5. What should you know about a clinical facility to be prepared in case of fire?

   _____

   _____

   _____

6. Give the acronym for remembering the four basic steps to follow in case of fire. Write the meaning of each letter in the acronym.

   _____

   _____

   _____

   _____

225

7. Write the steps for safe use of a fire extinguisher as indicated by the acronym PASS.

P: _____

A: _____

S: _____

S: _____

8. Being cautious about avoiding electric shock is especially important when using electricity around _____

_____.

9. List steps that should be taken to provide safety in the case of a hazardous chemical spill, such as a concentrated bleach or fixer solution.

_____

_____

_____

_____

EXERCISE 2

Answer the following questions.

1. The principles of proper body alignment, movement, and balance are referred to as

_____.

2. (*Circle the correct phrase.*) When lifting a heavy object from the floor, you should (bend your body at the waist/bend at the hips and knees).

3. (*Circle the correct phrase.*)When moving a heavy object that is on wheels, you should (push it/pull it).

4. Label the names of the body positions shown in Fig. 21.1.

A. _____

B. _____

C. _____

D. _____

E. _____

F. _____

G. _____

H. _____

I. _____

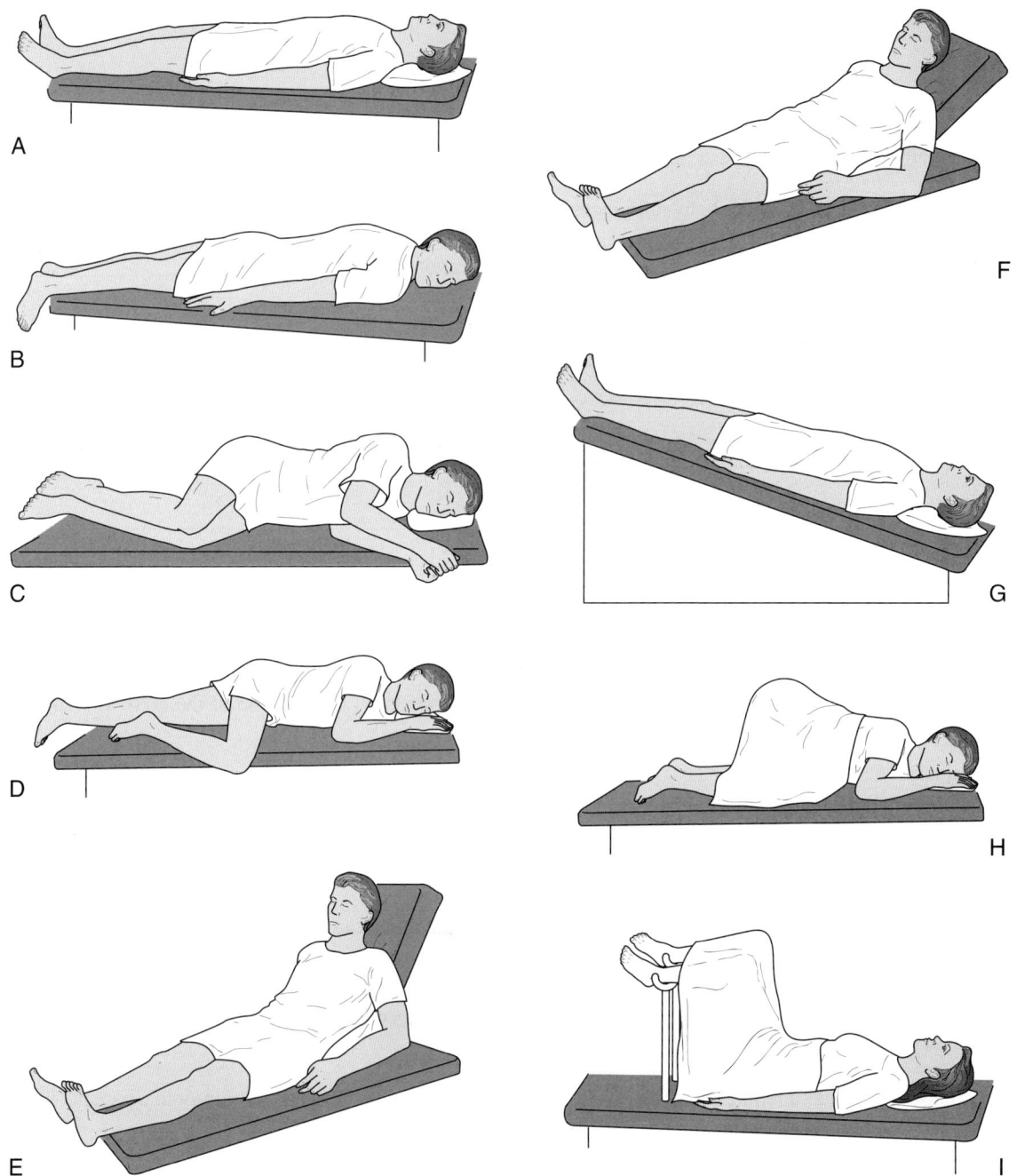

Fig. 21.1 Body positions.

5. To relieve lumbosacral stress or abdominal strain when a patient is supine, a bolster is placed under the

_____.

6. Inability to breathe when lying down is termed _____.

7. Check the positions listed below that are appropriate for nauseated patients to provide safety from possible aspiration of vomitus.

_____ Fowler   _____ Trendelenburg   _____ Supine

_____ Sims   _____ Lateral recumbent

8. Padding should be placed under bony prominences such as the sacrum, heels, or midthoracic curvature of older or debilitated patients for comfort and to prevent the development of _____.

9. When assisting a patient to lie down, place one arm under the _____ and the other under the

_____.

10. It is preferable for patients suffering from recent back injuries and those recovering from spinal surgery to sit up from

the _____ position.

11. A temporary state of low blood pressure that causes patients to feel light-headed or faint when they first sit up is

termed _____.

12. (*Circle the correct phrase.*) When assisting a patient who has weakness on one side of the body to walk, position yourself on the patient's (strong side/weak side).

13. The most common type of fall associated with wheelchair transfer occurs when _____

_____.

14. (True/False) The use of sandbags to immobilize trembling extremities can assist in minimizing motion, even when the area of interest does not involve the extremity.

15. (True/False) The application of physical restraints to the arms or legs of an adult patient without the patient's consent requires a physician's order.

16. (True/False) An incident report must be completed only for occurrences that result in injury to a patient.

EXERCISE 3

Answer the following questions.

1. The four principal factors involved in the spread of disease, sometimes called the *cycle of infection*, are:

A. _____

B. _____

C. _____

D. _____

2. Match the following terms referring to microorganisms and other infectious agents with their definitions.

1. _____ Normal flora

2. _____ Pathogens

3. _____ Bacteria

4. _____ Viruses

5. _____ Endospores

6. _____ Fungi

7. _____ Prions

8. _____ Protozoa

A. The smallest and least understood of all infectious agents

B. Very small subcellular organisms that cause influenza, chickenpox, and the common cold

C. Bacterial forms that are resistant to heat, cold, and drying and can live without nourishment

D. Agents that cause disease

E. Complex single-cell animals that generally exist as free-living organisms

F. Microorganisms that live on or within the body without causing disease

G. Very small single-cell organisms with a cell wall and an atypical nucleus that lacks a membrane; named for their shapes, including bacilli, cocci, spirochetes, and spirilla

H. Occur as single-celled yeasts or as filament-like structures called molds

3. Describe the five indirect routes of disease transmission, and give an example of each.

1. Fomite: _____

_____

2. Vector:_____

_____

3. Vehicle:_____

_____

4. Airborne contamination: _____

_____

5. Droplet contamination _____

_____

4. The infectious agent that causes acquired immunodeficiency syndrome (AIDS) is

_____.

5. In the list below, check the types of contact that may result in the transmission of human immunodeficiency virus (HIV).

_____ Shaking hands   _____ Sharing contaminated needles

_____ Sexual intercourse   _____ Contact with drinking fountains

_____ Eating food prepared by an infected individual   _____ Contact with toilets

6. (True/False) There is no known cure for AIDS.

7. (True/False) The patient's right to confidentiality regarding AIDS diagnosis or HIV status may prevent you from being informed about the patient's status.

8. (True/False) There are thousands of documented, confirmed cases of HIV infection in health care workers resulting from accidental needlesticks.

9. The hepatitis B virus (HBV) is spread through contact with _____.

10. The types of hepatitis that are spread through contact with food or water contaminated with feces are type_____

_____ and type _____.

11. Vaccine is available to protect health care workers from infection by which hepatitis virus?

_____.

12. If postexposure prophylaxis (PEP) is recommended following a needlestick injury, how soon after the injury should this therapy be administered?

_____

13. The microbe that causes COVID-19 is a:
   A. bacterium.
   B. protozoon.
   C. virus.
   D. prion.

14. COVID-19 is transmitted by means of _____

_____.

15. Pulmonary tuberculosis is spread by means of _____

_____

16. (True/False) Most of those who become infected with tubercle bacilli develop a clinical disease and become infectious to others.

17. (True/False) Lowered resistance because of immunodeficiency, malnutrition, other illness, or old age may cause reactivation of a tuberculosis infection.

18. The simplest and most common method of testing for tuberculosis infection is the _____

_____.

19. The standard precautions defined by the Centers for Disease Control and Prevention (CDC) call for the use of barriers whenever contact is anticipated with four things, which are:

    1. _____

    2. _____

    3. _____

    4. _____

20. List three pathogens that are commonly responsible for health care-associated infections.

    1. _____

    2. _____

    3. _____

EXERCISE 4

Answer the following questions.

1. The destruction of pathogens by chemical agents is called _____.

2. Treating items with heat, gas, or chemicals to make them germ free is called _____.

3. Decontamination of the hands using soap and water, an antiseptic hand wash, or an alcohol-based hand rub is called

_____.

4. (True/False) Alcohol hand rubs are effective against most microorganisms.

5. (True/False) Hand hygiene is not necessary when gloves are worn.

6. When should washing with soap and water be used for hand hygiene instead of an alcohol rub? _____

_____

7. As a cleaning agent for decontaminating environmental surfaces, the CDC recommends either a disinfectant regis

tered by the Environmental Protection Agency as effective against HIV, HBV, and the tuberculosis bacterium or _____

_____.

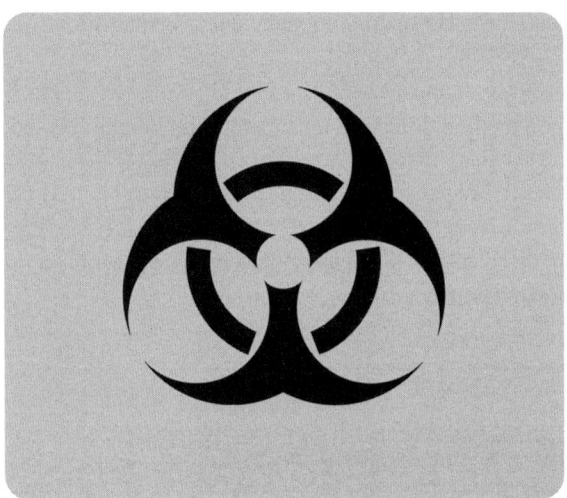

Fig. 21.2 Symbol.

8. Fig. 21.2 is a symbol that indicates_____.

9. (True/False) You should not remove anything from a hazardous waste container once it has been placed inside.

10. (True/False) To prevent needlestick injuries, you should always recap needles.

11. A receptacle for the disposal of needles, syringes, and contaminated items capable of puncturing the skin is called a

_____.

12. The quickest and most convenient means of sterilization for items that can withstand heat is _____

_____.

13. The type of sterilization that is used for telephones, stethoscopes, blood pressure cuffs, and other equipment that

cannot withstand heat is _____.

14. A germ-free area prepared for the use of sterile supplies and equipment is called a _____

_____.

15. The first step in preparing a sterile field is to confirm the sterility of packaged supplies and equipment. List the criteria that indicate when packages are considered sterile.

1. _____

2. _____

3. _____

16. (*Circle the correct phrase.*) When opening a sterile pack, open the first corner (toward you/away from you).

17. (True/False) It is alright to reach across a sterile field as long as you do not touch anything that is sterile.

18. (True/False) Any sterile object or field touched by an unsterile object or person becomes contaminated.

19. (True/False) Before adding a liquid to a sterile tray, you should discard a small amount from the container to rinse the container's lip.

20. (*Circle the correct word.*) The (application/removal) of a dressing is a procedure that requires sterile technique.

CHALLENGE EXERCISE

This exercise does not have to be completed at the same time as the other exercises in this workbook chapter. The exercise is designed to assess retention of the essential information contained in the corresponding textbook chapter. It is recommended that you complete this exercise when you begin to study for the state limited licensure examination. This will help determine what you know and which information should be further reviewed.

1. Why is it important to observe special fire safety precautions in areas where oxygen is in use?

   _____

2. What is the name of the position in which a patient is recumbent on the left lateral aspect of the body with the right knee flexed? _____

3. What is the name of the position in which a patient is supine with the head lower than the feet?

   _____

4. Orthopnea is a condition in which _____.

5. Microorganisms that cause disease are termed _____.

6. When assisting a patient to walk who has weakness on one side of the body, on which side should you position yourself? _____.

7. Name a disease that requires the use of personal respirator equipment, isolation rooms with negative air pressure and special ventilation or circulation, and annual training about the disease. _____ How is this disease transmitted? _____

8. Name the two principal means by which the human immunodeficiency virus is spread.

   1._____

   2._____

9. The CDC recommends a system of infection control that calls for the use of barriers whenever contact with blood,

body fluids, or mucous membranes is anticipated. This system is called _____

_____.

10. Under what circumstances is the use of an alcohol hand rub an inadequate form of hand hygiene?

_____

22 Assessing Patients and Managing Acute Situations

EXERCISE 1

Answer the following questions.

1. List the three skills that will help you adequately determine patients' needs.

   1. _____

   2. _____

   3. _____

2. List steps you can take to reassure and comfort patients who feel anxious.

   _____

   _____

   _____

3. List considerations that might help meet patients' physiologic needs.

   _____

   _____

4. Loss of bladder control is termed _____.

5. List the six characteristics of a patient's chief complaint that should be addressed in the questions used to elicit a preliminary medical history of the complaint.

   1. _____

   2. _____

   3. _____

   4. _____

   5. _____

   6. _____

Answer the following questions.

1. When a patient exhibits a bluish coloration in the mucous membranes of the lips and in the nail beds, the patient is

    said to be _____.

2. When a patient is described as diaphoretic, this means that the patient is _____.

3. Hot, dry skin may indicate that the patient has _____.

4. *(Circle the correct word.)* Rectal temperatures are (higher/lower) than oral temperatures.

5. *(Circle the correct word.)* Axillary temperatures are (higher/lower) than oral temperatures.

6. When is it *not* appropriate to take a patient's temperature orally?

    _____

    _____

7. A rapid pulse, when the heart beats more than 100 times per minute, is called _____.

8. A pulse that is described as thready is one that is both _____ and _____.

9. *(Circle the correct word.)* The first or upper number in a blood pressure value is the (diastolic/systolic) pressure.

10. *(Circle the correct word.)* The term *hypertension* refers to (high/low) blood pressure.

11. The cuff and gauge for measuring blood pressure are called a(n):

    A. stethoscope.

    B. sphygmomanometer.

    C. tympanic thermometer.

    D. aneroid barometer.

12. List two steps you should take to ensure that emergency supplies are ready for use when an emergency arises.

    1. _____

    2. _____

EXERCISE 3

Answer the following questions.

1. *(Circle the correct term.)* In an emergency situation, oxygen is usually administered by means of a (mask/nasal cannula).

2. The usual flow rate for oxygen administration by face mask is _____.

3. *(Circle the correct word.)* Patients suffering from emphysema should receive an oxygen flow rate that is (greater/less) than the usual or average rate.

4. When a patient is unable to swallow or to cope with secretions, blood, or vomitus, you should prepare to assist with

   _____.

5. If a patient complains of sudden intense pain under the sternum, you should assume until proven otherwise that the

   patient might be having _____.

EXERCISE 4

Answer the following questions.

1. When a patient suddenly loses consciousness, the first thing you should do is _____

   _____.

2. Lack of effective circulation to the central nervous system for 5 minutes can cause _____

   _____.

3. A rapid, weak, and ineffective heartbeat caused by the interruption of electric signals that control the heart is called

   _____.

4. When bleeding or swelling occurs inside the skull, seizures, loss of consciousness, or respiratory arrest may occur

   because of increased _____.

5. When a blow to the head causes damage on the side of the head opposite the side of the blow, this is termed a

   _____.

6. List the four levels of consciousness.

   1. _____

   2. _____

   3. _____

   4. _____

7. A fracture in which the bone protrudes through the skin is called a _____.

8. Continuous, abnormal blood flow is called _____.

9. Redness of the skin is termed _____.

10. A severe allergic reaction is termed _____ or _____.

11. An antihistamine medication, such as diphenhydramine, may be given as a treatment for _____

    _____.

12. Anaphylaxis is a type of shock caused by _____.

13. An individual who is terribly thirsty, urinates copious amounts frequently, and has fruity-smelling breath may be

    approaching a state of _____.

14. An enzyme normally produced in the pancreas that aids in the digestion of glucose is _____.

15. A cerebrovascular accident (CVA) is also called a _____.

16. The American Stroke Association recommends the use of the acronym FAST as a guide in the event of a suspected
    CVA. State the meaning of each letter in this mnemonic device and the steps recommended for each.

    1. F _____

       _____

    2. A _____

       _____

    3. S _____

       _____

    4. T _____

       _____

17. A transient ischemic attack is a mild temporary form of a _____.

18. In the event of a seizure, your first duty is to _____.

19. A brief loss of consciousness (absence) during which the patient stares or may lose balance and fall is a type of ___

    _____.

20. When an anxious patient hyperventilates and complains of feeling faint or dizzy, what should you do?

_____

_____.

21. Syncope is another term for _____.

22. A sensation of dizziness in which the patient feels as if the room is moving or whirling is termed _____

_____.

23. Squeezing firmly against the nasal septum for 10 mins is a treatment for _____.

CHALLENGE EXERCISE

This exercise does not have to be completed at the same time as the other exercises in this workbook chapter. The exercise is designed to assess retention of the essential information contained in the corresponding textbook chapter. It is recommended that you complete this exercise when you begin to study for the state limited licensure examination. This will help determine what you know and which information should be further reviewed.

1. A bluish coloration of the skin, mucous membranes, and/or nail beds is termed _____.

2. The normal pulse rate for an adult is _____.

3. Name the equipment needed to measure blood pressure: _____

_____

4. Compare the usual oxygen flow rate for patients who have dyspnea with that which is best for patients who suffer

from emphysema, and explain the reason for the difference. _____

_____

5. A contrecoup injury is a specific type of injury to the _____.

6. A type of shock that is caused by a severe allergic reaction is called _____.

7. The medical term for a stroke, or loss of circulation to a portion of the brain, is _____

_____.

8. When the body is unable to produce sufficient insulin, the resulting disease is called

_____.

9. Which blood chemical is most affected by the condition in Question 8?

_____

10. How does a compound fracture differ from other fractures?

_____

11. List symptoms that might alert you to the onset of a myocardial infarction.

_____

12. What is the lay term for the condition in Question 11?

_____

Chapter **22** **Assessing Patients and Managing Acute Situations**

© 2026 Elsevier Inc. All rights are reserved, including those for text and data mining, AI training, and similar technologies.

23 Medications and Their Administration

Answer the following questions.

1. List duties related to medication administration that a limited operator may perform, even if not permitted to actually administer the medication.

   1. _____

   2. _____

   3. _____

   4. _____

   5. _____

2. Whose duty is it to determine the route of administration for a medication? _____

3. (True/False) A standing order might allow a nurse to administer a specific dose of nitroglycerin to a patient experiencing angina when the physician is not present.

4. (True/False) Checking expiration dates on medication supplies is not important in physicians' offices and clinics because such supplies are used infrequently.

5. The name of a drug that identifies its specific chemical composition is called its_____.

6. The brand name given to a product by its manufacturer is called its_____

   _____ or _____name.

7. Match the following types of medication effects with their definitions.

   1. _____ Toxic   A. Produces a specific action that promotes a desired effect

   2. _____ Agonistic   B. Causes an unusual or peculiar effect, or the opposite of the expected effect

   3. _____ Antagonistic   C. Effect of two or more drugs whose combined effect is beyond the individual effects of each drug alone

   4. _____ Synergistic   D. Has poisonous consequences

   5. _____ Idiosyncratic   E. Prevents or reverses the effects of other drugs

8. The government agency that sets standards for the control of drugs is the_____.

9. The efficacy of a drug refers to its _____.

10. The potency of a drug refers to its _____.

EXERCISE 2

Answer the following questions.

1. Match the following routes of administration with their definitions.

   1. _____ Topical   A. Inside the cheek

   2. _____ Intradermal   B. Under the skin

   3. _____ Intramuscular   C. Between the skin layers

   4. _____ Sublingual   D. Within a vein

   5. _____ Buccal   E. Under the tongue

   6. _____ Subcutaneous   F. Within the muscle

   7. _____ Intravenous   G. By mouth, swallowed

   8. _____ Oral   H. On the skin

2. Match the following drug classes with their applications.

   1. _____ Antihistamine   A. Antimicrobial, prevents or treats infection

   2. _____ Antibiotic   B. Antiinflammatory, treats inflammation, including that caused by allergic reactions

   3. _____ Nonsteroidal antiinflammatory drug C. Tranquilizer, sedates

   4. _____ Anesthetic   D. Analgesic, relieves pain

   5. _____ Corticosteroid   E. Antiallergic, relieves symptoms of allergic reactions

   6. _____ Benzodiazepine   F. Eliminates sensation

3. Medication effect is determined to some degree by the water content of body tissues, which is termed_____

   _____.

4. Match the following terms related to pharmacokinetics with their definitions.

   1. _____ Excretion   A. The process by which the body transforms drugs into an inactive form that can be eliminated from the body

   2. _____ Absorption   B. The process by which the drug enters the systemic circulation to provide a desired effect

   3. _____ Metabolism   C. The elimination of drugs from the body

   4. _____ Distribution   D. The means by which drugs travel to the site of action

5. The most common mechanism of drug action is the binding of drugs to_____

   _____.

6. Drugs are administered to produce a predictable physiologic response called the_____

  _____.

7. Opioids and other substances whose availability is strictly regulated or outlawed because of their potential for abuse or

  addiction are called_____substances.

8. Life-threatening respiratory depression is a possible side effect following the administration of_____

  _____.

9. A specific drug that treats a toxic effect is called a(n)_____.

EXERCISE 3

Answer the following questions.

1. If a child weighs 30 pounds, what is the child's weight in kilograms? _____

2. If a drug is supplied in a strength of 5 mg/mL, and you want to administer 15 mg, you will need_____ mL.

3. If 5 mL of a drug has been administered and the strength is 30 mcg/mL, what dose was given?

  _____

4. (True/False) The Occupational Safety and Health Administration regulations now require the use of engineering controls to decrease the risk to healthcare workers from contaminated needlesticks.

5. (True/False) A 22-gauge needle is larger around than an 18-gauge needle and delivers a given volume of fluid more rapidly.

6. For intramuscular injection in small children, the preferred muscle site is the_____.

7. (True/False) You should wear protective gloves when giving injections.

8. (True/False) Aseptic technique should always be followed for injection procedures.

9. List the information that must be included when the administration of a medication is charted.

  _____

  _____

  _____

24 Medical Laboratory Skills

EXERCISE 1

Answer the following questions.

1. Standard precautions were developed to protect healthcare workers from infection with

   _____.

2. The essence of standard precautions is embodied in the statement that

   _____.

3. List the three essential aspects of the standard precautions as they relate to handling blood and urine.

   1. _____

   2. _____

   3. _____

4. Any refuse that is poisonous or dangerous to living creatures is termed

   _____.

5. Objects that can puncture the skin, such as needles, glass tubes, glass slides, and finger lancets, must be disposed of in a(n)

   _____.

EXERCISE 2

Answer the following questions.

1. The technique of entering a vein with a needle to withdraw a blood sample is termed

   _____.

2. The veins most commonly used for obtaining blood samples are located in the

   _____.

3. The evacuated plastic tubes used for blood specimen collection have color-coded stoppers that indicate

   _____.

245

4. List two ways in which the handling of blood specimen tubes that have additives differs from the handling of those that do not.

    1. _____

    2. _____

5. (True/False) An evacuated blood specimen tube cannot be used a second time following an unsuccessful venipuncture.

6. State the needle gauge and length for routine venipuncture:

    _____ gauge, _____ inches in length.

7. A standard venipuncture needle is actually two needles attached to a threaded plastic hub. The needle mounted to

    the threaded side of the hub is designed to puncture _____. The other needle,

    mounted to the nonthreaded end of the hub, is for puncturing _____.

8. (True/False) Special venipuncture needles with engineered sharps injury protection are available to minimize the risk of needlestick injury to personnel and to comply with the requirements of the Occupational Safety and Health Administration.

9. (True/False) Venipuncture needle holders (barrels) are reusable items.

10. A tight band placed around the arm to facilitate distention of the vein for venipuncture is called a(n)

    _____

11. Alcohol preparation wipes are generally used to cleanse the skin for venipuncture, but povidone-iodine wipes must

    be used if the specimen is being collected for _____ or _____

    _____.

12. (True/False) Some manufacturers produce evacuated tubes with stoppers covered by plastic caps to minimize aerosol production; these caps eliminate the need to use a shield when opening specimen tubes.

13. List three sites that should be avoided when selecting a site for venipuncture.

    1. _____

    2. _____

    3. _____

14. Choice of a vein for venipuncture is based on _____.

15. (*Circle the correct word.*) When obtaining a blood specimen, you should engage the vacuum tube on the internal needle (before/after) the external needle is properly situated in the vein.

16. (*Circle the correct word.*) When all blood specimens have been obtained, you should remove the last tube from the needle holder (before/after) removing the needle from the vein.

17. Failure of the tube to fill with blood during venipuncture means that _____
_____.

EXERCISE 3

Answer the following questions.

1. The physical, microscopic, and/or chemical examination of urine is termed _____.

2. List the three components of a routine urinalysis.

   1. _____

   2. _____

   3. _____

3. What should you do to maintain the quality and accuracy of reagent strips?

_____

_____

4. (True/False) *Urinalysis tube* is another term for a urine specimen collection cup.

5. When should a urine specimen be collected to obtain the greatest amount of diagnostic information?

_____

6. Urine collected regardless of the time of day is termed a(n) _____.

7. The correct method for collecting a urine specimen is called the _____.

8. (*Circle the correct phrase.*) When a female cleanses the labia for a clean-catch midstream specimen, the cleansing sponge or towelette is wiped in a(n) (anterior to posterior/posterior to anterior) direction.

9. If a urine specimen cannot be analyzed promptly, how should the specimen be handled when first obtained and before analysis?

_____

_____

_____

10. List the two characteristics to be assessed in a macroscopic (visual) examination of urine.

    1. _____

    2. _____

11. (True/False) When a urine reagent strip is read, timing is critical, and the test result must be read at the time indicated by the manufacturer.

12. When the color of a urine reagent strip does not match any of the reference colors, and the test has been repeated with the same results using a strip from a different bottle, what should you do?

    _____

13. When multiple end-point colors are noted within the test area for blood, revealing a green speckled pattern overlying an orange background, the result is reported as

    _____.

14. If it is necessary to perform a urinalysis during the menstrual period, what method is used to prevent contamination of the specimen with menstrual blood?

    _____

    _____

15. List the abnormal results from analyses of the chemical and physical characteristics of urine that indicate the need for a microscopic examination of the urine sediment.

    _____

16. A special electrical device in laboratories that spins the urine tubes rapidly to separate solids from liquid for the

    microscopic evaluation of sediment is called a(n) _____.

25 Additional Procedures for Assessment and Diagnosis

EXERCISE 1

Answer the following questions.

1. What should be the setting of a balance scale before the patient steps on it to be weighed?

   _____

   _____

2. (*Circle the correct word.*) When a patient is weighed on a balance scale, the weight on the (upper/lower) calibration bar should be adjusted first.

3. When a patient is standing on a balance scale and the scale is in balance, how is the patient's weight determined?

   _____

   _____

4. When a digital electronic scale is used, if the weight readout keeps changing or does not appear promptly, this is most

   likely an indication that_____.

5. (*Circle the correct word.*) When the height of a patient is measured using the calibration rod of a balance scale, the rod should be raised and the measuring bar unfolded into the horizontal position (before/after) the patient steps onto the platform.

6. A patient's weight should be recorded to the nearest_____.

7. A patient's height should be recorded to the nearest_____.

EXERCISE 2

Answer the following questions.

1. Define the following conditions, which can be identified by simple vision screening tests.

   Myopia: _____

   Hyperopia: _____

   Presbyopia: _____

2. For children who have not learned the alphabet or patients who are unfamiliar with the English alphabet, distance

   vision is tested using the_____ chart.

3. Distance vision assessment is usually made at a distance of_____.

4. Write the abbreviations for the following terms used to chart the results of vision tests.

Right eye:_____

Left eye:_____

5. The classic method of evaluating color perception is the_____ test.

EXERCISE 3

Answer the following questions.

1. A graphic representation of tiny electrical currents generated within the heart is a diagnostic tool used to assess heart disease and is called a(n)_____.

2. Label the waves that represent a complete cardiac cycle in the electrocardiogram (ECG) tracing in Fig. 25.1.

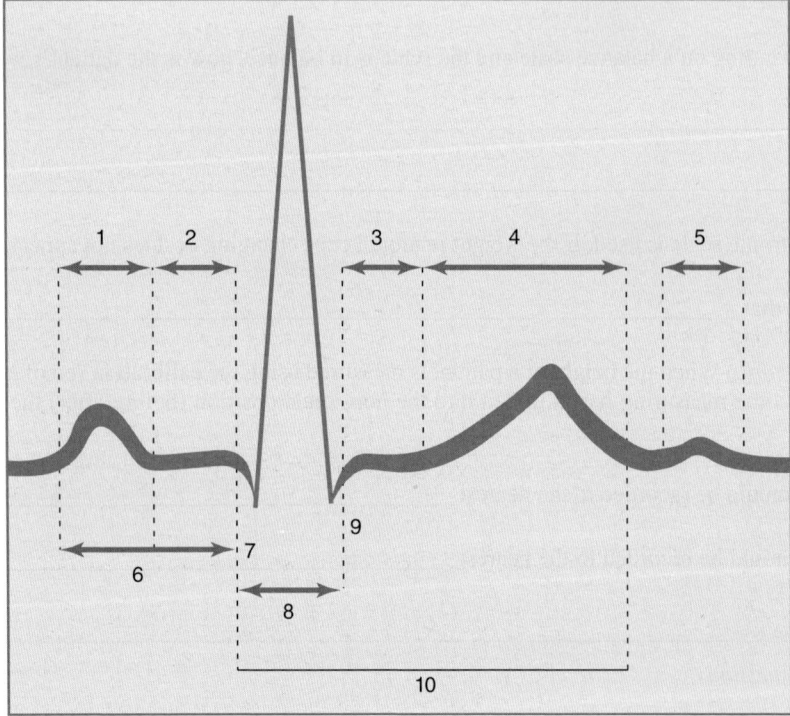

Fig. 25.1 ECG waves.

1. _____

2. _____

3. _____

4. _____

5. _____

6. _____

7. _____

8. _____

9. _____

10. _____

3. List the three types of leads that are used in a routine diagnostic ECG study. In each of the three categories, state the abbreviation or designation of each specific lead.

    1. _____

    2. _____

    3. _____

4. What aspect of the recording is controlled by the standard (STD) settings on an ECG machine?

    _____

5. If the amplitude of the QRS complex on an ECG is so great that it causes the stylus to move off the paper, what should you do?

    _____

6. The speed of the paper feed must be standardized for the tracing to be interpreted accurately. The universal recording

    speed is_____.

7. (*Circle the correct phrase.*) When connecting the patient cable to the electrodes, each lead wire (may be connected to any electrode/must be connected to a specific electrode).

8. Match the features and artifacts on the following ECG tracings with their descriptions.

    1. _____

A. Subtle wandering baseline

B. Lead codes

C. Interrupted baseline

D. Standardization marks

E. Alternating current artifact

F. Major wandering baseline

G. Muscle artifact

2. _____

.

..

...

_

_ _

_ _ _

_.

_..

_...

_....

_.....

_......

3. _____

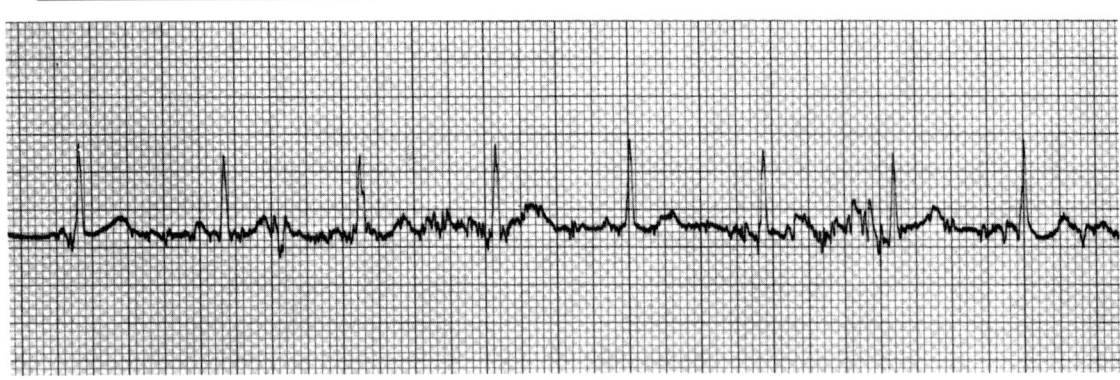

4. _____

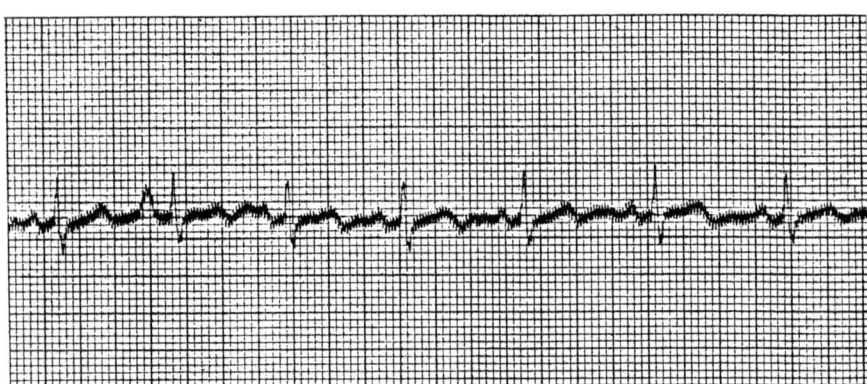

5. _____

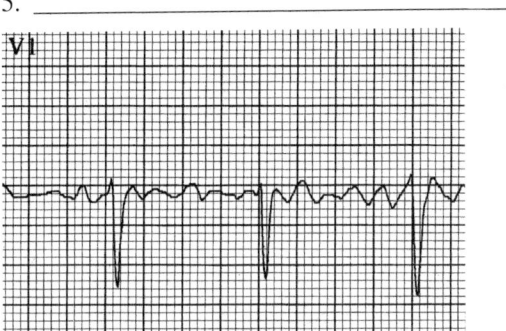

6. _____

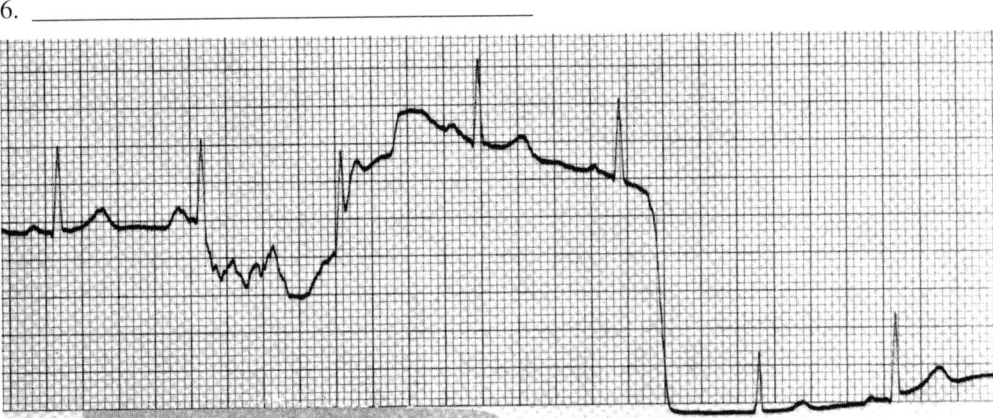

7. _____

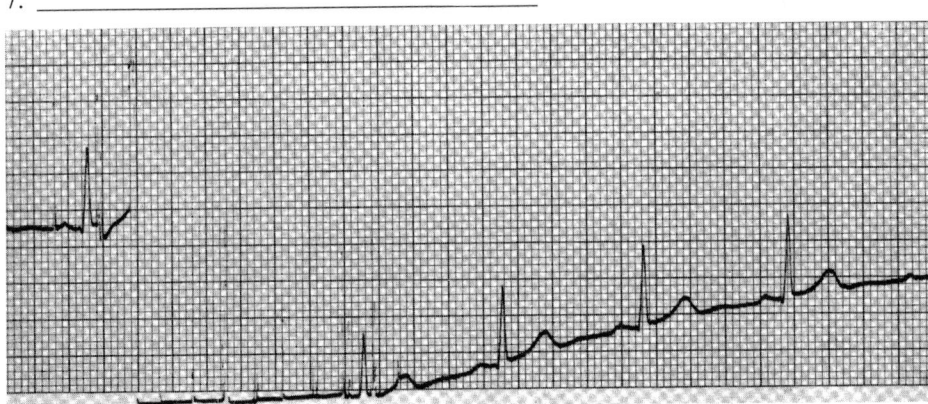

9. What type of compound is used to enhance the electrical contact between ECG electrodes and the patient's skin?

_____

10. (True/False) When the electrodes are all connected in preparation for an ECG, you should arrange the cords so that they lie on the patient's body.

11. Recording of ECG tracings during strenuous exercise is called a(n)

_____.

Answer the following questions.

1. The measurement of lung air flow using a special machine is called_____.

2. List the two basic types of spirometers.

   1. _____

   2. _____

3. Identify the two types of spirometric graphs in the following figures.

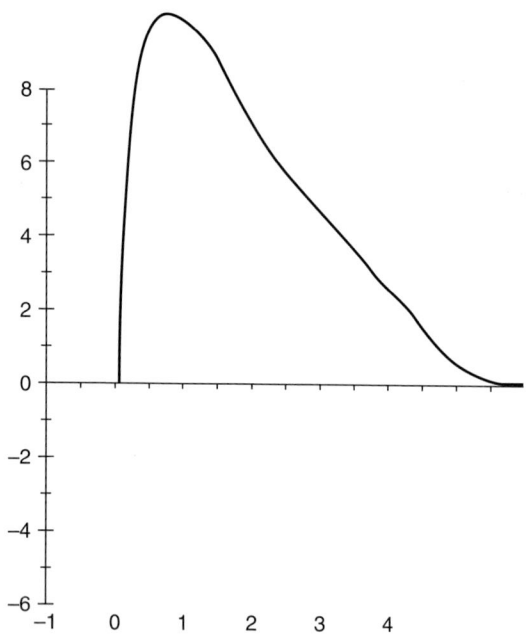

1. _____

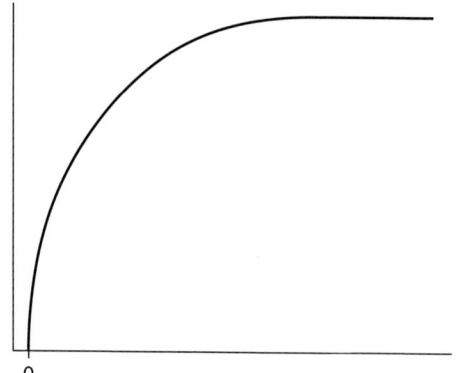

2. _____

4. List the three characteristics of a satisfactory forced expiration maneuver.

1. _____

2. _____

3. _____

5. How many satisfactory forced expiration graphs constitute a complete test?

_____

6. What is the maximum number of attempts that should be made to obtain the required number of satisfactory forced expiration graphs?

_____

7. List five contraindications to forced expiration spirometry.

1. _____

2. _____

3. _____

4. _____

5. _____

26 Bone Densitometry

NOTE TO THE STUDENT

The following four exercises provide a very comprehensive block of information to challenge you in every aspect of bone densitometry that can be tested on the ARRT Bone Density examination.

EXERCISE 1

Answer the following questions by selecting the best choice.

1. The bone measurement values from a dual-energy x-ray absorptiometry (DXA) scan are used to assess:
    1. bone strength
    2. diagnose disease associated with low bone density
    3. predict risk of future fractures
    A. 1 and 2
    B. 1 and 3
    C. 2 and 3
    D. 1, 2, and 3

2. DXA is of value in diagnosing which of the following diseases?
    A. Diabetes
    B. Osteoporosis
    C. Osteomalacia
    D. Osteogenic sarcoma

3. Which of the following would <u>not</u> be an advantage of using DXA for assessing bone density?
    A. Low radiation dose
    B. Short scan time
    C. Good precision
    D. Comfort during the scanning

4. DXA is scanned at two different energy levels to:
    A. eliminate the soft tissue that is scanned
    B. reduce the radiation dose to the patient
    C. create higher resolution images
    D. allow greater precision in the Z-score

5. The scanned x-ray images that are produced during a DXA scan are used for what purpose?
    A. To confirm the correct bone is scanned
    B. To confirm the correct positioning
    C. To allow measurement of the bone mineral density
    D. To allow measurement of the bone mineral volume

6. Which of the following are the most widely used sites for measuring bone density?
    1. Spine
    2. Shoulder
    3. Proximal femur (hip)
    A. 1 and 2
    B. 1 and 3
    C. 2 and 3
    D. 1, 2, and 3

7. Bone mass increases in youth until the age of:
    A. 12 years
    B. 18 years
    C. 20 to 30 years
    D. 30 to 40 years

8. Which of the following are true for cortical bone?
    1. It accounts for 50% of skeletal mass.
    2. It resists bending and twisting.
    3. The outer shell is very dense.
    A. 1 and 2
    B. 1 and 3
    C. 2 and 3
    D. 1, 2, and 3

9. Where is trabecular bone found?
    A. At the ends of long bones
    B. In the large areas of the ilium
    C. In the hip primarily
    D. In the spine primarily

10. The equivalent of a new skeleton is formed by the human body every:
    A. 4 years
    B. 7 years
    C. 10 years
    D. 20 years

11. Bone destroying cells are called:
    A. epithelial cells
    B. neutrophils
    C. osteoclasts
    D. osteoblasts

12. The purpose of the skeleton in our body is to:
    1. support the body and protect organs
    2. manufacture red blood cells
    3. store minerals necessary for life—calcium and phosphate
    A. 1 and 2
    B. 1 and 3
    C. 2 and 3
    D. 1, 2, and 3

13. At what age does bone mass start to decrease in the females?
    A. 40 years
    B. 50 years
    C. 60 years
    D. 70 years

14. What medical condition is an indication for performing a DXA scan of the forearm?
    A. Hyperparathyroidism
    B. Cushing disease
    C. Type 2 osteoporosis
    D. Osteopenia

15. Osteoporosis is a disease characterized by:
    1. bone necrosis
    2. low bone mass
    3. structural deterioration of bone architecture
    A. 1 and 2
    B. 1 and 3
    C. 2 and 3
    D. 1, 2, and 3

16. All of the following would be associated with patients who have diagnosed osteoporosis, *except*:
    A. increased red blood cell counts
    B. decreased life quality
    C. deformity and disability
    D. increased risk of morbidity, especially from hip fractures

17. Increased risk factors for developing osteoporosis would include:
    1. female gender
    2. family history
    3. smoking tobacco
    A. 1 and 2
    B. 1 and 3
    C. 2 and 3
    D. 1, 2, and 3

18. Which of the following accounts for 70% of the peak bone mass?
    A. Genetics
    B. Nutrition
    C. Exercise
    D. Calcium level

19. Type II osteoporosis occurs in aging males and females because of:
    A. decreased calcium levels and other blood factors
    B. decreased ability of the body to build bone
    C. maternal family history
    D. environmental issues

20. Which of the following would be a cause of secondary osteoporosis?
    1. Hyperparathyroidism
    2. Multiple myeloma
    3. Rheumatoid arthritis
    A. 1 and 2
    B. 1 and 3
    C. 2 and 3
    D. 1, 2, and 3

21. Hip fractures account for what percentage of osteoporosis fractures?
    A. 10%
    B. 15%
    C. 20%
    D. 30%

22. The most common osteoporotic fracture occurs in which bone?
    A. Vertebrae
    B. Femoral neck of the hip
    C. Proximal humerus
    D. Ribs

23. The majority of osteoporotic fractures occur because of:
    A. living conditions
    B. genetics
    C. falls
    D. nutrition

24. The Surgeon General's recommendations for bone health and osteoporosis include:
    1. engage in physical activity
    2. obtain daily amounts of calcium and vitamin D
    3. reduce hazards in the home
    A. 1 and 2
    B. 1 and 3
    C. 2 and 3
    D. 1, 2, and 3

25. The Surgeon General's recommendation for intake of vitamin D for adults over age 50 is:
    A. 500 IU/day
    B. 800 IU/day
    C. 1000 IU/day
    D. 2000 IU/day

26. High-energy and low-energy x-rays are used together during a DXA scan. These energy levels are picked up by a detector and sent to a computer for processing. This process results in the:
    A. patient receiving a very low radiation dose
    B. soft tissues being subtracted, producing a profile of the bone
    C. the image of the bone having high resolution
    D. production of a three-dimensional image

27. Bone mineral density (BMD) is calculated by the following equation:
    A. bone mineral content (BMC) times the area
    B. BMC divided by the area
    C. area divided by BMC
    D. area times BMC

28. The sum of the data values obtained during a DXA scan, which is divided by the number of values, is calculated as the:
    A. mean
    B. precision
    C. standard deviation (SD)
    D. coefficient of variation (%CV)

29. The measure of the variability of the spread of the data values from a DXA scan is referred to as the:
    A. mean
    B. precision
    C. SD
    D. %CV

30. The percent of %CV that is used to determine the accuracy of the DXA scan is the:
    A. difference in values of the two energy levels used
    B. sum of the data values obtained during the scan
    C. variability of the spread of the data values from a scan
    D. comparison of variability between different data sets obtained during the scan

31. The ability of a DXA system to reproduce the same results in repeat measurements of the same patient is known as:
    A. mean
    B. standard deviation
    C. precision
    D. accuracy

32. The precision of a DXA scanner can be measured using:
    1. in vitro (a phantom)
    2. in vivo (a live body)
    3. a radiation detector device
    A. 1 and 2
    B. 1 and 3
    C. 2 and 3
    D. 1, 2, and 3

33. Each DXA laboratory should determine its "precision error." This calculation is known as the:
    A. T-score
    B. Z-score
    C. standard deviation
    D. least significant change

34. In order to detect drifts or shifts in calibration on a DXA machine, what test should be performed as part of its quality control?
    A. Standard deviation of 10 scans
    B. Quantitative measurement using software
    C. In vivo scan on a live patient
    D. In vitro scan with a phantom

35. The precision error for each operator should be done using which of these procedures?
    1. Measure 15 patients three times
    2. Measure 30 patients two times
    3. Measure 50 patients one time
    A. 1 and 2
    B. 1 and 3
    C. 2 and 3
    D. 1, 2, and 3

36. Every operator should perform an in vivo precision assessment after:
    1. basic scanning skills have been learned
    2. after having performed at least 50 patient scans
    3. after having performed at least 100 patient scans
    A. 1 and 2
    B. 1 and 3
    C. 2 and 3
    D. 1, 2, and 3

37. The ISCD Precision Assessment tool provides precision values for individual technologists/operators. The minimum acceptable precision value for the lumbar spine is:
    A. 1.9%
    B. 2.5%
    C. 2.8%
    D. 3.2%

38. A facility performing DXA should perform "cross-calibration" whenever:
    1. changing hardware
    2. changing to a new machine
    3. changing to a system from a new manufacturer
    A. 1 and 2
    B. 1 and 3
    C. 2 and 3
    D. 1, 2, and 3

39. Which DXA examination serves as a database to provide reference information for all manufacturing of DXA machines?
    A. Forearm
    B. Shoulder
    C. Hip
    D. Lumbar spine

40. The number of SDs a patient's BMD is from the average BMD for the patient's age and sex group is called the:
    A. T-score
    B. Z-score
    C. precision assessment
    D. accuracy indicator

41. The number of SDs a patient's BMD is from the average BMD of young, normal, and sex-matched individuals is referred to as the:
    A. T-score
    B. Z-score
    C. precision assessment
    D. %CV

42. Which of the following will be used to indicate if a patient needs an evaluation for secondary osteoporosis?
    A. T-score
    B. Z-score
    C. precision assessment
    D. %CV

43. According to the World Health Organization, a patient has osteoporosis if their BMD or BMC T-score is:
    A. 1
    B. 2
    C. > –2.5
    D. < –2.5

44. The three factors that directly relate to radiation safety in DXA scanning are:
    A. time, distance, and shielding
    B. time, distance, and monitoring
    C. time, exposure, and monitoring
    D. time, exposure, and shielding

45. How far should the technologist's/operator's working console be from the DXA's x-ray source?
    A. 3 ft
    B. 4 ft
    C. 5 ft
    D. 6 ft

46. The operator should have an individual dosimetry device (radiation badge) placed at:
    A. a table within 3 ft from the scanner
    B. their sleeve on the side closest to the scanner
    C. the waist on the side closest to the scanner
    D. the collar on the side closest to the scanner

47. The radiation dose to the patient for a DXA scan from various sites would be:
    A.   1 Sv
    B.   2 Sv
    C. 1 to 5 mSv
    D. 2 to 8 mSv

48. Patients who have a DXA scan may be frail or have increased risk for fragility fractures. Which of the following should be adhered to in the scanning room?
    1. The location of floor-level cables should be checked in the scan room to avoid tripping.
    2. All external artifacts should be removed on the patient clothing.
    3. Provide a simple explanation of the expected action of the scan-arm and proximity of the scan-arm to the patient's face.
    A. 1 and 2
    B. 1 and 3
    C. 2 and 3
    D. 1, 2, and 3

49. Which of the following would not need to be asked on the patient questionnaire?
    A. Are you a smoker?
    B. Are you able to lie on your back for several minutes?
    C. Have you had any previous fractures or surgery on the hip, spine, abdomen, or forearm?
    D. Do you have any medical conditions affecting the bone, such as osteoporosis, curvature of the spine, or arthritis?

50. In order to provide Medicare coverage, a patient must meet all of the following, *except*:
    A. be estrogen deficient
    B. have a low red blood cell count
    C. have hyperthyroidism
    D. have vertebral abnormalities

51. Which of the following applies to the patient data and DXA scan results on a patient?
    A. HIPAA rules must apply.
    B. The institution can decide how this information is kept.
    C. The questionnaire and scan results should be kept electronically and continually.
    D. The questionnaire can be kept in a paper file but the scan results must be kept electronically.

52. The operator must be proficient and able to do which of the following for DXA work?
    1. Be proficient at direct patient care and education.
    2. Provide accurate recordkeeping and confidentiality.
    3. Be computer literate.
    A. 1 and 2
    B. 1 and 3
    C. 2 and 3
    D. 1, 2, and 3

53. *Longitudinal quality control* procedures are done on the DXA scanner to:
    A. meet ISCD Precision Assessment guidelines
    B. provide a safe examination for the patient
    C. ensure the radiation dose is kept to a minimum
    D. ensure the equipment is functioning properly and has stable calibration

54. What device is used to provide *longitudinal quality control* scans to ensure proper calibration?
    A. Patient equivalent water phantoms
    B. Semianthropomorphic and aluminum phantoms
    C. A radiation dosimeter and software to detect errors
    D. Sheets of plexiglass of various thickness to simulate different-sized patients

55. When not recommended by the manufacturer, the ISCD advises that a quality control scan should be performed at least:
    A. once per day
    B. once per week
    C. twice per week
    D. once each month

56. How many phantom scans should be performed and plotted before and after a scanner has preventative maintenance, relocation, or software upgrades?
    A. 5 scans
    B. 10 scans
    C. 15 scans
    D. 20 scans

57. Who is required to maintain service logs, compliance with government inspections, radiation surveys, and regulatory requirements?
    A. Operator
    B. Department manager
    C. Hospital vice president
    D. Service person from the machine's manufacturer

58. One of the most important things that needs to be done to ensure that the DXA baseline and serial scans are as accurate as possible is:
    A. the patient must be scanned once per year
    B. ensure the longitudinal quality control procedures have been performed
    C. patient positioning on the scanner needs to be exactly the same for each scan
    D. the pre-scan instructions given to the patient

59. Which of the following can falsely elevate a patient's BMD for the posteroanterior (PA) lumbar spine?
    1. Degenerative changes in the spine
    2. Compression fractures
    3. Amount of calcium and vitamin D taken daily
    A. 1 and 2
    B. 1 and 3
    C. 2 and 3
    D. 1, 2, and 3

60. To ensure the inclusion of all of L4 on a PA lumber spine scan, which area of anatomy must be seen on the scan?
    A. Both hips
    B. Iliac crests
    C. Sacrum
    D. All five lumber vertebrae

61. Compared to the PA spine scan, the proximal femur (hip) scan is more difficult to perform properly and precisely because of:
    A. the specifics of placing the femur and legs in the correct position
    B. the overall density of the proximal femur area
    C. the time it takes to scan both hips
    D. variations in anatomy and the small region of interest (ROI)

62. How much should the legs be internally rotated for a DXA scan of the hips?
    A. 12 degrees
    B. 20 degrees
    C. 15 to 25 degrees
    D. 20 to 30 degrees

63. For a DXA scan of the hip the femurs must be positioned accurately. Which of the following describes the important position of the femurs?
    A. They must be straight and parallel to the long axis of the table.
    B. They must be touching each other at the knees.
    C. The ankles must be touching each other.
    D. The knees should be raised 2 in. so the femurs are parallel to the tabletop.

64. The limits of technology are challenged for DXA scans on which patients?
    1. Those who are very thin
    2. Those who are very thick
    3. Those who have very low bone mass
    A. 1 and 2
    B. 1 and 3
    C. 2 and 3
    D. 1, 2, and 3

65. How should the lesser trochanter appear on a hip scan?
    A. In full profile
    B. Totally invisible
    C. At least 50% should be seen
    D. Very diminished in size and only slightly visible

66. Which of the following are the ROIs for the forearm DXA scan?
    1. Ultradistal region
    2. Proximal region
    3. Mid-forearm (33% region)
    A. 1 and 2
    B. 1 and 3
    C. 2 and 3
    D. 1, 2, and 3

67. Each of the following is a reason that a patient should not have a DXA scan of the forearm, *except*:
    A. internal hardware from surgery
    B. history of wrist fracture
    C. having hyperparathyroidism
    D. deformity resulting from arthritis

68. For a DXA scan of the forearm, the one-third, or 33%, ROI is determined by:
    A. using computer software to mathematically measure the distance
    B. taking an anteroposterior (AP) radiograph before the scan
    C. measuring the radius from the radial styloid to the head
    D. measuring the ulna from the styloid process to the olecranon process

69. The most common problem that occurs during the DXA scan of the forearm is:
    A. motion of the forearm
    B. patient's fear radiation because their head is close to the source
    C. sitting in an uncomfortable chair designed for forearm scanning
    D. difficulty holding the position for the length of the scan

70. Placement for the ultradistal ROI should be:
    A. at the distal 1-in. of the ulna
    B. just below the end plate
    C. between the 33% region and the radial styloid
    D. between the 33% region and the ulnar styloid

71. VFA is a special technique used for the sole purpose of detecting:
    A. vertebral fractures
    B. subtle fractures that may not be seen in general spine imaging
    C. BMD in pediatric and adolescent patients
    D. curvature changes in the entire spine due to osteoporotic fractures

72. Which patient position is used in scanning for VFA?
    A. AP
    B. PA
    C. lateral
    D. PA and lateral

73. The greatest challenge in using VFA for bone densitometry is:
    A. cost since a regular DXA has to also be done
    B. concern about the radiation dose
    C. length of time of the scan
    D. if the patient has scoliosis

74. Children and adolescents are diagnosed with osteoporosis if they have the following:
    1. clinically significant skeletal fragility
    2. a BMD Z-score less than or equal to -2.0
    3. clinically significant history of fracture
    A. 1 and 2
    B. 1 and 3
    C. 2 and 3
    D. 1, 2, and 3

75. The PA spine and total body less head DXA are the preferred skeletal sites for performing BMC and areal BMD in which group of patients?
    A. Adults
    B. Teenagers
    C. Adolescents
    D. Most pediatric patients

76. According to ISCD 2019, which of the following should <u>not</u> be reported in pediatric DXA reports?
    1. The term "osteopenia"
    2. The term "osteoporosis"
    3. T-scores
    A. 1 and 2
    B. 1 and 3
    C. 2 and 3
    D. 1, 2, and 3

77. What does the FRAX tool provide in bone densitometry?
    A. A computerized assessment of osteoporosis using a patient's Z-scores
    B. An estimate of the 10-year probability risk of a major osteoporotic fracture
    C. An estimate of risk of fracture in females over age 70 and in males over age 75
    D. An assessment of pediatric risk of fracture

78. One element the FRAX tool looks at for risk is the BMD at which scanning site?
    A. Femoral neck
    B. Lumbar spine
    C. Forearm ultradistal region
    D. Forearm 33% region

79. The ISCD has issued a "Best Practices" document which states quality standards for bone densitometry. Which of the following is not one of the published standards?
    A. DXA technologists should be educated and competent.
    B. The DXA facility must comply with radiation safety requirements for the patient and technologist.
    C. The person interpreting the DXA scans should be a radiologist holding special certification.
    D. The DXA facility should have a detailed SOP for the procedures and all personnel should follow.

80. Bone density operators must adhere to ethical and professional statements from which of the following?
    1. Code of Ethics for Radiologic Technologists
    2. ASRT Bone Density Practice Standards
    3. HIPAA of 1996
    A. 1 and 2
    B. 1 and 3
    C. 2 and 3
    D. 1, 2, and 3

EXERCISE 2

Answer the following questions

1. What are the two types of bone?

   _____

2. Bone is constantly going through the process of replacing old bone with new bone. This is called:

   _____

3. Bone-building cells are called:

   _____

4. At what age do males start to lose bone mass?

   _____

5. Osteoporosis will create what type of fracture?

   _____

6. What is the percentage of males who have osteoporosis?

   _____

7. What causes type I osteoporosis in females?

   _____

8. Secondary osteoporosis can be caused by the use of prescription drugs. Name four of those drugs.

_____

_____

_____

_____

9. The five most common bones that get fractured as a result of having osteoporosis are:

_____

_____

_____

_____

10. What is the mortality rate for an osteoporotic person who suffers a hip fracture?

_____

11. How much calcium should a females over age 50 take per day and a male over age 51 take per day?

_____

12. Name the three statistics that are important in bone densitometry:

_____

_____

_____

13. From the DXA scan data, is a smaller standard deviation (SD) or a larger SD better?

_____

14. Is a smaller or a larger percent coefficient of variation (%CV) preferred from a DXA scan?

_____

15. The two important performance measures in bone densitometry are:

_____

16. In DXA scanning, the accuracy is determined by the:

_____

17. Name three of the six factors that will affect the precision of a DXA scan:

_____

_____

_____

18. A BMD measurement from a patient is most useful when it is compared statistically with an appropriate sex matched:

_____

19. Two standardized scores have been developed to compare a patient's BMD with a reference population. These two scores are the:

_____

20. The definition of *osteopenia* is:

_____

21. To diagnose fracture risk, osteoporosis, and osteopenia, which BMD score is used?

_____

22. What is the term used when there are different T-scores at anatomic sites within a patient?

_____

23. Compared to conventional radiography, is the radiation dose for a DXA scan higher or lower?

_____

24. A scan should be postponed on a patient for what four reasons?

_____

_____

_____

_____

25. A normal osteoporosis report would result when the BMD or BMC T-score is:

_____

26. The control limit for a longitudinal quality control scan is:

_____

27. Why are serial DXA scans done on patients?

_____

28. What is the purpose of using the leg positioning bloc for the PA lumber spine scan?

_____

29. Name the six items that should be on the checklist for an accurate DXA PA lumber spine.

_____

_____

_____

_____

_____

_____

30. Why is the DXA hip scan considered the most important?

_____

31. How should a fractured hip with hardware installed be scanned?

_____

32. Name the six items that should be on the checklist for an accurate DXA hip scan.

_____

_____

_____

_____

_____

_____

33. Which of the two forearms is used for the DXA forearm scan?

_____

34. An indication or scanning the forearm using DXA would be if a patient has documented:

_____

35. Name the six items that should be on the checklist for an accurate DXA scan of the forearm.

_____

_____

_____

_____

_____

_____

266

Chapter **26** **Bone Densitometry**

36. In contrast to traditional lateral spine x-rays, the VFA technique for visualizing the spine is:

_____

37. DXA can be done on infants as young as age:

_____

38. Why is the hip not a preferred measurement site for scanning growing children?

_____

39. What is the preferred term for pediatric DXA reports when BMC or areal BMD Z-scores are less than or equal to −2.0 SD?

_____

40. The FRAX tool is used for risk assessment of osteoporosis in patients between the ages of:

_____

EXERCISE 3

Match the following with their definition.

1. Precision   A. Coefficient of variation

2. PA lumbar spine   B. Comparison with young adult normal values

3. %CV   C. Milliamperage. The rate of current flowing in the x-ray tube

4. Mean   D. Disease- or medication-induced osteoporosis

5. Secondary osteoporosis   E. Postmenopausal or age-related osteoporosis

6. 33%   F. The technologist/operator's ability to reproduce the same positioning

7. Serial scanning   G. Kilovoltage. Measure of x-ray voltage

8. T-score   H. Region of interest on the forearm

9. Z-score   I. Position of the patient for a lumbar spine DXA scan

10. Primary osteoporosis   J. Measure of absorbed dose radiation in the body

11. kVp   K. Age-related BMD

12. mA   L. Average

13. Gray   M. DXA scans performed after the baseline scans

Answer the following questions.

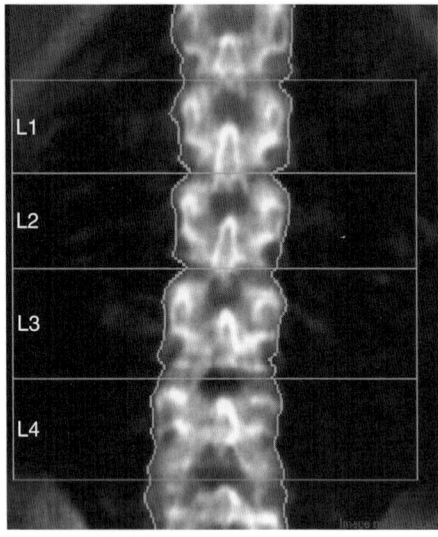

Fig. 26.1 Lumbar spine. (Courtesy of Erickson Retirement Bone Health Program, 2008.)

1. Has this lumbar spine image been acquired correctly?
   A. Yes
   B. No

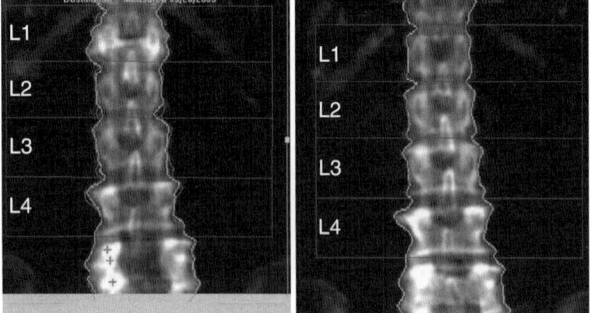

Fig. 26.2 Serial scan showing densitometric changes. (Courtesy Erickson Retirement Bone Health Program, 2008.)

2. Serial scan showing densitometric changes.

   A. Describe the changes that have occurred between the two scans in Fig. 26.2 and how they will affect the analysis of the lumbar spine scan.

   _____

   _____

   _____

B. Describe the steps the operator must take to ensure proper comparison with the baseline lumbar spine scan.

_____

_____

_____

_____

_____

_____

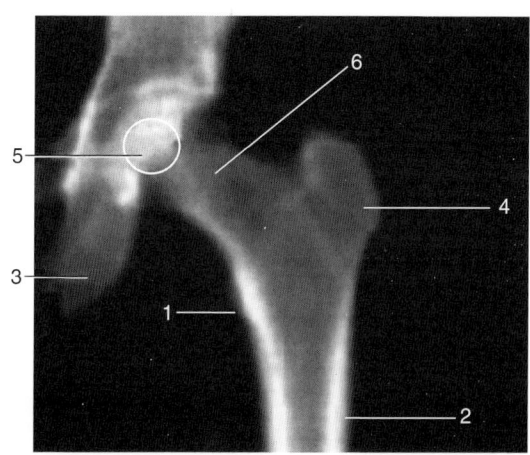

Fig. 26.3 Image of femur. (Courtesy Erickson Retirement Bone Health Program, 2008.)

3. Match the following parts of this proximal femur image with the corresponding number.

Greater trochanter   _____

Femoral neck   _____

Femoral head   _____

Pelvic ischium   _____

Lesser trochanter   _____

Femoral shaft   _____

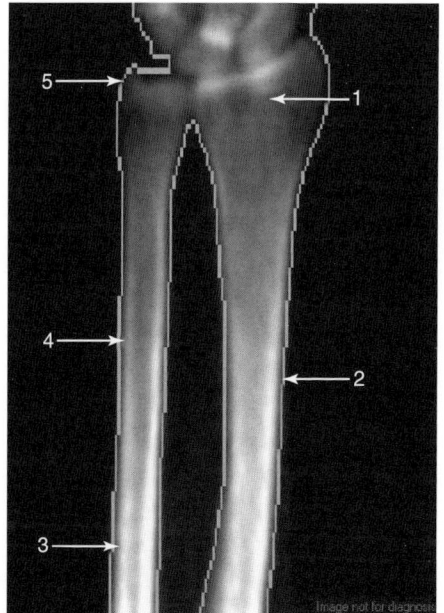

Fig. 26.4 Anatomy of the forearm. (Courtesy Erickson Retirement Bone Health Program, 2008.)

4. Match the following parts of this forearm image with the corresponding number.

Ulna   _____

Radius   _____

Distal radius   _____

Proximal ulna   _____

Ulnar styloid   _____

Answers to Section One

CHAPTER 01: ROLE OF THE LIMITED X-RAY MACHINE OPERATOR

Workbook Answer Keys

Exercise 1

1. D
2. A
3. C
4. True
5. A
6. B
7. D
8. D
9. A
10. C
11. B
12. B
13. C
14. B
15. B
16. B
17. False
18. True

Exercise 2

1. X-rays were discovered in 1895 by Wilhelm Conrad Roentgen at the University of Würzburg in Germany.
2. Purpose: Establish qualifications, administer examinations, and provide certification for professional radiologic technologists. This organization also provides limited-scope examinations to states that provide certifications for limited-scope x-ray machine operators. In addition, ARRT publishes the Code of Ethics and Rules of Ethics for professional radiographers, which are the existing standard of practice for radiography. Although these standards do not apply directly to limited operators, they should be seen as the prevailing standards for appropriate conduct by limited operators and radiographers.
3. Licenses or permits may be suspended or revoked. Fines and/or imprisonment may be levied against the limited operator and/or the employer.
4. The professional credential is RT(R), and it stands for "registered technologist (radiography)."
5. Reciprocity is the recognition of credentials acquired in one state by other states. Reciprocity facilitates the ability of limited radiographers to qualify to practice when moving from state to state.
6. Front office activities: Patient waiting, making appointments, handling payments, handling insurance and billing, and filing records. Back office activities: Consultation, examination, treatment, laboratory tests, and radiography.

7. a. Explain radiographic procedures to patients.
   b. Measure parts to be radiographed.
   c. Determine exposure factors and set the control panel.
   d. Position the patient correctly for the examination.
   e. Position the x-ray tube correctly for the examination.
   f. Position the IR correctly for the examination.
   g. Process the image in the reader device.
   h. Evaluate the image for quality.
   i. File and store images for reading by the physician.
8. 1. Basic x-ray machine operator
   2. Practical x-ray machine operator
   3. Limited radiologic technologist
9. Bone mineral content and density of various bones in the body

Exercise 3

1. D
2. G
3. H
4. E
5. C
6. F
7. A
8. B

Exercise 4

1. F
2. B
3. A
4. E
5. C
6. D
7. H
8. G
9. I
10. A

CHAPTER 02: INTRODUCTION TO RADIOGRAPHIC EQUIPMENT

Workbook Answer Keys

Exercise 1

1. C
2. D
3. C
4. B
5. D
6. A
7. B
8. A

9. C
10. A
11. D
12. B
13. C
14. A
15. D
16. D

Exercise 2

1. Turn on the collimator light. The crosshair in the center of the illuminated radiation field indicates the location of the central ray.
2. Between the patient and the IR, on the side of the patient opposite that of the x-ray tube
3. *Attenuation* is the term used to refer to absorption of the x-ray beam. Attenuation results in the production of scattered radiation.
4. The control console, also called the control panel
5. Release the appropriate lock(s).
6. On the underside of the x-ray tube housing
7. By reading the scale on the face of the collimator
8. Before making an exposure, be certain that:
   The x-ray room door is closed.
   No nonessential persons are in the x-ray room.
   All persons in the control booth are completely behind the lead barrier.
   No cassettes are in the room except the one in use.
9. Immediately. X-rays travel at the speed of light and do not linger in the room. They are present only during an exposure.
10. Primary radiation is defined as the x-ray beam that leaves the tube and is unattenuated, except by air. Its direction and location are predictable and controllable. Remnant radiation is what remains of the primary beam after it has been attenuated by matter. Because the pattern of densities in the matter results in differential absorption of the radiation, this pattern will be inherent in the remnant radiation. The pattern of the remnant radiation creates the IR image.
11. 8×10 inches, 10×12 inches, 14×14 inches, 14×17 inches, and 14×36 inches.
12. The patient is placed on the x-ray table, and the table is tilted so the head is lower than the feet. The angle is typically at least 15 degrees.
13. The latent image is the unseen image that is on the IR after exposure.
14. Upright cassette holder

Exercise 3

1. C
2. F
3. A
4. G
5. B
6. D
7. E

Challenge Exercise

1. Port
2. Tube housing
3. Central ray
4. Radiation field
5. Remnant or exit
6. Latent image
7. Primary beam
8. Attenuation
9. Patient
10. Scattered radiation
11. Scattered radiation has less energy
12. Scatter radiation fog
13. All directions, or 360 degrees
14. Cassette and phosphor plate
15. Computed radiography (CR)
16. CR Reader
17. Falling
18. 1. Test the footboard and shoulder guards to ensure they are securely attached.
    2. Be certain the spaces under the table are clear before tilting the table.
19. The Bucky
20. Upright cassette holder
21. Trendelenburg
22. 1. Close the x-ray room door.
    2. Ask nonessential persons to leave the room.
    3. Ensure all persons in the x-ray room are behind the control booth.
    4. Ensure that no IRs are in the room.

CHAPTER 03: BASIC MATHEMATICS FOR LIMITED OPERATORS

Workbook Answer Keys

Exercise 1

1. C
2. F
3. B
4. G
5. D
6. E
7. A

Exercise 2

1. Denominator
2. Numerator
3. Whole number, fraction
4. The numerator of the fraction, the denominator of the fraction
5. A. 8
   B. 20
   C. 60
   D. 75
   E. 56
6. A. 2/5
   B. 1/4
   C. 1/3

D. 3/5
E. 1/3
F. 3/5
G. 3/4

Exercise 3

1. Whole numbers
2. Tenths (10ths); hundredths (100ths); thousandths (1000ths)
3. True
4. False
5. A.
$$\begin{array}{r} 21.70 \\ +5.39 \\ \hline 27.09 \end{array}$$

   B.
$$\begin{array}{r} 33.06 \\ +30.20 \\ \hline 63.26 \end{array}$$

   C.
$$\begin{array}{r} 14.911 \\ +208.700 \\ \hline 223.611 \end{array}$$

   D.
$$\begin{array}{r} 29.844 \\ 3.300 \\ +27.600 \\ \hline 60.744 \end{array}$$

   E.
$$\begin{array}{r} 285.200 \\ 46.910 \\ +11.402 \\ \hline 343.512 \end{array}$$

6. A.
$$\begin{array}{r} 335.65 \\ -46.23 \\ \hline 289.42 \end{array}$$

   B.
$$\begin{array}{r} 456.33 \\ -3.87 \\ \hline 452.46 \end{array}$$

   C.
$$\begin{array}{r} 9.800 \\ -6.323 \\ \hline 33.477 \end{array}$$

   D.
$$\begin{array}{r} 21.00 \\ -7.51 \\ \hline 13.49 \end{array}$$

   E.
$$\begin{array}{r} 19.042 \\ -4.120 \\ \hline 14.922 \end{array}$$

7. Count the total number of decimal places in the numbers that are being multiplied. This is the number of decimal places that should be in the product before any zeros are dropped. For example, when a number with one decimal place is multiplied by a number with two decimal places, the product should have three decimal places.

8. A.
$$\begin{array}{r} 29.5 \\ \times 5 \\ \hline 147.5 \end{array}$$

   B.
$$\begin{array}{r} 17.6 \\ \times 40 \\ \hline 704.0 \end{array}$$

   C.
$$\begin{array}{r} 341.225 \\ \times 48.33 \\ \hline 10.23675 \\ 102.3675 \\ 2729.800 \\ 13649.00 \\ \hline 16491.40425 \end{array}$$

   D.
$$\begin{array}{r} 0.2213 \\ \times 82.7 \\ \hline 15491 \\ 4426 \\ 17704 \\ \hline 18.30151 \end{array}$$

   E.
$$\begin{array}{r} 83.22 \\ \times 906.1 \\ \hline 8322 \\ 49932 \\ 748980 \\ \hline 75405.642 \end{array}$$

9. A.
$$\begin{array}{r} 6.9 \\ 5\overline{)34.5} \end{array}$$

   B.
$$\begin{array}{r} 72.035 \\ 10\overline{)720.350} \\ \underline{70} \\ 20 \\ \underline{20} \\ 03 \\ \underline{0} \\ 35 \\ \underline{30} \\ 50 \\ \underline{50} \\ 0 \end{array}$$

10. Numerator; denominator
11. A. 0.125
    B. 0.375
    C. 0.0166
    D. 0.1333
    E. 1.25

12. Right to left
13. 5; 4
14. A. 1.67
    B. 0.7414
    C. 0.25
    D. 3.255
    E. 10.44
15. A. $1/4 = 0.25$ $1/20 = 0.05$ $2/3 = 0.667$
       $0.25 + 0.05 + 0.667 = 0.967$
    B. $3/10 = 0.3$ $1/5 = 0.2$ $1/2 = 0.5$
       $0.3 + 0.2 + 0.5 = 1.0$
    C. $3/4 = 0.75$ $3/8 = 0.375$ $0.75 - 0.375 = 0.375$
    D. $2/15 = 1.333$ $1.333 \times 200 = 266.6$
    E. $3/5 = 0.6$ $1/2 = 0.5$ $0.6 \div 0.5 = 1.2$

Exercise 4

1. False
2. True
3. A. 0.2
   B. 0.713
   C. 0.85
   D. 0.69
   E. 1.72
   F. 8
4. A. 33%
   B. 40%
   C. 6%
   D. 189%
   E. 230%
   F. 600%
5. A. $73\% + 27\% = 100\%$
   B. $50\% + 25\% = 75\%$
   C. $30\% - 3\% = 27\%$
   D. $20\% \times 60\% = 0.2 \times 0.6 = 0.12 = 12\%$
   E. $79\% \times 30\% = 0.79 \times 0.3 = 0.237 = 23.7\%$
   F. $25\% \div 10\% = 0.25 \div 0.1 = 2.5 = 250\%$
   G. $48\% \div 2\% = 0.48 \div 0.02 = 24 = 2400\%$
6. A. $30\% = 0.3$ $0.3 \times 27 = 8.1$
   B. $95\% = 0.95$ $0.95 \times 320 = 304$
   C. $50\% = 0.5$ $0.5 \times 31 = 15.5$
   D. $170\% = 1.7$ $1.7 \times 60 = 102$
   E. $200\% = 2$ $2 \times 20 = 40$
7. A. $11 \div 64 = 0.1718 = 17.2\%$
   B. $71 \div 90 = 0.7888 \ldots = 78.9\%$
   C. $50 \div 300 = 0.1666 \ldots = 16.7\%$
   D. $40 \div 200 = 0.2 = 20\%$
   E. $70 \div 35 = 2 = 200\%$
8. A. $100\% + 15\% = 115\% = 1.15$
      $1.15 \times 75 = 86.25$
   B. $100\% + 100\% = 200\% = 2$
      $2 \times 30 = 60$
   C. $100\% + 20\% = 120\% = 1.2$
      $1.2 \times 12 = 14.4$
   D. $100\% - 10\% = 90\% = 0.9$
      $0.9 \times 85 = 76.5$
   E. $100\% - 12\% = 88\% = 0.88$
      $0.88 \times 50 = 44$

Exercise 5

1. Equation
2. True
3. Divided
4. True
5. Ratio
6. Proportion
7. A. $2x + 9 - 9 = 11 + 3 - 9$
      $2x = 5$
      $2x \div 2 = 5 \div 2$
      $x = 2.5$
   B. $16/x \times x = (12 - 4) \times x16 = 8x$
      $16 \div 8 = 8x \div 8$
      $2 = x$
   C. $x - 61 + 61 = 12 + 61$
      $x = 73$
   D. $45 + 15 = 4x - 15 + 15$
      $60 = 4x$
      $60 \div 4 = 4x \div 4$
      $15 = x$
   E. $3x \times 3 = 9/3 \times 3$
      $9x = 9$
      $9x \div 9 = 9 \div 9$
      $x = 1$
   F. $64 \div 8 = 8x \div 8$
      $64 = 8x$
      $8 = x$
   G. $10x = 2 \times 25$
      $10x = 50$
      $10x \div 10 = 50 \div 10$
      $x = 5$
   H. $12 \times x = 3 \times 48$
      $12x = 144$
      $12x \div 12 = 144 \div 12$
      $x = 12$
   I. $72x = 8 \times 80$
      $72x = 640$
      $72x \div 72 = 640 \div 72$
      $x = 8.889$
   J. $4x = 6 \times 10$
      $4x = 60$
      $4x \div 4 = 60 \div 4$
      $x = 15$

Exercise 6

1. 4^3
2. 5^5
3. A. $3^2 = 3 \times 3 = 9$
   B. $3^3 = 3 \times 3 \times 3 = 27$
   C. $2^4 = 2 \times 2 \times 2 \times 2 = 16$
   D. $9^2 = 9 \times 9 = 81$
   E. $40^2 = 40 \times 40 = 1600$
4. A. 3
   B. 4
   C. 5
   D. 9
   E. 12

274

Answers to Section One

Exercise 7

1. 1. C
   2. H
   3. F
   4. D
   5. B
   6. E
   7. G
   8. A
2. A. 3
   B. 12
   C. 16
   D. 2000
   E. 16
3. A. 100
   B. 1000
   C. 1000
   D. 0.001
4. A. 70,000 V
   B. 500 cm
   C. 0.03 L
   D. kg
   E. 0.002 g
5. A. 18 inches ÷ 12 = 1.5 ft   1.5 ft ÷ 3 ft = 0.5 yd
   B. 1 qt × 2 = 4 pt   4 pt × 16 = 48 oz.
   C. 68 inches ÷ 12 = 5.67 ft
   D. 20 qt ÷ 4 = 5 gal
   E. 3.5 lb × 16 = 56 oz.
6. A. 5 fl. oz. × 30 = 150 mL
   B. 100 lb × 0.45 = 45 kg
   C. 14 inches × 2.54 = 35.36 cm
      35.36 ÷ 100 = 0.354 m
   D. 50 mm ÷ 10 = 5 cm
      5 cm × 0.39 = 1.95 inches
   E. 100 g × 0.0022 = 0.22 lb
      0.22 × 16 = 3.52 oz.
7. A. 1/60 s = 0.0167 s
      0.0167 × 1000 = 16.7 ms
   B. 260 s ÷ 60 = 4.3333 min
      4.3333 min ÷ 60 = 0.0722 h
   C. 2.4 days × 24 h/day = 57.6 h
   D. 75 − 32 = 43
      43 ÷ 1.8 = 23.89 °C
   E. 25 °C × 1.8 = 45
      45 + 32 = 77 °F

Exercise 8

1. The total quantity of the exposure
2. mA × Time (s) = mAs
3. mAs ÷ mA = Time (s)
4. A. 10 mAs
   B. 75 mAs
   C. 70 mAs
   D. 25 mAs
   E. 15 mAs
   F. 187.5 mAs
   G. 0.8 mAs
5. A. 0.2 s (or 1/5 s)
   B. 0.2 s (or 1/5 s)
   C. 0.02 s (or 20 ms)
   D. 0.02 s (or 20 ms)
   E. 0.188 s

Exercise 9

1. $mAs_1/mAs_2 = SID_1^2/SID_2^2$
2. A. 25%, or 1/4 of the original intensity
   B. 225%, or 21/4 times the original density
   C. 36 mAs
   D. 40.83 mAs
   E. 38.88 mAs

Exercise 10

1. 2; 3
2. 30%; 20%
3. A. 81 kVp
   B. 78 kVp
   C. 16 mAs
   D. 84.5 mAs
   E. 19.5 mAs
4. Divide

Exercise 11

1. Dose ÷ Strength = Volume
2. 4 tablets
3. 3 mL
4. 4 mL
5. 2 tablets
6. 2000 mg (2 g)
7. Body weight = 40 lb × 0.45 = 18 kg (metric body weight)
   2 mg/kg × 18 kg = 36 mg prescribed dose
   36 mg ÷ 4 mg/mL = 9 mL volume to administer

Challenge Exercise

1. Quotient
2. 97.75
3. 50%
4. mAs
5. 1.5 mAs
6. 1000
7. 6 mL
8. $mAs_1/mAs_2 = SID_1^2/SID_2^2$

CHAPTER 04: BASIC PHYSICS FOR RADIOGRAPHY

Workbook Answer Keys

Exercise 1

1. A
2. C
3. B
4. C
5. B
6. C
7. D
8. A
9. C
10. B
11. B

275

12. A
13. A
14. C
15. D
16. C
17. D
18. B
19. A
20. D
21. B
22. True
23. False
24. True
25. True
26. False
27. True

Exercise 2

1. When AC current is converted by a rectifier to flow in one direction and is changed DC current.
2. K-shell
3. Ultraviolet rays
   Visible light
   Infrared rays
   Microwaves
   Radar waves
   Television waves
   Radio waves
4. The shorter the wavelength, the more penetrating the beam.
5. Ionization is the creation of one or more charged particles that occurs when an electron is added or subtracted from a neutral atom. The ionizing ability of electromagnetic radiation is determined by wavelength. Wavelengths shorter than 1 nm have sufficient energy to remove an electron from its orbit.
6. Have no mass
   Are highly penetrating and invisible
   Are electrically neutral
   Are polyenergetic and heterogeneous
   Travel in straight lines at the speed of light
   Can ionize matter
   Produce biologic changes in tissues
   Produce secondary and scatter radiation
7. The velocity of x-rays is approximately 186,000 miles per second (3×10^{10} cm/s). All electromagnetic energy has the same velocity.
8. Current: amperes (A)
   Potential difference: volts (V)
9. Step-up transformer, where it is rectified and changed to DC.
10. Rectified and changed to direct current (DC)
11. The process by which an electric current in one circuit influences a current to flow in a second circuit. Induction occurs because of movement between the magnetic field surrounding wire in the first circuit and coils of wire in the second circuit. No other connection exists between the two circuits.
12. To change voltage

Exercise 3

1. G
2. I
3. F
4. E
5. C
6. H
7. B
8. D
9. J
10. A

Challenge Exercise

1. Solids, liquids, gases
2. Photon
3. Electrons
4. K-shell
5. Binding energy
6. Tungsten
7. Ionization
8. Electromagnetic
9. Wavelength
10. Wavelength and frequency
11. X-rays cause ionization in the atoms in the human body. This has the potential to create cancer.
12. Ionizing
13. Very short
14. Very high
15. 1. Have no mass
    2. Are highly penetrating and invisible
    3. Are electrically neutral
    4. Travel in straight lines
    5. Can ionize matter
16. Amps or milliamps
17. Volts or kilovolts
18. 40 to 125 kV
19. 50 to 500 mA
20. Alternating
21. Rectification
22. 6000 Hz
23. Electromagnetic induction
24. Transformer
25. Step-up and step-down
26. When a metal conductor is placed in a magnetic field and there is movement between the lines of magnetic force and the conductor, an electrical current will flow in the conductor. The magnetic field will induce a current in the conductor.

CHAPTER 05: X-RAY PRODUCTION

Workbook Answer Keys

Exercise 1

1. D
2. A
3. A
4. D
5. B

6. D
7. C
8. C
9. A
10. B
11. B
12. B
13. D
14. D
15. D
16. C
17. B
18. D
19. A
20. C
21. C
22. D
23. B
24. B
25. B

Exercise 2

1. Tungsten is a metal element. It can be readily formed into wire (as for the filament) or a smooth, hard surface (as in the target). It is an excellent target material because it has a high melting point and it is efficient at conducting heat away from the anode. Tungsten is a good filament material because it has a high atomic number, so there are many electrons available to provide a source of electrons for x-ray production.

2. Thermionic emission refers to the process of applying heat to the filament of the x-ray tube. Negatively charged particles (electrons) are given off by the tungsten filament material, supplying a source of free electrons for x-ray production.

3. Heterogeneous, as referred to in the x-ray tube, means the x-ray beam has a wide range of wavelengths. Bremsstrahlung interactions in the anode produce a heterogeneous x-ray beam. Characteristic interactions in the anode always produce the same wavelength.

4. A dual-focus tube has two filaments and two focal spots. A single-focus tube has only one of each.

5. Target angulation of at least 12 degrees is necessary in a general-purpose tube to create a primary x-ray beam that is large enough to cover a standard 35 × 43 cm IR at a 40-inch SID, which is one of the standard distances for radiography work.

6. Increased kVp results in an x-ray beam with greater energy and greater penetrating power. A kVp increase will cause a decrease (shortening) of the shortest wavelengths in the x-ray beam and therefore a shorter average wavelength in the beam.

7. An increase in mA might be desirable to increase the quantity of the exposure or to permit a shorter exposure time. Increased mA increases tube load and anode heat. Consistent use of the highest mA settings causes the tube to deteriorate more rapidly.

8. $100\,mA \times 0.25\,s = 25\,mAs$. Other possible combinations of mA and time that will produce 25 mAs include 50 mA and 0.50 s; 200 mA and 0.125 s; 500 mA and 0.05 s.

9. 0.5 mm inherent + 1.25 mm additional = 1.75 mm present. The total required is 2.5 mm. Therefore 0.75 mm Al equivalent filtration must be added (2.5 − 1.75 = 0.75).

10. 3600 rpm is the standard anode rotation speed.

11. None. Characteristic radiation can only be produced above 70 kVp.

12. 45%

13. Reduce patient dose.

14. 1. Oil
    2. Pyrex glass
    3. Mirror

15. Anode

16. The amount of radiation, or x-rays, that are absorbed in the patient's body.

Exercise 3

Simple x-ray tube:
1. Tungsten target
2. Heated tungsten filament
3. Pyrex glass envelope
4. Cathode
5. Anode

Effective focal spot:
1. Electron stream size
2. Actual focal spot size
3. Effective focal spot size

Exercise 4

1. 20
2. 5
3. 75
4. 75
5. 50
6. 400
7. 200
8. 100
9. 1
10. ½
11. 2
12. ¾

Challenge Exercise

1. Tungsten
2. Tungsten
3. Aluminum filtration
4. Thermionic emission
5. Negative
6. Positive
7. To dissipate the higher heat generated when high technical factors are used
8. 3600 and 10,000 rpm
9. Bremsstrahlung
10. 70 kVp

277

11. Heat
12. Bremsstrahlung
13. Effective focal spot
14. There is a greater volume or intensity of radiation on the cathode side of the tube. Or, x-ray intensity gradually increases from anode to cathode.
15. The cathode, or more intense x-rays, should always be placed on the thicker side of the body part.
16. kVp, or kilovoltage
17. mA, or milliamperage
18. Total quantity of exposure
19. kVp, or kilovoltage
20. 1. Has a very high melting point.
    2. Is efficient at conducting heat away from the anode.
21. 2.5 mm of aluminum equivalent
22. It absorbs the low energy and allows the higher energy x-ray to pass through to the patient.
23. 1. Oil
    2. Pyrex glass
    3. The mirror
24. Spatial resolution
25. Induction motor
26. Larger patients, or thick and dense body parts
27. 14 × 17 inches IR
28. 1. Tube heat capacity, 2. Spatial resolution, 3. Size of the x-ray beam.

CHAPTER 06: X-RAY CIRCUIT AND TUBE HEAT MANAGEMENT

Workbook Answer Keys

Exercise 1
1. A
2. A
3. C
4. C
5. A
6. D
7. B
8. D
9. C
10. C
11. B
12. B
13. C
14. C
15. B
16. D
17. C
18. C
19. True
20. False
21. True
22. True
23. False

Exercise 2
1. 3
2. 1
3. 3
4. 3
5. 2
6. 1

Exercise 3
1. 1. Warm up the anode according to instructions.
    2. Do not hold down the rotor for long periods.
    3. Use low mA settings whenever possible.
    4. Use the low-speed rotor whenever possible.
    5. Do not make repeated exposures near the tube heat limits.
2. To vary the voltage to the primary side of the step-up transformer.
3. 1. Prevent overexposure to the patient.
    2. Prevent damage to the x-ray tube.
4. 40 to 125 kVp
5. 1. High-frequency generators produce a more efficient and constant voltage.
    2. More constant voltage permits shorter exposure times and reduces patient dose.
6. Activate and hold rotor switch.
   On signal, activate and hold exposure switch.
   Observe exposure indicator to validate exposure and to determine when it is complete.
   Release rotor and exposure switches.
7. The anode begins to rotate.
   Full heat is applied to the filament.
8. The copper mass incorporated in the anode conducts heat from the target.
   The rotating anode spreads heat over a greater area.
   The structural layers of the rotating anode are designed to handle heat effectively.
   Oil in the tube housing dissipates heat from the glass envelope.
9. 80%
10. 600 mAs
11. The center detector is always located in the center of the IR at the central ray.
12. 200 mA
13. 1. Autotransformer
    2. Step-up transformer
    3. Step-down transformer
14. 1. kVp
    2. mA
    3. Exposure time
    4. AEC detectors
    5. Body habitus
15. To terminate the exposure if the AEC system fails.
16. It will cause the anode to crack.
17. Three
18. Overexposure or underexposure
19. Patient positioning

Challenge Exercise

1. 1. Low-voltage circuit
   2. Filament circuit
   3. High-voltage circuit
2. Vary the voltage on the primary side of the transformer.
3. Heat the filament of the cathode to provide thermionic emission of electrons.
4. Supply the x-ray tube with voltage high enough to create x-rays.
5. 1. Autotransformer
   2. Step-down transformer
   3. Step-up transformer
6. Filament circuit
7. High-voltage circuit
8. Rectification
9. Three
10. It will cause the anode to crack.
11. 1. Single-phase
    2. Three-phase
    3. High-frequency
12. To terminate the exposure if the AEC system fails.
13. Three
14. High-frequency
15. High-frequency
16. 6000 Hz
17. 1. Produce x-rays more efficiently than single or three-phase generators
    2. A single source of AC current is all that is needed to power the generator.
    3. Less exposure time is needed because of the higher output.
    4. Produce the greatest amount of x-rays for the same exposure technique.
18. Electronic
19. Manual exposure control
20. The exposure time
21. Patient positioning
22. Light, or underexposed (because the exposure time was reduced)
23. Exposure time, kVp, mA, AEC detectors, body habitus, Bucky, and SID
24. 600 mAs
25. Multiply the mA, kVp, and exposure time (mA × kVp × time = HU).
26. High-frequency: 2730 HU
27. 80% or less
28. 1 ms or less
29. Three low technique exposures should be made at least 30 seconds apart to warm the tube.
30. 1. Warm up the anode.
    2. Do not hold down the rotor switch.
    3. Use low mA settings when possible.
    4. Use the low-speed rotor whenever possible.
    5. Do not make repeated exposures near the tube limit.
31. Patient positioning

CHAPTER 07: PRINCIPLES OF EXPOSURE AND IMAGE QUALITY

Workbook Answer Keys

Exercise 1

1. A
2. D
3. A
4. C
5. C
6. D
7. B
8. C
9. A
10. B
11. D
12. B
13. C
14. A
15. D
16. C
17. C
18. A
19. B
20. B
21. D
22. C
23. B
24. A
25. True
26. False
27. True
28. False
29. True
30. False

Exercise 2

1. C
2. G
3. B
4. A
5. F
6. J
7. D
8. I
9. E
10. L
11. H
12. K
13. M

Exercise 3

1. Both milliamperage (mA) and exposure time (s) are directly proportional to the quantity of exposure.
2. Milliampere-seconds (mAs) are directly proportional to the total quantity of exposure and are used to indicate it.

3. $300\,\text{mA} \times 0.3\,\text{s} = 90\,\text{mAs}$
4. The mAs should be reduced to make the image lighter. This could be accomplished by reducing either the mA or the time. Time is usually the factor that is altered.
5. A short scale of contrast (obtained with lower kVp) provides greater differences between tissue densities that are similar; that is, greater contrast. A short scale of contrast is more desirable.
6. The standard mA and exposure time must be changed. An increase in mA, followed by a corresponding decrease in exposure time to maintain mAs and density, will significantly reduce motion.
7. The scale of contrast is too long (the kVp is too high).
   Fog is causing decreased contrast. This could be due to fog from any source.
8. Increased SID or decreased focal spot size, or both, would improve the image.
9. Image blur affects the radiographic image sharpness or spatial resolution. A shorter exposure time might solve the problem.
10. A stable position
    Positioning aids for comfort, such as radiolucent sponges
    Positioning aids for stability, such as sandbags or a table restraint
    Effective communication; clear instructions with ample time to comply
    Shorter exposure time
11. Subject contrast
    kVp
    Collimation
    Fog
12. OID
    SID
    Alignment of the body part
    CR angulation, direction, and degree
    IR position in relation to the body part
13. Geometric factors (increase SID, decrease OID)
    Reduce motion
    Reduce quantum mottle
    Use the small focal spot
14. 1. mA
    2. kVp
    3. Exposure time
    4. SID
15. Brightness
16. Window level
17. Contrast
18. Penetrometer
19. Short-scale contrast
20. Long-scale contrast
21. 1. kVp
    2. Tissue density
22. Fog
23. 1. Size
    2. Shape
24. Magnification
25. Shape distortion
26. 1. Elongation
    2. Foreshortening
27. The kVp or the mA is set too low and not enough photons reach the IR.
28. Density, contrast, radiographic distortion, spatial resolution

Challenge Exercise

1. mA, kVp, exposure time, and SID
2. mA, kVp, and filtration
3. kVp and filtration
4. Number of photons produced per second, or the quantity of x-rays
5. Double
6. Double
7. mAs
8. Energy of the x-ray beam increases when kVp is increased; vice versa
9. mA, exposure time, mAs, kVp
10. mAs
11. Four times more photons will be emitted.
12. kVp
13. kVp
14. SID, or source-to-indicator distance
15. SID and intensity (or volume) of radiation
16. Will be reduced to one-fourth (1/4) of the original density
17. It will be increased four times (4×).
18. 40 inches and many departments are going to 48 inches.
19. The overall blackness or darkness of the radiograph
20. The difference in radiographic density between adjacent portions of the image
21. A geometric property that refers to the differences between the actual subject and its radiographic image
22. A geometric property that refers to the sharpness or detail in the image
23. Overexposure
24. Underexposure
25. The mass density of a body part; also, the atomic number of a body part
26. Brightness
27. A decrease in kVp will increase contrast. An increase in kVp will decrease contrast.
28. A solid aluminum tool or device shaped like a step-wedge; when x-rayed, it simulated the densities found in a human body.
29. Short-scale contrast is when there is a short number, or range, of densities shown. Long-scale contrast is when there is a long number, or range, of densities shown.
30. Subject contrast
31. The presence of fog and collimation
32. Fog is unwanted exposure on the radiographic image.

33. When collimation is close or tight, there is less fog on the radiograph. Vice versa.
34. Window-width.
35. High-contrast or short-scale contrast
36. Low-contrast or long-scale contrast
37. Magnification
38. OID
39. When an object in the image projects, or appears longer than it actually is
40. When an object in the image projects, or appears shorter than it actually is
41. Patient motion, OID, SID, focal spot, and quantum mottle
42. Penumbra
43. Less recorded detail
44. Greater magnification and less recorded detail
45. Blurring of the radiographic image, or lack of recorded detail
46. Decreased exposure time with increased mA (keeping mAs the same)
47. Involuntary and voluntary
48. Effective communication with the patient
49. Reduce the exposure time
50. Quantum mottle
51. When there is a lack of photos at the IR to create a diagnostic image. Usually this is from too low kVp or mA, or both.
52. Ensure the body part is parallel to the IR and ensure that the CR is perpendicular. This is, however, for those body parts that require this. Some body parts may, for example, require an angle; therefore, ensure that particular angle is used.
53. 1. Reduce motion.
    2. Use the maximum allowed SID.
    3. Use the shortest OID.
    4. Use the small focal spot.
54. Density, contrast, radiographic distortion, and spatial resolution

CHAPTER 08: DIGITAL IMAGING

Workbook Answer Keys

Exercise 1
1. E
2. B
3. G
4. A
5. F
6. D
7. C

Exercise 2
1. G
2. B
3. A
4. D
5. H
6. F
7. C
8. E

Exercise 3
1. D
2. B
3. D
4. C
5. B
6. A
7. A
8. C
9. A
10. C
11. D
12. D
13. D
14. B
15. D
16. C
17. B
18. A
19. C
20. D
21. A
22. B
23. D
24. A
25. C
26. B
27. A
28. A
29. D
30. D
31. C
32. B
33. C

Exercise 4
1. Laser light
2. 10,000
3. DR
4. 1. Ability to see images very fast, or
   2. A wide dynamic range of exposures is available
   3. Image density and contrast can easily be adjusted
5. Quantum mottle
6. Picture archiving and communications systems
7. Compensating filters
8. kVp
9. Covered with lead
10. Scatter radiation
11. 1 second
12. Quantum mottle
13. Two
14. 1. Subtraction
    2. Contrast enhancement
15. DICOM grayscale function

16. 1. Moire
    2. Decreased quantum mottle
    3. Light spots
    4. Scratches
    5. Phantom or ghost images
    6. Extraneous line patterns
17. Smoothing
18. Rescaling
19. CCD and CMOS
20. The more signal that is sampled, the more information is obtained and spatial resolution is improved.
21. Detectors with high fill factors present higher spatial and contrast resolution.
22. MTF is used to measure the capacity or accuracy of the digital detector to pass its spatial resolution characteristics to the final image.
23. The histogram is basically a graph of the minimum and maximum signals in the image. Each x-ray image has a histogram as a part of its electronic file.
24. The LUT is a file of stored images for each projection. These files are referenced during processing.
25. Preexposure collimation by the operator
26. *White line* artifacts appear along the length of travel on the image due to dust on the light guide.
27. Fill factor
28. Light spots
29. CR reader
30. Rescaling
31. Radiation fog
32. Full spine x-rays done for scoliosis

Exercise 5
1. F
2. T
3. T
4. F
5. T
6. F

Exercise 6
1. B
2. E
3. C
4. A
5. F
6. D

Challenge Exercise
1. Computed radiography (CR)
2. Barium fluorohalide with europium
3. CR reader
4. 10,000 times
5. The IP is very sensitive to scatter radiation and must be protected before and after exposure.
6. Laser light
7. An intense white light
8. DR or digital radiography
9. DR

10. *White line* artifacts appear along the length of travel on the image due to dust on the light guide.
11. 17×17 inches
12. 1. Indirect conversion, two-step process
    2. Direct conversion, one-step process
13. 3 to 5 seconds
14. Process and see x-ray images very fast.
15. 1. X-ray energy is converted to light.
    2. X-ray energy is then converted to an electrical signal.
16. An electrical signal
17. Matrix
18. Pixel
19. Spatial resolution
20. 1,440,000 pixels
21. Smaller pixels means the spatial resolution will be greater.
22. Pixels will be smaller.
23. Contrast resolution
24. Dynamic range
25. Quantum mottle
26. Signal-to-noise ratio (SNL)
27. A greater electrical signal, or SNL, means the noise will be reduced and the image quality, or spatial resolution, will be greater.
28. Window "level" controls density or brightness.
29. Window "width" controls contrast.
30. The Joint Commission and the State Department of Health
31. ALARA
32. kVp (which controls penetration)
33. Analog-to-digital converter (ADC)
34. CCD and CMOS
35. Postprocessing
36. DICOM, or Digital Imaging and Communications in Medicine
37. DICOM grayscale function
38. Subtraction and contrast enhancement
39. Inadequate exposure technique, usually low mAs or low kVp
40. When the grid lines are not aligned with the laser scanning frequency
41. Incomplete imaging plate erasure
42. Background radiation most likely due to sensitivity to x-ray scatter
43. Noise in the CR reader electronics
44. PACS
45. Patient's name or institution ID, birth date or institution ID, date of the examination, and name and location of the x-ray facility
46. Slightly increase the kVp
47. Compensating filter
48. Conventional x-ray images, CT, MRI, and ultrasound image
49. In the center
50. A lead shield
51. The exposure indicator number
52. Four. At least two should be seen on every image.

53. 25%
54. Dust, scratches, and interactions between materials
55. Edge enhancement
56. Smoothing
57. Automatic rescaling
58. The LUT is a file of stored images for each projection. These LUT files are referenced during processing. The LUT is used as a base image reference when adjustments are made on an image.
59. MTF is used to measure the capacity or accuracy of the digital detector to pass its spatial resolution characteristics to the final image.
60. *White line* artifacts appear along the length of travel on the image due to dust on the light guide.
61. *Histogram analysis error* may be due to any of the following: improper collimation, improper technique, beam alignment error, scatter, and extreme subject density differences.
62. Electronic cropping also known as *masking* or *cropping*, is used to blacken out the white collimation borders. This eliminates the glare to the eyes.

CHAPTER 09: SCATTER RADIATION AND ITS CONTROL

Workbook Answer Keys

Exercise 1
1. C
2. D
3. B
4. D
5. A
6. B
7. B
8. A
9. A
10. A
11. B
12. B
13. A
14. C
15. D
16. A
17. B
18. C
19. D
20. D
21. A
22. A
23. D
24. A
25. A
26. D

Exercise 2
1. T
2. T
3. F
4. F
5. T
6. F
7. T
8. T
9. T
10. T
11. F
12. T
13. T
14. F
15. F

Exercise 3
1. Photoelectric interactions produce characteristic scatter radiation.
2. Part thickness
   Field size
3. The quantity of fog is increased because the scatter produced with higher kVp has greater energy.
4. The patient is the principal source of scattered radiation fog in radiography.
5. 1. Volume of tissue
   2. kVp
   3. Density of matter
   4. Field size
6. Volume of tissue irradiated
7. Because the x-rays are absorbed in the part, or there is more photoelectric absorption
8. Maintaining the correct field size, or collimating
9. 1. Collimator template
   2. Beam alignment cylinder
10. It leaves the atom.
11. It is totally absorbed, causing dose to the patient.
12. The grid oscillates.
13. Decrease
14. 60 kVp
15. Increase
16. Focused
17. Dose is increased

Challenge Exercise
1. 1. Compton effect
   2. Photoelectric effect
2. All directions, or 360 degrees
3. Backscatter
4. It scatters outside the body.
5. It scatters outside the body.
6. It is totally absorbed in the body part.
7. The energy is decreased.
8. Increased
9. Decreased
10. Fog
11. 1. Volume of tissue
   2. kVp
   3. Density of matter
   4. Field size
12. Volume of tissue irradiated
13. Scatter is increased.

14. 10 or greater
15. Scatter radiation fog is increased.
16. Scatter is decreased.
17. Maintaining the correct field size, or collimation
18. A grid
19. 1. Use a grid for body parts over 10 cm.
    2. Reduce field size and collimation to only the body part.
    3. Reduce kVp.
20. 10 to 12 cm or kVp is over 60.
21. Increases contrast as a result of less scatter radiation
22. Cone-down image
23. 1. Collimator
    2. Central ray alignment
24. 1. Collimator template
    2. Beam alignment cylinder
25. 2% of the SID
26. 1 degree of perpendicular

CHAPTER 10: FORMULATING X-RAY TECHNIQUES

Workbook Answer Keys

Exercise 1

1. D
2. C
3. C
4. B
5. D
6. D
7. C
8. C
9. A
10. C
11. A
12. C
13. D
14. C
15. B
16. B
17. A
18. B
19. C
20. A
21. D
22. A
23. True
24. False
25. True
26. True
27. False

Exercise 2

1. 100 mAs
2. 7.5 mAs

Exercise 3

1. ↑
2. ↑
3. ↓

4. ↑
5. ↑
6. ↓
7. ↑
8. ↓
9. ↓
10. ↓
11. ↑
12. ↓
13. ↑
14. ↑

Exercise 4

1. The highest kVp setting that will produce sufficient contrast for acceptable image density
2. An x-ray caliper is used to measure body part thickness in units of centimeters (cm). 200 mA and below
3. Higher contrast and greater spatial resolution
4. The exposure and image will have more latitude for exposure error and radiation exposure will be lower.
5. In increments of doubling or halving.
6. 10 mAs ÷ 100 mA = 1/10 (or 0.1) s
7. Conditions requiring an *increase:*
   Chest conditions: atelectasis, cardiomegaly, congestive heart failure (CHF), pleural effusion, pneumonia, malignancy. Conditions of bone: arthritis (rheumatoid), osteochondroma, hydrocephalus, metastasis, Paget disease. Abdomen: ascites, cirrhosis of liver. Generalized conditions: abscess, edema.
   Conditions requiring a *decrease:*
   Chest conditions: chronic obstructive pulmonary disease (COPD, emphysema), pneumothorax. Conditions of bone: arthritis (degenerative), gout, metastasis, multiple myeloma, osteoporosis. Abdomen: bowel obstruction, free air. Generalized conditions: advanced age, atrophy, emaciation.
8. Increased latitude and decreased dose are obtained by increasing kVp. To change kVp without altering radiographic density, the 15% rule is used (increase kVp by 15% and divide mAs by 2). The new exposure is 200 mA, 0.15 s, and 81 kVp.
9. The formula needed here is $mAs_1/mAs_2 = SID_1^2/SID_2^2$. The result is 65 mAs.
10. 1. The x-ray machine is not calibrated.
    2. The digital processor may not be working properly.
    3. The limited operator may not be referring to it and instead memorizing the techniques.
11. 100% if the image is too light and 50% if the image is too dark
12. Either doubling the mAs or reducing the mAs by half (50%)
13. When a body part contains areas of significantly variable tissue density
14. AP thoracic spine, axio-lateral hip, AP shoulder, C7–T1 cervico-thoracic area, AP foot, and AP and lateral full-spine standing

15. Entire spine is on one image, reduction in radiation exposure to the patient (mostly young patients)
16. To ensure the filter does not fall onto the patient
17. Simply measure the cast and use the measured cm from the technique chart.

Challenge Exercise

1. Exposure technique chart
2. The Joint Commission
3. Exposure time, kVp, mAs, SID
4. Manual technique chart
5. Anatomically programmed radiography, or APR
6. Measuring caliper
7. 1. Variable kVp
   2. Fixed kVp
8. Using the highest kVp setting that will produce sufficient contrast for acceptable image quality. This also lowers the dose to the patient.
9. A 15% change in kVp will produce the same change in radiographic density as a doubling or halving of the mAs.
10. If the exposure was low, double the mAs. If the exposure was high, halve the mAs.
11. The highest mA should be used with the shortest exposure time and keeping the mAs the same.
12. 1. The limited operator may not be following the posted exposure techniques for body parts.
    2. The generator could be out of calibration.
13. 1. Cardiomegaly
    2. Congestive heart failure
    3. Edema
    4. Pleural effusion
    5. Pneumonia
    6. Rheumatoid arthritis
14. 1. Pneumothorax
    2. Degenerative arthritis
    3. Osteoporosis
    4. Bowel obstruction
    5. Advanced age
    6. Atrophy
15. 1. Pediatric patients
    2. Obese patients
16. Inadequate penetration of the body part (kVp does not go high enough)
17. Increasing the kVp
18. 30%
19. 100% if the image is too light; 50% if the image is too dark
20. $mAs_1/mAs_2 = D_1^2/D_2^2$
21. A body part that has two very widely varying thicknesses that have to be included on one x-ray image
22. 1. AP shoulder
    2. Lateral C7–T1 cervical-thoracic area
    3. AP foot
    4. AP thoracic spine
23. Compensating filters can be placed between the radiographic tube and the IR.

CHAPTER 11: RADIOBIOLOGY AND RADIATION SAFETY

Workbook Answer Keys

Exercise 1

1. B
2. C
3. D
4. C
5. D
6. D
7. A
8. A
9. B
10. C
11. D
12. B
13. A
14. C
15. C
16. B
17. C
18. B
19. D
20. C
21. C
22. A
23. D
24. C
25. C
26. C
27. D
28. B
29. D
30. C
31. A
32. B
33. D
34. False
35. True
36. True
37. False
38. True
39. False
40. True
41. False
42. True
43. True

Exercise 2

1. B
2. F
3. E
4. H
5. G
6. J
7. I

8. C
9. D
10. A
11. K

Exercise 3

1. 1. Reduce repeat x-rays.
   2. Use collimation.
   3. Increase the kVp.
   4. Use the 40-inch SID.
2. 0.5-mm lead equivalent
3. 1. Mobile radiography
   2. Fluoroscopy
4. Long-term (latent) effects usually occur 5 to 30 years after exposure. They are random and unpredictable and the severity is not related to dose. They include malignant diseases, such as cancer and leukemia. Short-term effects result from higher doses. They include loss of function of organs and tissue, especially blood cells, and syndromes, such as radiation sickness and CNS effect, which involve seizures, coma, and death. The severity of short-term effects is directly related to dose.
5. 1. Time
   2. Distance
   3. Shielding
6. At a dose of 250 mSv, you would see blood changes.
7. 1. Can measure small doses more precisely.
   2. Are accurate over a wide range.
   3. Have excellent long-term stability.
8. 1. Double-check the requisition and the patient identification.
   2. Explain the procedure and obtain the patient's cooperation.
   3. Use established procedures for IR placement, tube placement, and patient positioning to prevent overlooking details.
   4. Collimate to include only the anatomic area of clinical interest.
   5. Shield gonads and any sensitive organs near the radiation field.
   6. Measure the patient correctly, and check the technique chart precisely.
   7. Consider whether any variations in the usual technique are needed for this particular patient.
   8. Be certain that the computer processor is operating correctly, and use standard procedures for imaging processing.
   9. Maintain equipment, digital processor, and accessories in good condition.
   10. Use low-dose techniques.
9. Low-dose techniques involve using optimum kVp (the highest kVp consistent with acceptable contrast), appropriate collimation, careful use of a grid, a minimum SID of 40 inches, and nongrid techniques when appropriate.
10. Be sure that a policy exists for this purpose and that you are familiar with it. Possible considerations include the posting of warning signs and discussing the possibility of pregnancy with female patients of childbearing age. Neither the 10-day rule nor an early pregnancy test can guarantee that the patient is not pregnant, but these can greatly decrease the likelihood of pregnancy.
11. The shielding provided by the control booth
12. 1. Aprons: 0.5-mm lead equivalency
    2. Gloves: 0.25-mm lead equivalency
13. As low as reasonably achievable
14. Ionizing radiation is radiation that, when passing through the body, produces positively and negatively charged particles.
15. Radiation protection is the measures taken to safeguard patients, personnel, and the public from unnecessary exposure to ionizing radiation.
16. Radiation badges should be worn in the region of the collar and on the anterior surface of the body. They should be on the outside of the lead apron when an apron is worn for holding patients or during fluoroscopy.
17. Gonads of reproductive males and females
18. 5.5 mSv
19. The purpose of the "control" badge is to measure any radiation exposure that might occur to the entire batch of personnel monitors while in transport to and from the company.
20. The children and grandchildren of the irradiated individual.
21. Computed tomography (CT scans).
22. Lumbar spine and pelvis.
23. At the waist level for all radiography procedures and under a lead apron if one is worn.
24. Cleft palate, spina-bifida, polydactyly and more.

Challenge Exercise

1. Gray-$_a$
2. Absorbed dose
3. Equivalent dose
4. 1
5. Exposure: Gray-$_a$
   Absorbed dose: Gray-$_t$
   Equivalent dose: Sievert
6. 100 mGy-$_a$
7. Radiation protection purposes
8. Entrance skin exposure
9. The relative sensitivity of cells in the body to radiation
10. 1. Age
    2. Differentiation
    3. Metabolic rate
    4. Mitotic rate
11. Younger patients, especially babies and children, are considerably more sensitive to the effects of radiation exposure than are adults.
12. Simple cells are more sensitive than highly specialized ones.
13. Blood cells, blood producing cells, thyroid gland, female breasts
14. Nerve cells, muscle cells, and cortical bone
15. 1. Short-term
    2. Long-term
    3. Somatic
    4. Genetic

16. Short-term effects
17. Not predictable
18. Long-term effects
19. Genetic effect
20. Erythema, or reddening of the skin
21. Lethal dose, or LD 50/30 means that 50% of the population would die in 30 days
22. 3000 to 4000 mGy
23. 2000 mSv
24. Long-term effects
25. 1. Cataracts
    2. Carcinogenesis
    3. Life-span shortening
    4. Leukemia
26. 10 to 15 years
27. Genetic effect
28. Gonads
29. 1. Cleft palates
    2. Spina bifida
    3. Polydactyly
30. 5.5 mSv per year
31. As low as reasonably achievable. This means our radiography work should be such that we are always giving the lowest dose to the patient.
32. Repeat x-rays.
33. 1. Reduce repeats.
    2. Use the smallest radiation field (collimation).
    3. Use the highest kVp permissible for a given body part.
    4. Never use less than a 40-inch SID.
34. Mutation, or high radiation doses to the gonads
35. 1. Contact shields
    2. Shadow shields
36. Within 5 cm of the gonads
37. 1. Mobile
    2. Fluoroscopy
38. 1. Time
    2. Distance
    3. Shielding
39. 6 months
40. Aprons: 0.5-mm lead equivalency
    Gloves: 0.25-mm lead equivalency
41. 1. Can measure small doses more accurately
    2. Are accurate over a wide range of exposures
    3. Have excellent long-term stability
42. The purpose of the "control" personnel dosimeter (or badge) is to measure any radiation exposure that might occur to the entire batch of dosimeters while being transported to and from the company.
43. In the region of the collar and on the anterior surface of the body; also, outside the apron if worn
44. Effective dose
45. Cumulative effective dose
46. 50 mSv
47. The formula is: Worker's age in years × 10 mSv.
48. 420 mSv
49. 150 mGy$_t$
50. First trimester
51. 0.5 mSv per month
52. 5.0 mSv
53. At the waist and under the apron
54. Patients become sick very fast because they receive whole-body doses in a very short period of time.
55. The amount of x-ray energy transferred on average, per the length of passage through the tissue.
56. When there is more oxygen in the tissues, it is more sensitive to radiation compared to tissues with low oxygen.
57. It reduces anxiety in the patient and increases the potential of success of the examination with no repeat exposures.
58. Published studies indicate the risk of a radiation-induced leukemia in children after a substantial dose of ionizing radiation is approximately *two times that of adults*. They also have longer lives and a greater chance of developing any cancer.

CHAPTER 12: INTRODUCTION TO ANATOMY, POSITIONING, AND PATHOLOGY

Workbook Answer Keys

Exercise 1
1. C
2. A
3. C
4. D
5. D
6. A
7. B
8. A
9. A
10. C
11. B
12. A
13. C
14. A
15. B
16. D
17. A
18. A
19. D
20. D
21. D
22. A
23. B
24. C
25. C

Exercise 2
1. C
2. K
3. E
4. I
5. G
6. A
7. D
8. B
9. H
10. F
11. J

287

Exercise 3

Top row, left to right:
1. Greenstick
2. Spiral
3. Overriding
4. Comminuted

Bottom row, left to right:
1. Transverse
2. Compression
3. Depressed
4. Avulsion

Exercise 4

1. When the central ray (CR) "skims" a body part.
2. The common positioning landmarks cannot be palpated.
3. 1. Sagittal plane, divides the body into right and left parts.
   2. Coronal plane, divided the body into anterior and posterior parts.
   3. Transverse or horizontal plane, divided the body into superior and inferior portions.
4. A rounded process on a bone, larger than a tubercle.
5. The skeletal system provides a rigid framework for the body.
6. The outer portion is the cortex. The inner portion is spongy bone, which may also be called *cancellous bone.*
7. Divides the body specifically into equal anterior and posterior parts.
8. Abduction: move away from center of body
   Adduction: move toward center of body
   Extension: straighten a hinge joint, straighten the spine (bend backward)
   Flexion: bend a hinge joint, bend the spine forward
   Pronate: rotate the forearm so the palm of the hand faces down
   Supinate: rotate the forearm so the palm of the hand faces up
9. Elbow
10. Left lateral position
11. Anteroposterior (AP)
12. Left lateral projection
13. Chest respiration: inspiration
    Abdominal respiration: expiration
14. LAO and RAO
15. When the x-ray tube is angled longitudinally 10 degrees or more
16. Set the SID to the standard level. Then lower the tube 1 inch for each 5 degrees of angle.
17. 1. Acute conditions are characterized by sudden onset, whereas chronic conditions are of long duration.
    2. Benign conditions are lesions that are limited in growth and remain at one site, whereas malignant conditions are cancers that grow more rapidly, invade surrounding structures, and can spread (metastasize) to distant sites.
18. The side closest to the IR, or touching the IR, is marked.
19. 1. C-5
    2. C-7, T-1
    3. T-2, T-3
    4. T-7
    5. L-4, L-5
    6. S-1, S-2
20. True
21. False
22. True
23. True
24. False

Challenge Exercise

1. Forward or front portion of the body or body part
2. Backward or back portion of the body or body part; the opposite of anterior
3. Pertaining to the head; toward the head; the opposite of caudal
4. Away from the head
5. Above, toward the head; the opposite of inferior
6. Below, farther from the head
7. Deep, near the center of the body or a part; the opposite of external
8. To the outside, at or near the surface of the body or a body part
9. Toward the center of the body or the center of a part; the opposite of lateral
10. Referring to the side, away from the center to the left or right
11. Toward the source or point of origin; the opposite of distal
12. Away from the source or point of origin; for example, the wrist is *distal* to the elbow, being farther from the point of origin of the arm, which is at the shoulder
13. Lying on the back
14. Lying face down
15. Lying down; the position is further described by adding the name of the body surface on which the patient is lying: *dorsal recumbent, lateral recumbent, ventral recumbent*
16. Erect, standing or seated
17. The patient is recumbent with the central ray (CR) horizontal, or parallel to the floor. This position is named according to the body surface on which the patient is lying: lateral decubitus (left or right), dorsal decubitus, or ventral decubitus.
18. Placement of the body or body part with the sagittal plane parallel to the IR. It is named according to the side adjacent to the radiographic table or IR.

19. Achieved when the body part or entire body is placed so that the coronal plane is not parallel with the radiographic table or IR. The description is usually stated as a degree of rotation, either from a body plane or toward the affected side.
20. Anteroposterior (AP) projection
21. Posteroanterior (PA) projection
22. Lateral projection
23. Oblique projection
24. Axial projection
25. Tangential projection
26. Divides the body into anterior and posterior parts.
27. Divides the body specifically into equal right and left halves.
28. The tube is adjusted to the standard SID. From there it is lowered 1 inch for every 5 degrees of tube angle.
29. On the side of the body that is up.
30. Right marker
31. *Acute*: Characterized by a sudden onset. *Chronic*: Characterized by a long duration.

CHAPTER 13: UPPER LIMB AND SHOULDER GIRDLE

Workbook Answer Keys

Exercise 1
1. C
2. B
3. C

4. D
5. C
6. A
7. C
8. D
9. D
10. D
11. B
12. A
13. B
14. D
15. C
16. A
17. C
18. D
19. A
20. A
21. C
22. C
23. C
24. D
25. A
26. B
27. B
28. D
29. A
30. C

Exercise 2

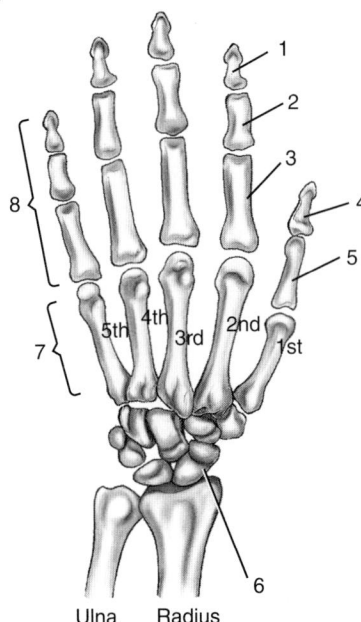

Fig. 13.1

1. Distal phalanx

2. Middle phalanx

3. Proximal phalanx

4. Distal phalanx

5. Proximal phalanx

6. Scaphoid

7. Metacarpals

8. Phalanges

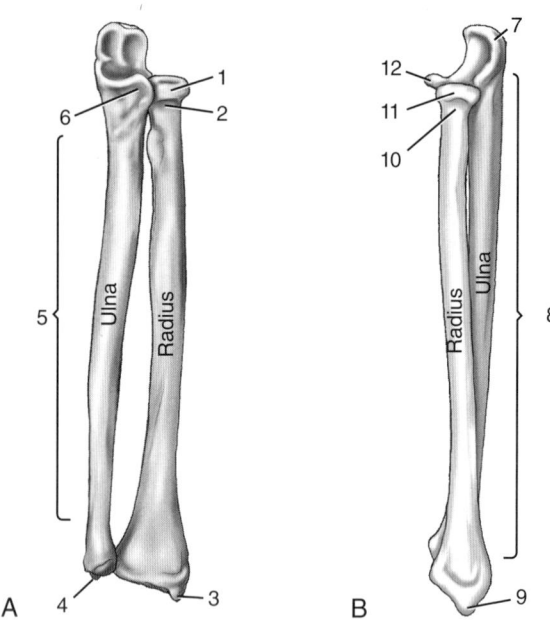

1. Head
2. Neck
3. Radial styloid process
4. Ulnar styloid process
5. Body
6. Coronoid process
7. Olecranon
8. Body
9. Radial styloid process
10. Neck
11. Head
12. Coronoid process

Fig. 13.2

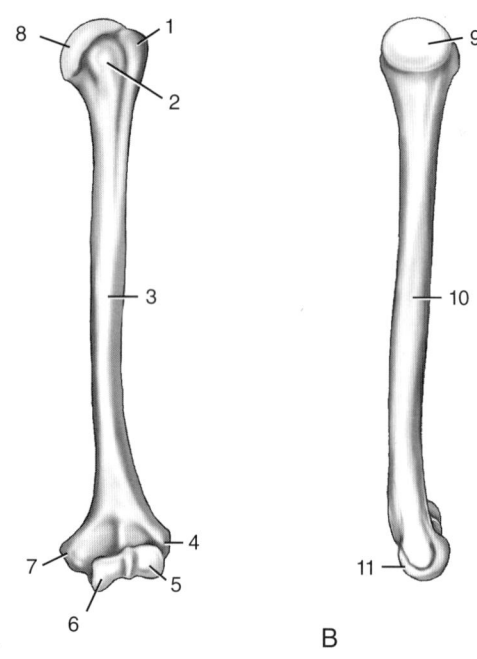

1. Greater tubercle
2. Lesser tubercle
3. Body
4. Lateral epicondyle
5. Capitulum
6. Trochlea
7. Medial epicondyle
8. Head of humerus
9. Head of humerus
10. Body
11. Medial epicondyle

Fig. 13.3

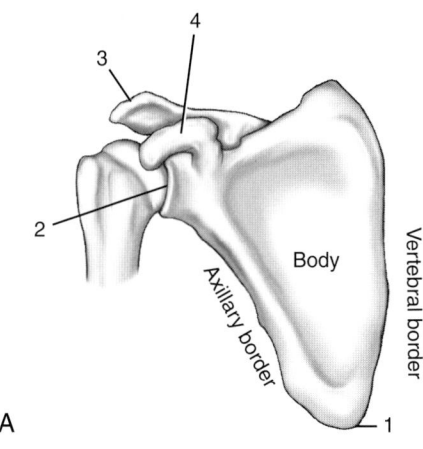

A

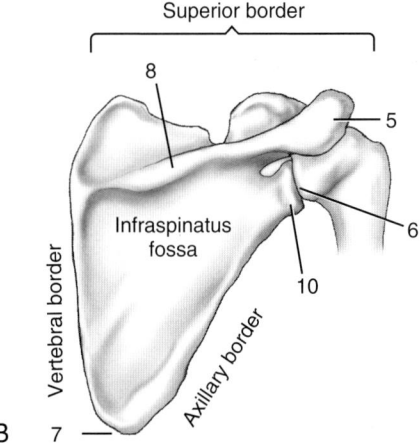

B

Superior border

Infraspinatus fossa

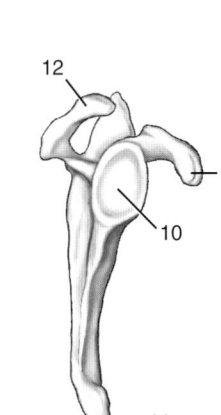

C

Fig. 13.4

1. Inferior angle
2. Glenoid fossa
3. Acromion
4. Coracoid process
5. Acromion
6. Glenoid fossa
7. Inferior angle
8. Spine
9. Corocoid process
10. Glenoid fossa
11. Inferior angle
12. Acromion

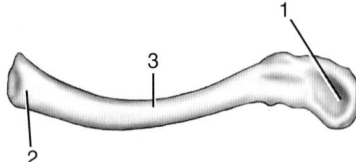

Fig. 13.5

1. Acromial extremity
2. Sternal extremity
3. Shaft

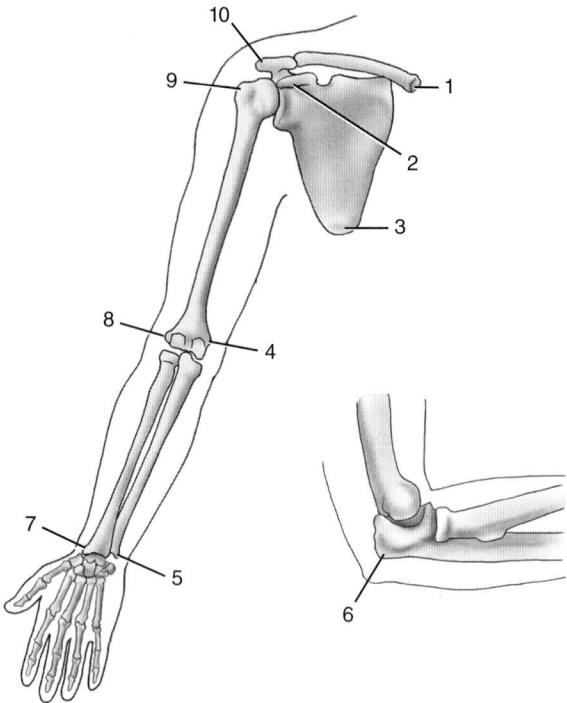

Fig. 13.6

1. Medial end of clavicle

2. Coracoid process

3. Inferior angle of scapula

4. Medial epicondyle

5. Ulnar styloid process

6. Olecranon process of ulna

7. Radial styloid process

8. Lateral epicondyle

9. Greater tubercle

10. Acromion

Exercise 3

1. The middle bone of the third digit is the middle phalanx. The carpal bone most easily fractured is the scaphoid.
2. The ulna is medial to the radius.
3. Capitulum (lateral humerus)
   Trochlea (medial humerus)
4. 1. AP, proximal forearm
   2. AP, distal humerus.
5. Hand is supinated.
6. The fingers are extended for a PA projection of the hand, but they are flexed into a loose fist for a PA projection of the wrist. The hand projection is centered at the third MCP joint, whereas the wrist is centered midway between the styloid processes (midcarpals).
7. PA, Ulnar deviation
   PA axial (Stecher method)

8. 1. AP
   2. Transthoracic lateral
   3. PA oblique (scapular Y)
9. 1. PA
   2. PA axial
10. The arm is abducted and the hand is supinated.
11. The coronal plane is placed perpendicular to the IR.
12. 45 to 60 degrees
13. Slow deep breaths during the exposure.
14. The CR is directed 2 inches medial and 2 inches inferior to the superolateral border of the shoulder.
15. Arm is abducted so the humerus is perpendicular to the body. The elbow is flexed 90 degrees.
16. Bilateral AP projections are required and, with and without weights on the arms.
17. Hand is placed in true lateral position.

Exercise 4

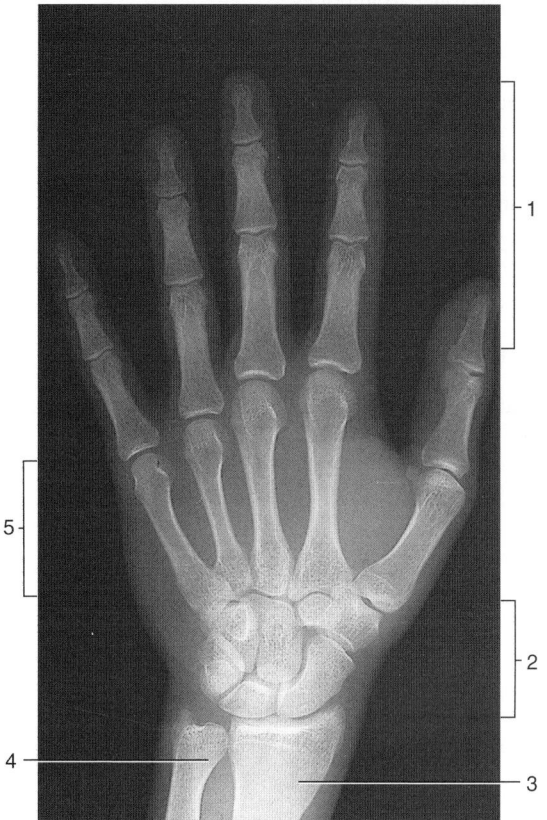

Fig. 13.7

1. Phalanges
2. Carpals
3. Radius
4. Ulna
5. Metacarpals

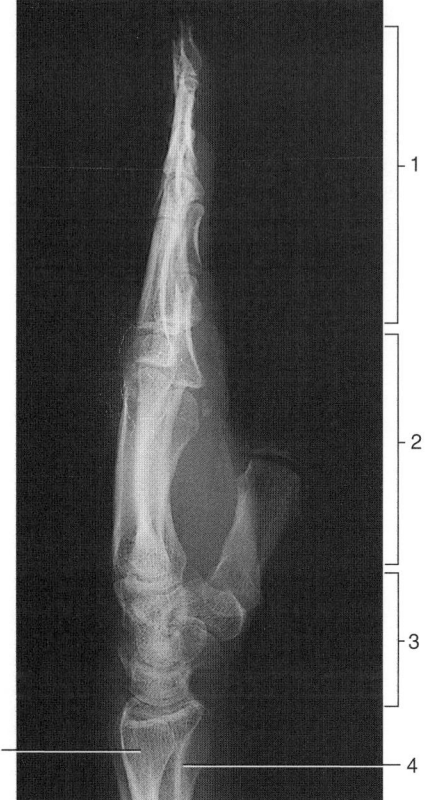

Fig. 13.8

1. Phalanges
2. Metacarpals
3. Carpal bones
4. Radius
5. Ulna

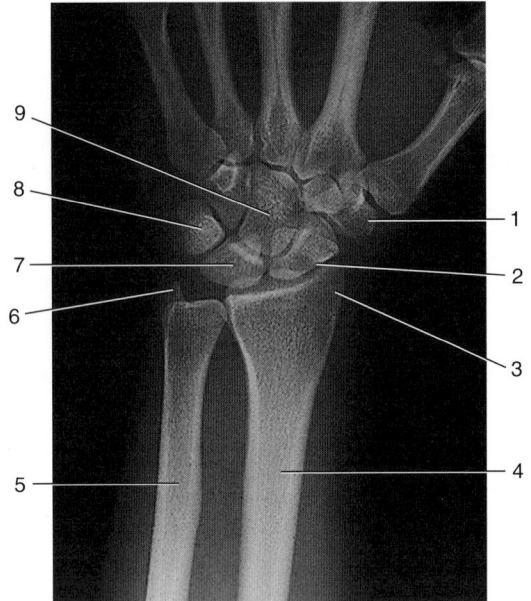

Fig. 13.9

1. Distal row carpal bones
2. Scaphoid
3. Radial styloid process
4. Radius
5. Ulna
6. Ulnar styloid process
7. Posterior row carpal bones
8. Carpal bone
9. Carpal bone

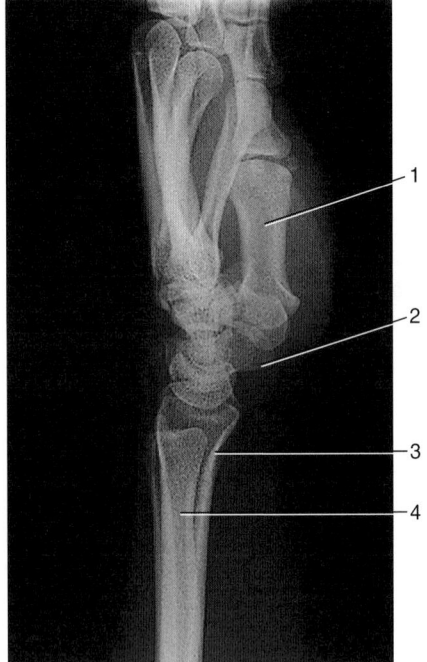

Fig. 13.10

1. First metacarpal
2. Scaphoid
3. Radius
4. Ulna

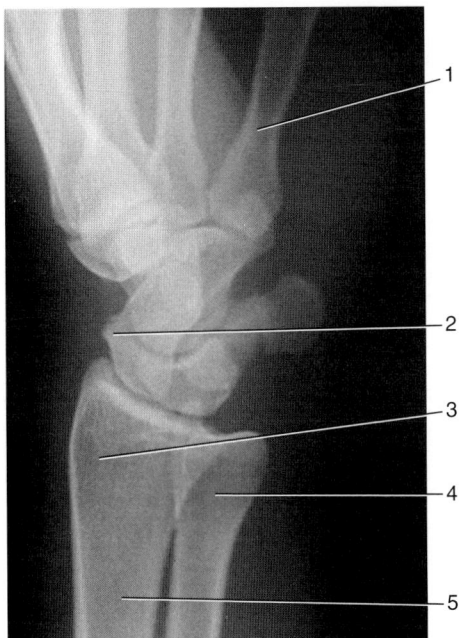

Fig. 13.11

1. Fifth metacarpal
2. Scaphoid
3. Radial styloid process
4. Distal ulna
5. Distal radius

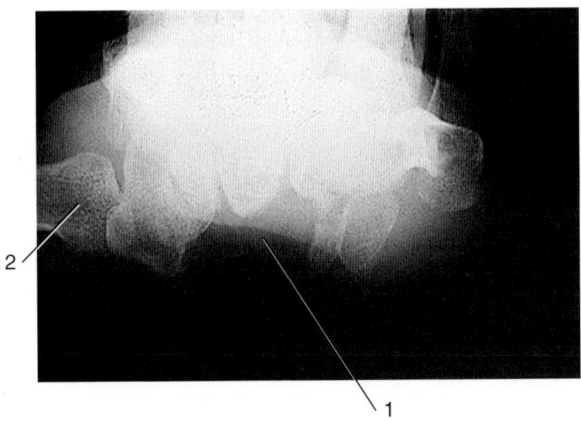

Fig. 13.12

1. Carpal canal
2. First metacarpal

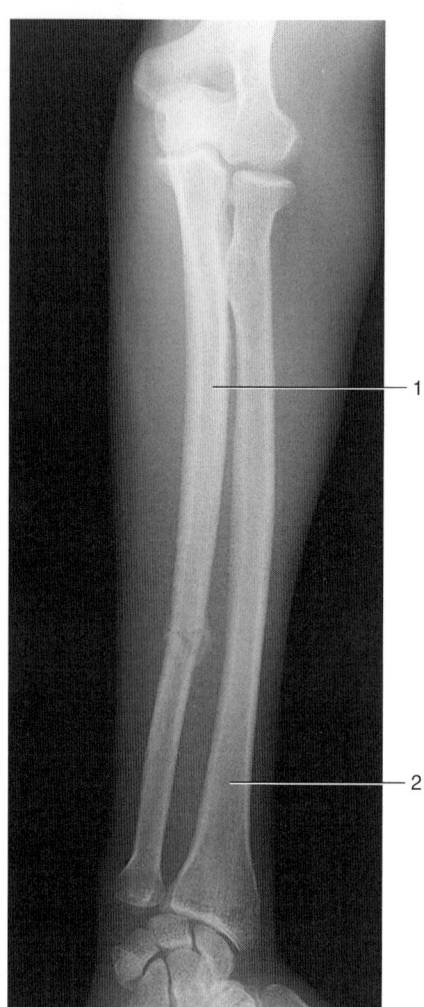

Fig. 13.13

1. Ulna

2. Radius

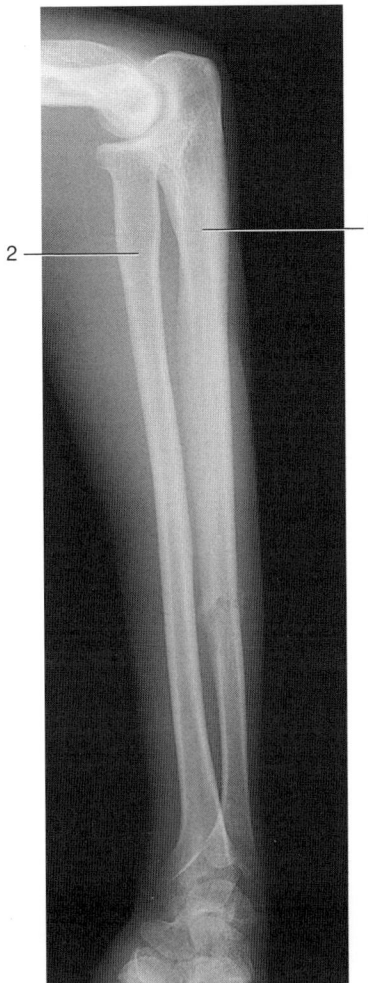

Fig. 13.14

1. Ulna

2. Radius

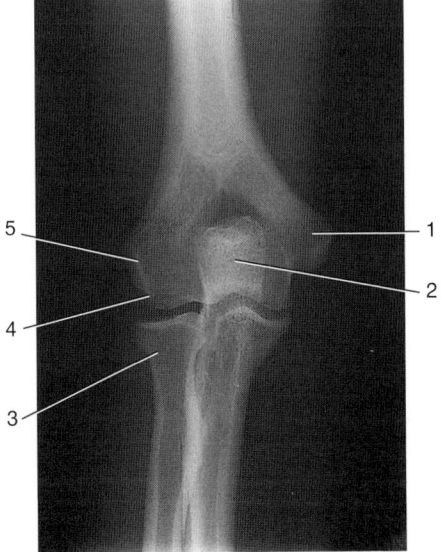

Fig. 13.15

1. Medial epicondyle

2. Olecranon process

3. Radial head

4. Capitulum

5. Lateral epicondyle

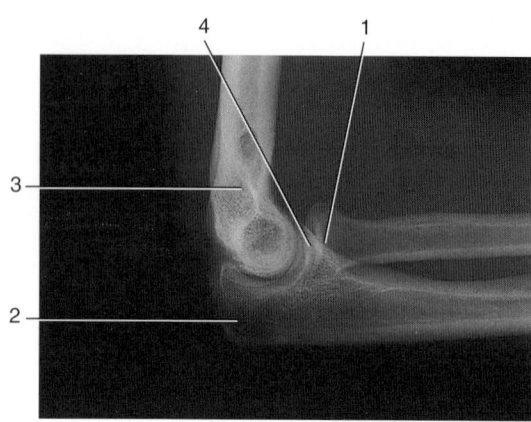

Fig. 13.16

1. Radial head

2. Olecranon process

3. Distal humerus

4. Coronoid process

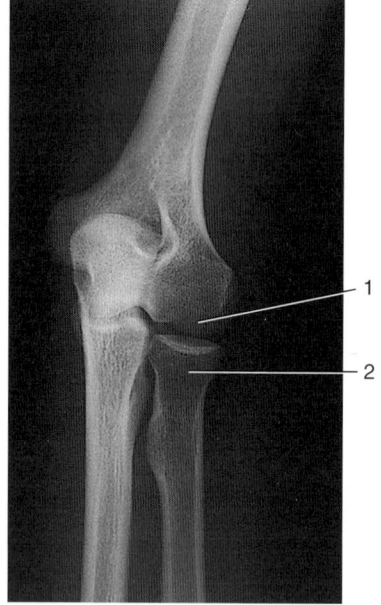

Fig. 13.17

1. Capitulum

2. Radial head

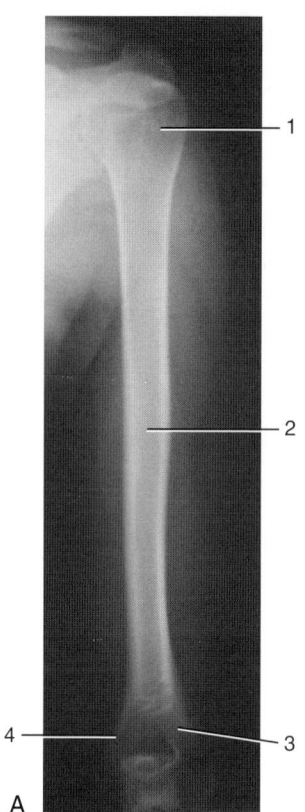

A

B

Fig. 13.18

1. Humeral head
2. Body
3. Lateral epicondyle
4. Medial epicondyle
5. Humeral head
6. Body
7. Olecranon
8. Body of scapula

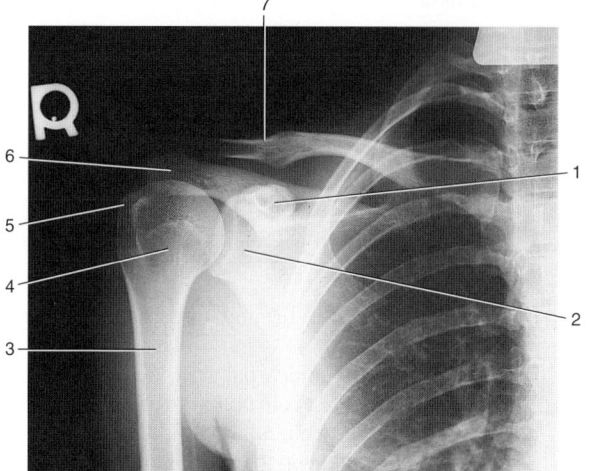

Fig. 13.19

1. Coracoid process
2. Glenohumeral joint
3. Body of humerus
4. Surgical neck
5. Greater tubercle
6. Acromion
7. Distal clavicle

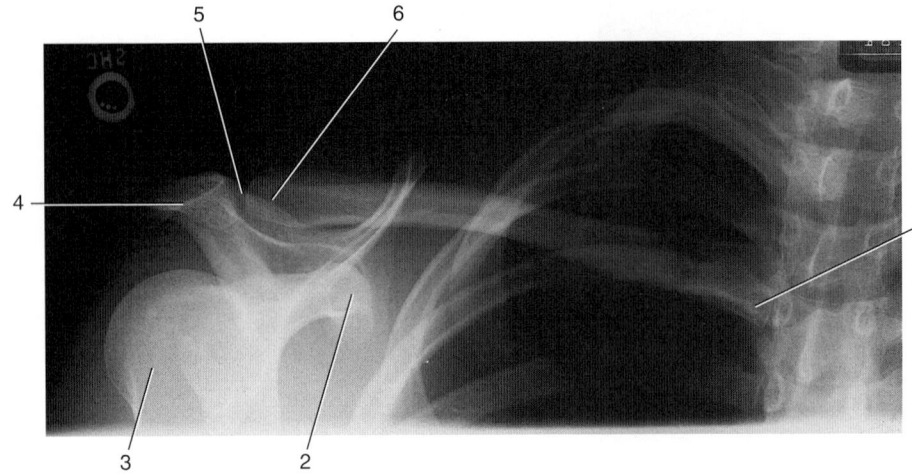

1. Proximal end of clavicle

2. Coracoid process

3. Humeral head

4. Acromion

5. Acromioclavicular (A-C) joint

6. Distal end of clavicle

Fig. 13.20

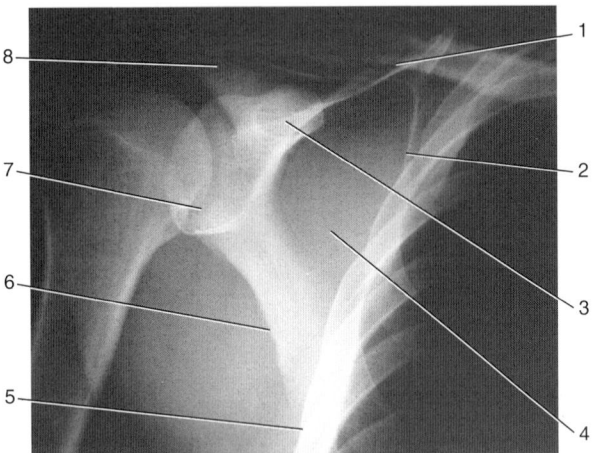

1. Scapular spine

2. Medial (vertebral) border

3. Corocoid process

4. Body

5. Inferior angle

6. Lateral border

7. Glenoid Fossa

8. Acromion

Fig. 13.21

Challenge Exercise

1. 40 inches
2. Hand open, fingers extended, with palmar surface in contact with IR, fingers moderately separated
3. Perpendicular to the third MCP joint
4. Coronal plane of hand forms 45-degree angle with IR
5. From the PA, hand is rotated lateral to place anteromedial (palmar/ulnar) surface in contact with IR. Coronal plane of fingers at 45-degree angle to IR. Fingers are supported by stair-step sponge.
6. The resulting image will have less detail than the AP projection image because the increased object-image receptor distance (OID) results in greater magnification distortion (geometric unsharpness).
7. Anterior surface of wrist is in contact with IR. Fingers are flexed to form a loose fist, placing wrist in close contact with IR and opening intercarpal joints.
8. Perpendicular to the midcarpal area.
9. Medial surface of wrist is in contact with IR. Coronal plane of wrist is perpendicular to IR.
10. Arm is fully extended with hand supinated and posterior surface in contact with IR. Both wrist and elbow are supinated with coronal plane of arm parallel to IR. This is achieved by adjusting the coronal plane of the humeral epicondyles parallel to the plane of the IR. A small sandbag in palm of hand can aid in maintaining position.
11. Arm is fully extended with hand supinated and posterior surface in contact with IR. Coronal plane of humeral epicondyles parallel to IR.
12. Elbow is flexed 90 degrees.

13. Arm slightly abducted with palm of hand supinated. Coronal plane of humeral epicondyles parallel to IR.
14. Arm slightly abducted with palm of hand supinated. Arm adjusted to place coronal plane of humeral epicondyles parallel to IR.
15. Humerus and arm rotated internally until back of hand is against thigh. Arm is adjusted to place coronal plane of humeral epicondyles perpendicular to IR.
16. 15 to 30 degrees cephalad
17. The purpose of attaching weights to the patient's wrists is to determine ligament integrity (a separation of the AC joint) by demonstrating change in relative positions of the acromion and clavicle when under stress.

CHAPTER 14: LOWER LIMB AND PELVIS

Workbook Answer Keys

Exercise 1, Limited-Scope

1. B
2. D
3. C
4. C
5. D
6. B
7. C
8. A
9. B
10. D
11. B
12. C
13. A
14. C
15. B
16. A
17. B
18. A
19. C
20. D
21. C
22. A
23. B
24. D
25. C
26. C
27. A
28. B
29. B
30. A
31. D
32. C
33. B
34. D
35. A
36. A
37. C
38. B
39. A
40. A
41. A
42. D

Exercise 2, Limited-Scope

1. Great toe: two phalanges
   Second toe: three phalanges
2. The fibula is lateral to the tibia.
3. The knee joint is formed by the articulation between the femur and the tibia.
4. Fibula
5. Medial malleolus
6. The entire leg is medially rotated with the sagittal plane of the foot and leg forming an angle of 15 to 20 degrees. The malleoli are parallel to the IR. The ankle is dorsiflexed.
7. 1. PA axial projection, Holmblad method.
   2. PA axial projection, Camp-Coventry method.
8. Dorsiflexion
9. Femur
10. Metatarsophalangeal (MTC)
11. Calcaneus
12. Behind the first MTP joint
13. Greater trochanter
14. Apex
15. Talus
16. Condyles
17. The MTP joint
18. Lateral
19. Femoral condyles
20. Base of the third metatarsal
21. 1-inch distal to the medial malleolus
22. ½ inch distal to the apex of the patella
23. Rotated 30 degrees
24. 3 to 5 degrees cephalad
25. 20 to 30 degrees

Exercise 1, Podiatry

Answer the following questions by selecting the best choice.

1. B
2. C
3. C
4. D
5. A
6. C
7. A
8. A
9. B
10. B
11. A
12. A
13. C
14. D
15. D

16. C
17. C
18. C
19. C
20. B
21. A
22. D
23. A
24. C
25. B
26. A
27. D
28. C
29. A
30. B
31. B
32. A
33. C
34. C

Exercise 2, Podiatry

Answer the following questions.

1. Forefoot, midfoot, and hindfoot
2. Two phalanges
3. Dorsiflexion
4. Perpendicular and tangential to first MTP joint, and going through the ball of the foot
5. DP and the axial-calcaneus (Harris-Beath method) projections
6. 45 degrees
7. Axial-calcaneus (Harris-Beath method) projection
8. AP oblique-mortise projection
9. Tibio-fibular joint
10. AP oblique-lateral rotation projection
11. Metatarsophalangeal (MTP) joint
12. Talus and calcaneus
13. Inversion and eversion
14. 30 degrees
15. Medial and intermediate cuneiforms and the navicular

Limited-Scope and Podiatry Students

Exercise 3

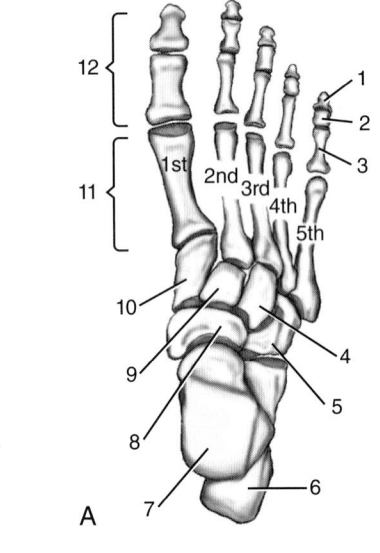

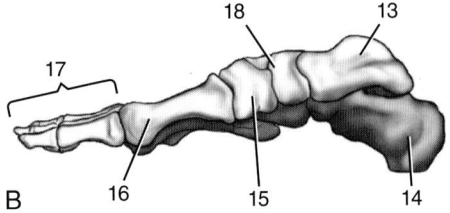

Fig. 14.1

1. Distal phalanx

2. Middle phalanx

3. Proximal phalanx

4. Lateral cuneiform

5. Cuboid

6. Calcaneus

7. Talus

8. Navicular

9. Intermediate cuneiform

10. Medial cuneiform

11. Metatarsals

12. Phalanges

13. Talus

14. Calcaneus

15. Medial cuneiform

16. First metatarsal

17. Phalanges

18. Navicular

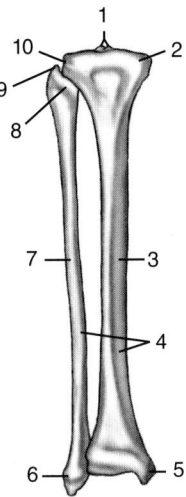

Fig. 14.2

1. Tibial plateau
2. Medial condyle
3. Tibia
4. Shafts
5. Medial malleolus
6. Lateral malleolus
7. Fibula
8. Head
9. Styloid
10. Lateral condyle

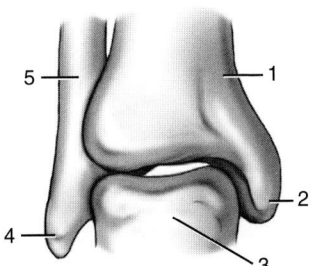

Fig. 14.3

1. Tibia
2. Medial malleolus
3. Talus
4. Lateral malleolus
5. Fibula

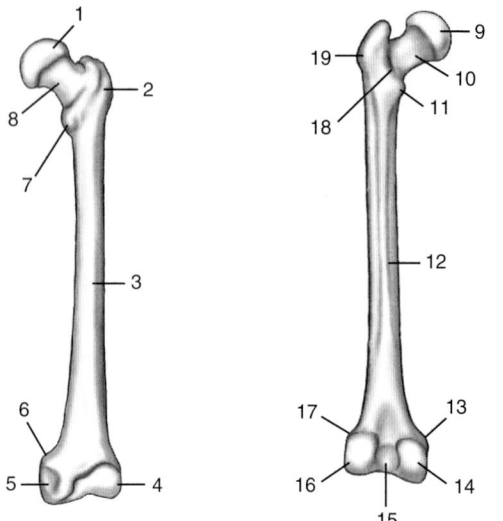

ANTERIOR ASPECT OF FEMUR   POSTERIOR ASPECT OF FEMUR

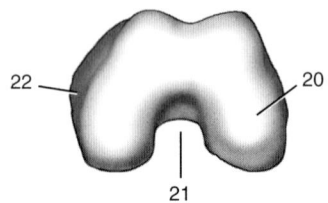

INFERIOR ASPECT OF FEMUR

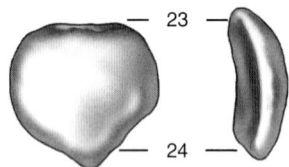

ANTERIOR ASPECT   LATERAL ASPECT
PATELLA

Fig. 14.4

1. Head
2. Greater trochanter
3. Shaft
4. Lateral condyle
5. Medial condyle
6. Medial epicondyle
7. Lesser trochanter
8. Neck
9. Head
10. Neck
11. Lesser trochanter
12. Shaft
13. Medial epicondyle
14. Medial condyle
15. Intercondylar fossa
16. Lateral condyle
17. Lateral epicondyle
18. Intertrochanteric crest
19. Greater trochanter
20. Lateral condyle
21. Intercondylar fossa
22. Medial condyle
23. Base
24. Apex

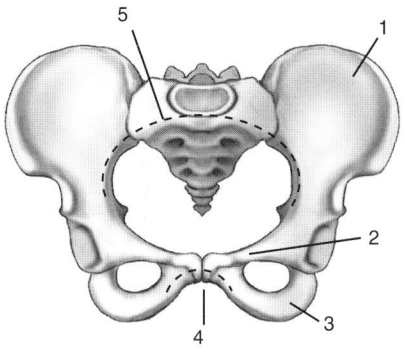

A   FEMALE PELVIS

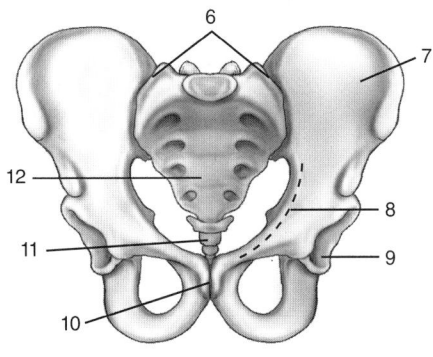

B   MALE PELVIS

Fig. 14.5

1. Ilium
2. Pubis
3. Ischium
4. Pubic arch
5. Brim of the lesser pelvis
6. Sacroiliac joints
7. Ilium
8. Arcuate line
9. Acetabulum
10. Pubic symphysis
11. Coccyx
12. Sacrum

Exercise 4

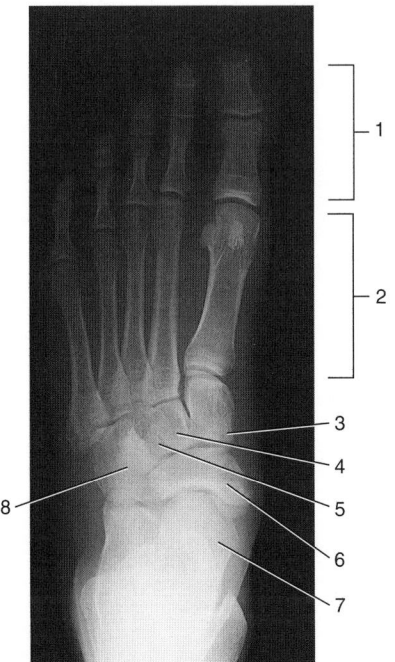

Fig. 14.6

1. Phalanges
2. Metatarsals
3. Medial cuneiform
4. Intermediate cuneiform
5. Lateral cuneiform
6. Navicular
7. Talus
8. Cuboid

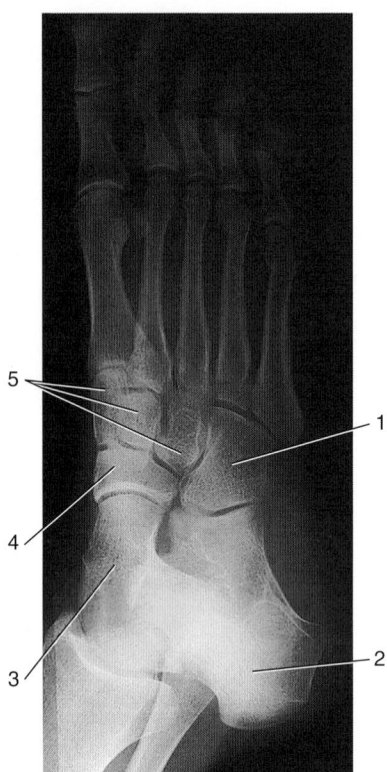

Fig. 14.7

1. Cuboid
2. Calcaneus
3. Talus
4. Navicular
5. Cuneiforms

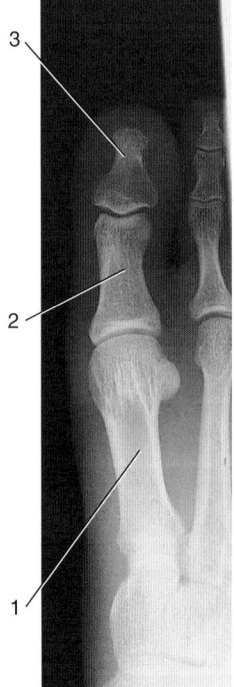

Fig. 14.8

1. First metatarsal
2. Proximal phalanx
3. Distal phalanx

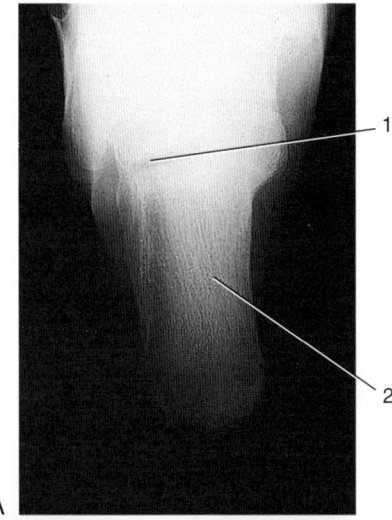

1. Calcaneocuboid articulation
2. Calcaneus
3. Talus
4. Calcaneus

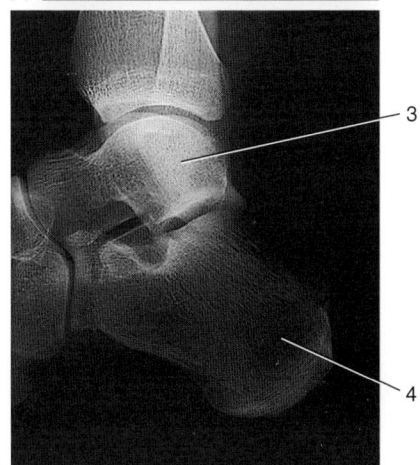

Fig. 14.9

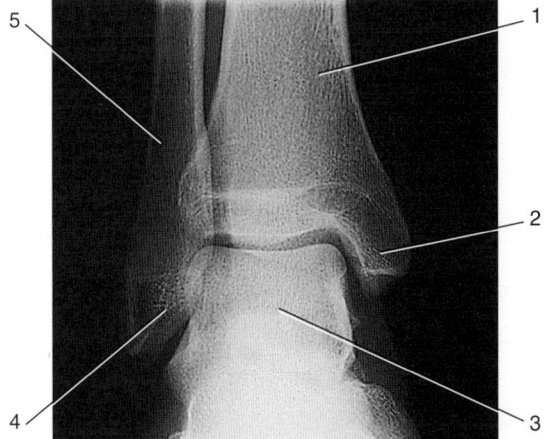

1. Distal tibia
2. Medial malleolus
3. Talus
4. Lateral malleolus
5. Distal fibula

Fig. 14.10

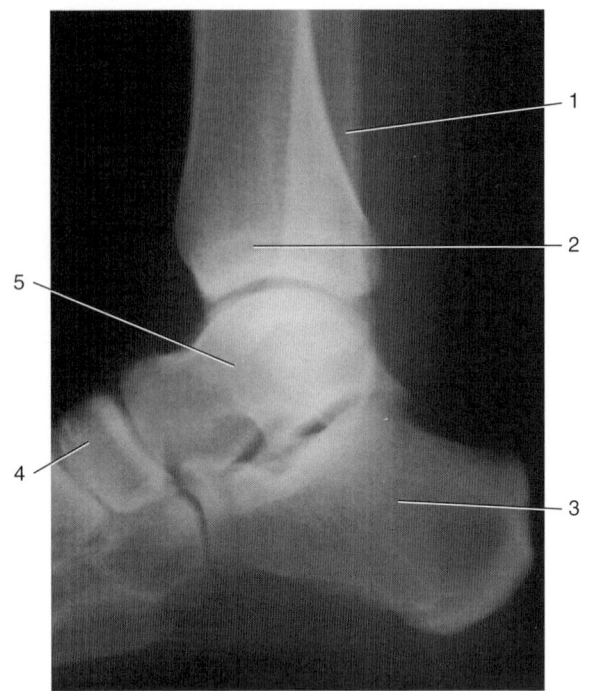

1. Distal fibula
2. Distal tibia
3. Calcaneus
4. Navicular
5. Talus

Fig. 14.11

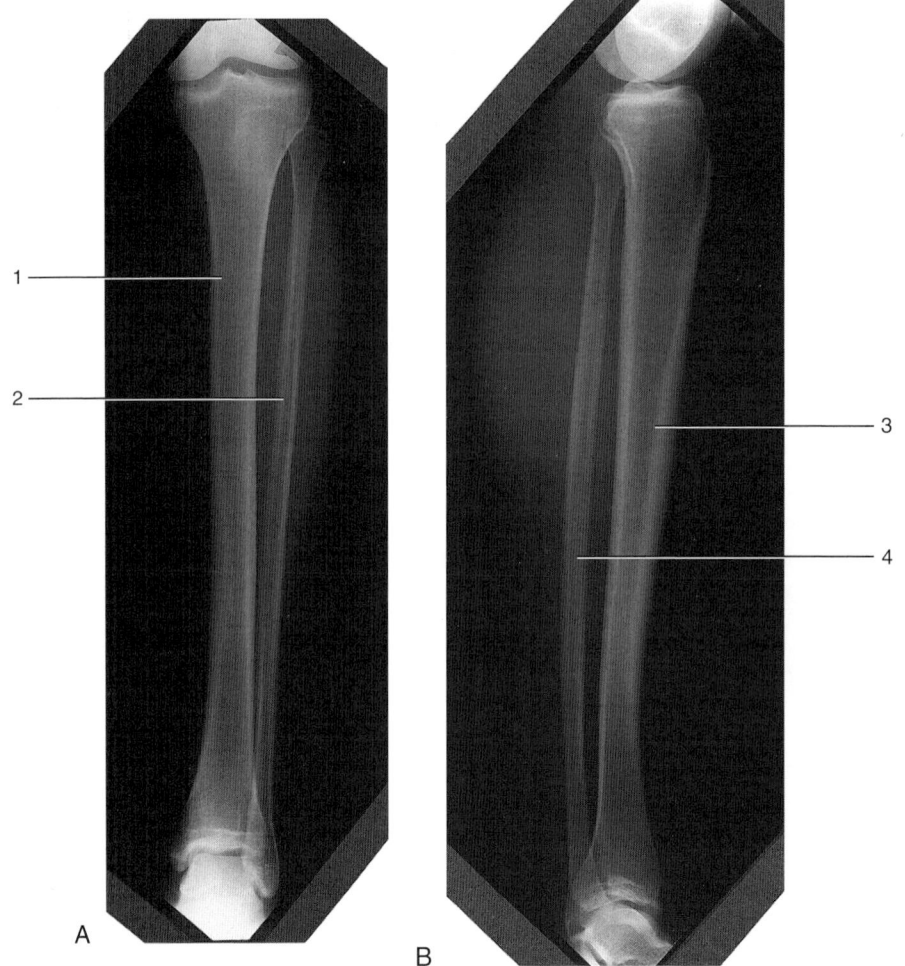

1. Tibia
2. Fibula
3. Fibula
4. Tibia

A

B

Fig. 14.12

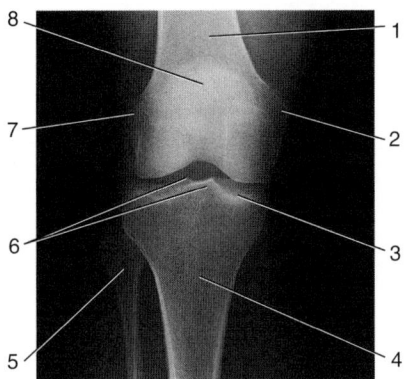

Fig. 14.13

1. Distal femur

2. Medial epicondyle

3. Tibial plateau

4. Proximal tibia

5. Head of fibula

6. Intercondylar eminences

7. Lateral epicondyle

8. Patella

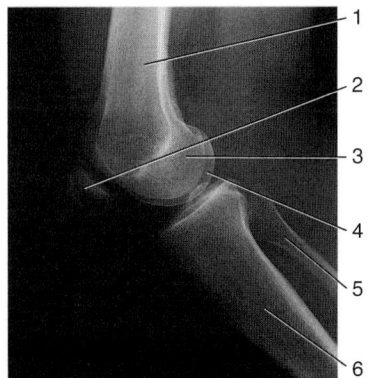

Fig. 14.14

1. Distal femur

2. Patella

3. Lateral condyle

4. Medial condyle

5. Fibula

6. Tibia

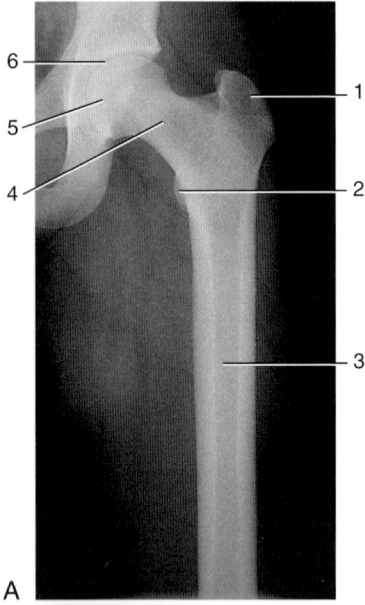

A

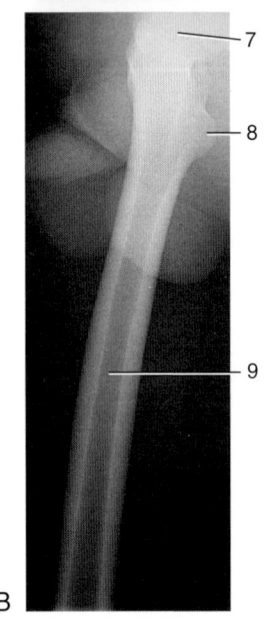

B

Fig. 14.15

1. Greater trochanter
2. Lesser trochanter
3. Shaft of femur
4. Femoral neck
5. Femoral head
6. Acetabulum
7. Femoral head
8. Greater trochanter
9. Shaft of femur

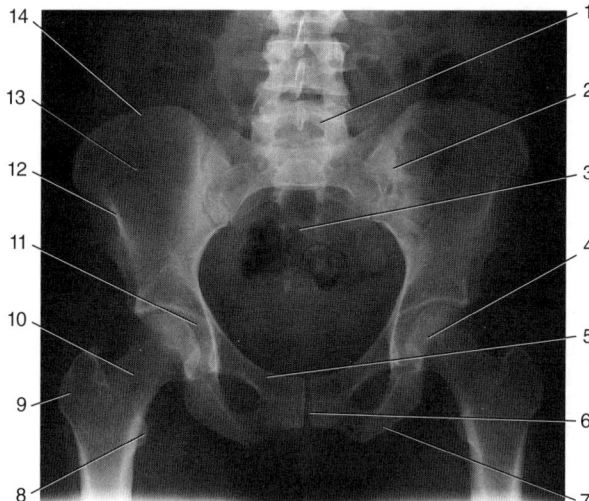

Fig. 14.16

1. L5
2. Sacroiliac joint
3. Sacrum
4. Femoral head
5. Pubis
6. Pubic symphysis
7. Ischium
8. Lesser trochanter
9. Greater trochanter
10. Femoral neck
11. Acetabulum
12. Anterior superior iliac spine
13. Ilium
14. Iliac crest

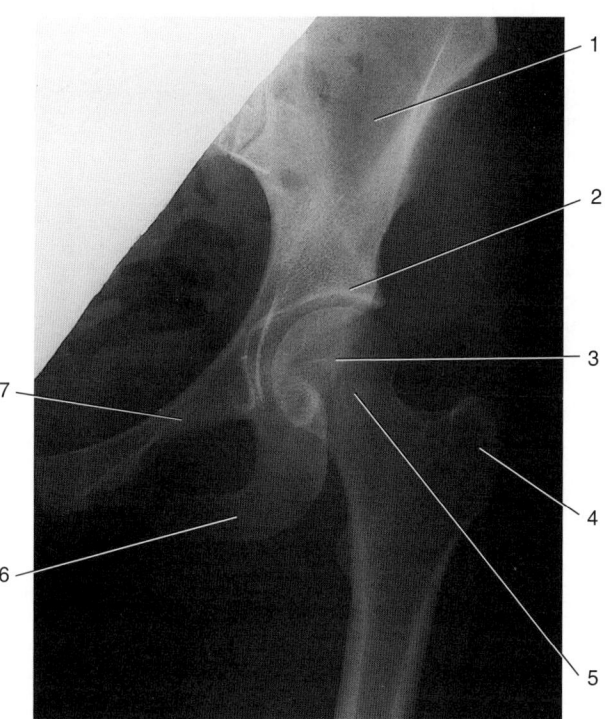

Fig. 14.17

1. Ilium
2. Acetabulum
3. Femoral head
4. Greater trochanter
5. Femoral neck
6. Ischium
7. Pubis

Challenge Exercise

1. 40 inches
2. Plantar surface of foot is in contact with IR. Foot is centered to IR so that toes, heel, and both malleoli are within field.
3. Angled 10 degrees posteriorly (toward heel) and entering base of third metatarsal
4. Plantar surface of foot forms a 30-degree angle with IR.
5. Angled 40 degrees cephalad to center of IR, entering at third metatarsal base
6. Posterior surface of heel and lower leg is in contact with IR. Midpoint between malleoli is centered to IR. Foot is dorsiflexed so that plantar surface of foot forms 90-degree angle with coronal plane of lower leg. Sagittal planes of leg and foot are perpendicular to IR. Foot may be held in position by patient using a strap or bandage.
7. Perpendicular to point midway between malleoli
8. Lateral surface of ankle is in contact with IR. Sagittal plane of foot and leg is parallel to IR. Foot is dorsiflexed so that plantar surface of foot forms 90-degree angle with coronal plane of lower leg.
9. Perpendicular to enter at the medial malleolus
10. From position for AP projection, entire leg is rotated medially 45 degrees. Sagittal planes of foot and leg must remain aligned to each other.
11. From position for AP projection, entire leg is rotated 15 to 20 degrees medially. Sagittal planes of foot and leg must remain aligned to each other.
12. Leg is fully extended with sagittal plane of leg perpendicular to IR.
13. Entering 0.5 inch distal to apex of patella. Angle is variable, depending on the measurement between the anterior superior iliac spine (ASIS) and the tabletop, as follows:
    <19 cm (thin patient) 3 to 5 degrees *caudad*
    19 to 24 cm 0 degrees (perpendicular)
    24 cm (large pelvis) 3 to 5 degrees *cephalad*
14. Knee is flexed 20 to 30 degrees. Sagittal plane of femur and lower leg is parallel to IR.
15. Angled 5 to 7 degrees cephalad entering 1 inch distal to medial epicondyle of femur
16. Superior margin of IR is placed at level of ASIS
17. Inferior margin of IR is placed 1 to 2 inches below the knee joint.
18. If there is no suspicion of recent fracture, femurs are rotated medially 15 to 20 degrees to place femoral necks parallel to IR.
19. Femur is medially rotated 15 degrees, the same as for the pelvis.
20. Hip is flexed as much as possible and femur abducted 45 degrees. If patient cannot abduct femur sufficiently from supine position, pelvis may be rotated toward affected side.

CHAPTER 15: SPINE

Workbook Answer Keys
Exercise 1

1. C
2. D
3. A
4. C
5. B
6. D
7. C
8. B
9. B
10. B
11. C
12. D
13. B
14. B
15. B
16. D
17. A
18. A
19. B
20. A
21. C
22. D
23. B
24. C
25. C
26. C
27. A
28. C
29. B
30. C
31. C
32. C
33. B
34. C
35. C
36. D
37. A

Exercise 2

1. Cervical spine: 7 vertebrae
   Thoracic spine: 12 vertebrae
   Lumbar spine: 5 vertebrae
   Sacrum: 5 segments
   Coccyx: 4 segments
2. The cervical and lumbar spines have a lordotic curve. The thoracic spine has a kyphotic curve.
   The sacrum and coccyx together form a kyphotic curve.
3. The atlas has no body, and its superior articular processes are set at a different angle from the superior articular processes of the other cervical vertebrae.

The axis has a superior projection from the body, called the *dens*, that passes through the ring of the atlas. The atlas has a far greater degree of rotation than is possible between any of the other vertebral bodies.

4. Twelve vertebrae make up the thoracic spine.
5. Extend the neck so that the line between the occlusal surface of the upper teeth and the base of the occipital bone is parallel to the floor.
6. On the oblique projection of the lumber spine.
7. The lateral projection in the neutral position should be taken and shown to the physician before proceeding with the flexion and extension positions.
8. This is caused by failure to use the anode heel effect by placing the patient's head toward the anode end of the x-ray tube. If the anode heel effect was used, a wedge compensating filter could be used to reduce the exposure to the upper thoracic area.
9. The patient should be instructed to disrobe except for underpants and put on a gown. Specifically, her bra must be removed. Shoes should be removed for upright examinations.
10. It helps overcome the magnification caused by the increased OID between the cervical spine and the IR.
11. Compression fractures.
12. Intervertebral foramina farthest from the IR
13. Sheet of lead, or lead rubber mask
14. Scoliosis
15. 3.5 inches posterior to the ASIS
16. The posteroanterior projection, PA

Exercise 3

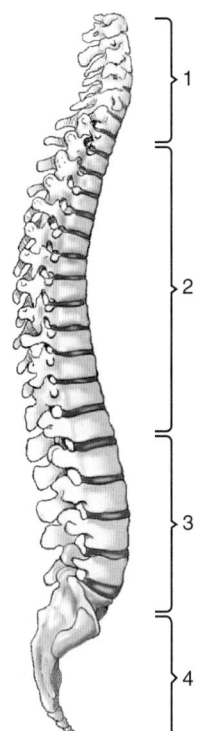

Fig 15.1

1. Lordotic curve
2. Kyphotic curve
3. Lordotic curve
4. Kyphotic curve

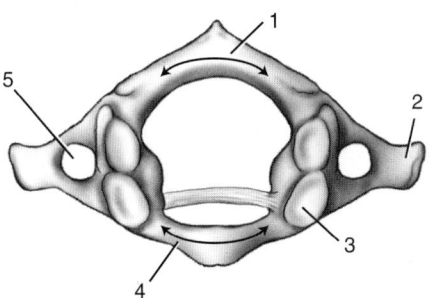

Fig. 15.2

1. Posterior arch
2. Transverse process
3. Superior articular process
4. Anterior arch
5. Transverse foramen

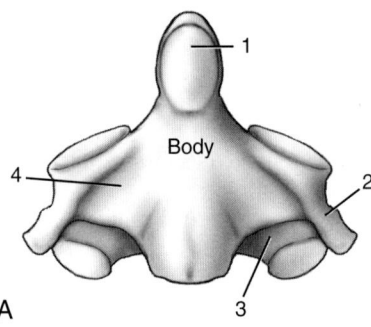

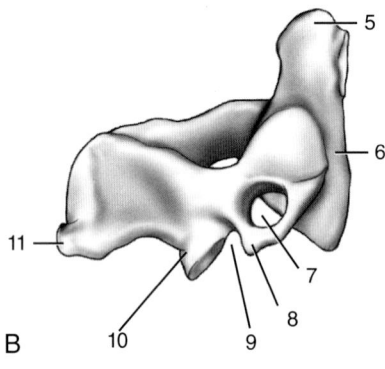

Fig. 15.3

1. Dens (odontoid process)
2. Transverse process
3. Inferior articular process
4. Superior articular process
5. Dens (odontoid process)
6. Body
7. Transverse foramen
8. Transverse process
9. Vertebral notch
10. Inferior articular process
11. Spinous process

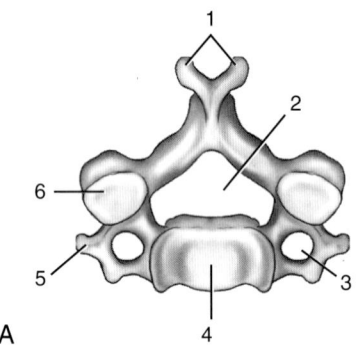

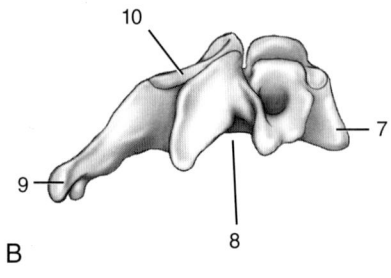

Fig. 15.4

1. Spinous process (bifid)
2. Vertebral foramen
3. Transverse foramen
4. Body
5. Transverse process
6. Superior articular process
7. Body
8. Vertebral notch
9. Spinous process
10. Superior articular process

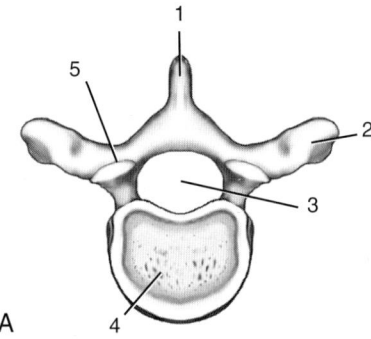

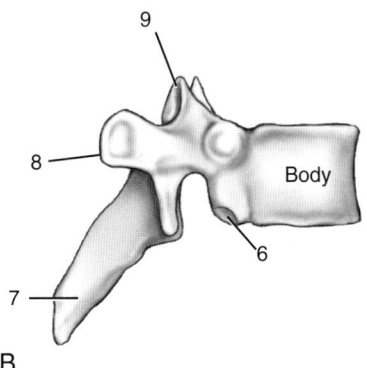

Fig. 15.5

1. Spinous process
2. Transverse process
3. Vertebral foramen
4. Body
5. Superior articular process
6. Vertebral notch
7. Spinous process
8. Transverse process
9. Superior articular process

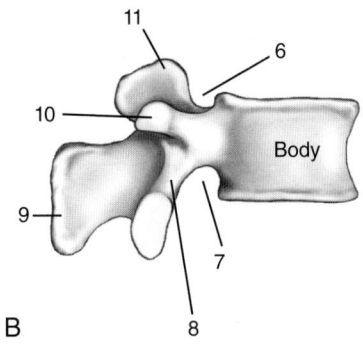

Fig. 15.6

1. Spinous process
2. Transverse process
3. Vertebral foramen
4. Body
5. Superior articular process
6. Vertebral notch
7. Vertebral notch
8. Inferior articular process
9. Spinous process
10. Transverse process
11. Superior articular process

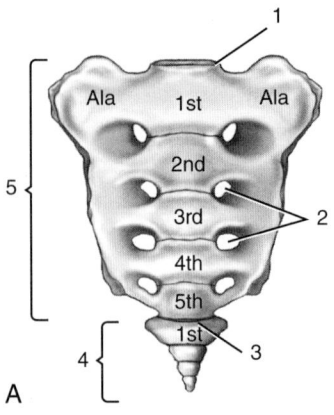

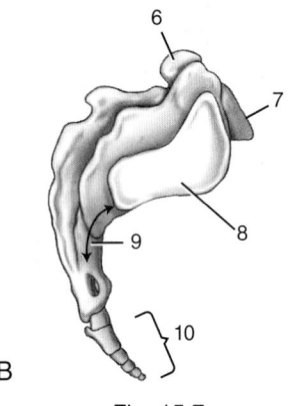

Fig. 15.7

1. Base
2. Pelvic sacral foramina
3. Base
4. Coccyx
5. Sacrum
6. Superior articular process
7. Base
8. Articular surface (sacroiliac joint)
9. Sacrum
10. Coccyx

Exercise 4

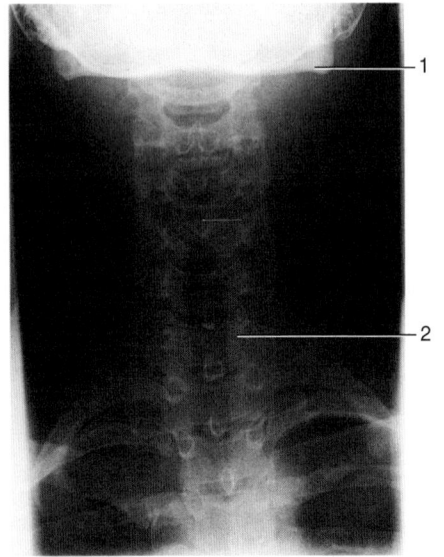

Fig. 15.8

1. Mandible and base of skull (superimposed)
2. C7

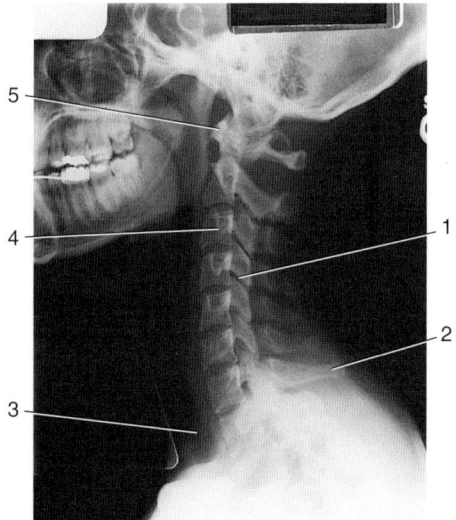

Fig. 15.9

1. C4–C5 zygapophyseal joint
2. Spinous process of C7
3. Trachea
4. Body of C3
5. Anterior arch of atlas (C1)

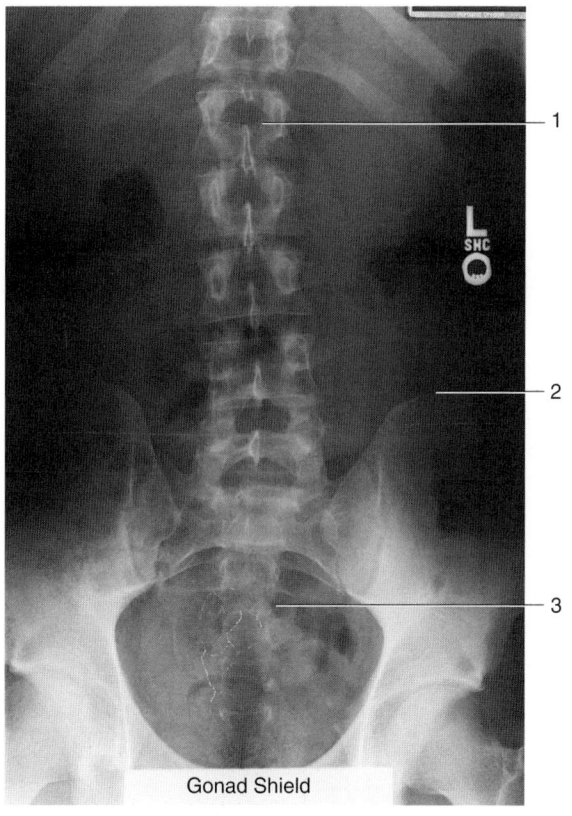

Gonad Shield

Fig. 15.10

1. L1
2. Iliac crest
3. Sacrum

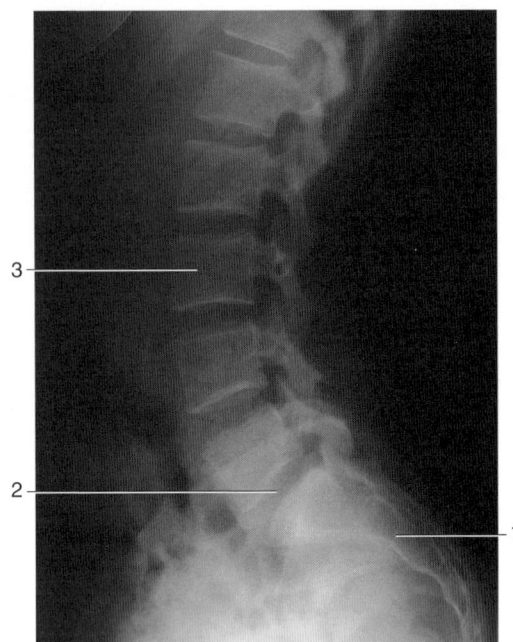

Fig. 15.11

1. Sacrum

2. Lumbosacral joint (L5–S1)

3. Body of L3

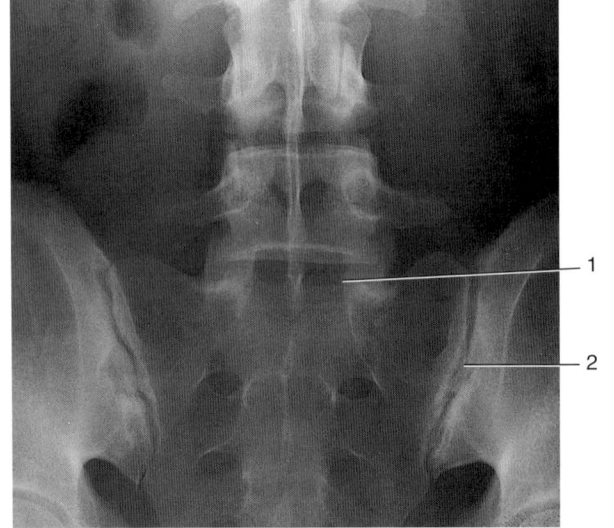

Fig. 15.12

1. Lumbosacral joint (L5–S1)

2. Sacroiliac joint

Challenge Exercise

1. Midsagittal plane of both body and head are aligned perpendicular to center of IR, with patient facing tube. Head position is adjusted so that a line between mental point and base of skull makes an angle of 15 degrees with horizontal plane.
2. Centered to IR at angle of 15 degrees cephalad through thyroid cartilage
3. Patient faces tube with midsagittal plane of both body and head perpendicular to center of IR. Position of head is adjusted so that a line between lower surface of upper teeth (occlusal plane) and base of skull is parallel to horizontal plane.
4. Perpendicular to center of IR, through midpoint of open mouth
5. Midsagittal planes of body and head are parallel to IR, with infraorbitomeatal line parallel to floor. Shoulders must be relaxed and depressed. IR is positioned so that upper margin is about 1 inch above the external auditory meatus (EAM).
6. Perpendicular to center of IR through body of C4
7. 60 to 72 inches
8. Coronal plane of body forms angle of 45 degrees with plane of IR. Sagittal plane of skull is perpendicular to coronal plane of body. Have patient elevate and, if necessary, protrude the chin so that mandible does not overlap spine.
9. Angled 15 degrees cephalad to center of IR through body of C4
10. Swimmer's technique
11. Patient is instructed to perform shallow breathing during exposure. A low milliamperage (mA) setting that provides the desired milliampere-seconds (mAs) with an exposure time of 1 to 3 seconds is necessary for best results with the breathing technique.
12. Patient faces tube with midsagittal plane perpendicular to IR and centered to it. Knees are flexed and may be supported with a bolster.
13. Perpendicular to center of IR through L4, in midline at level of iliac crest
14. In lateral recumbent position, spine is aligned parallel to center of Bucky with arms anterior to body. Radiolucent sponges may be used to elevate waist and/or hip to keep spine level. Knees are flexed. A pad between knees helps keep pelvis lateral and maintain lateral position of spine.
15. Perpendicular to center of IR through L4, in midaxillary line at level of iliac crest
16. From supine position, patient is rotated 45 degrees toward side being radiographed. Position may be supported by a large 45-degree-angle radiolucent sponge. Take care that there is no torsion (twist) of spine.
17. Perpendicular to center of IR through L3. Central ray enters at point 2 inches medial to ASIS farthest from IR and 1 1/2 inches superior to iliac crest.
18. A coned-down radiograph of the lumbosacral junction in the lateral projection is helpful when there is poor visualization of this area on the routine lateral projection. This may occur as a result of insufficient penetration of this dense area. This projection is important because this junction is a common site of chronic low back pain. Although this projection may be taken with the patient upright, the result is usually superior when the patient is recumbent.
19. From supine position, body is rotated so that coronal plane is aligned at angle of 25 to 30 degrees to IR. Side being radiographed is side that is elevated from IR. Position may be supported by radiolucent sponge under hip and lumbar area of elevated side. Take care that there is no torsion of spine.
20. Perpendicular to center of IR through point 1 inch medial to ASIS farthest from IR
21. Midsagittal plane is perpendicular to IR and centered to it. Knees are flexed and supported with a bolster.
22. Angled 15 degrees cephalad to center of IR through midsacrum. Central ray enters body at midline, 1 inch inferior to the ASIS.
23. Angled 10 degrees caudad and centered to IR. Central ray enters body in midline, 1 inch inferior to the ASIS.
24. Spine is aligned parallel to center of Bucky with arms anterior to body. Radiolucent sponges may be used to elevate waist and/or hips to keep spine level. Knees are flexed. A pad between knees helps keep pelvis lateral and maintain lateral position of spine.
25. Perpendicular to center of IR through center of sacrum. Central ray enters at point 3 1/2 inches posterior to ASIS.

CHAPTER 16: BONY THORAX, CHEST, AND ABDOMEN

Workbook Answer Keys

Exercise 1

1. C
2. B
3. B
4. D
5. C
6. A
7. B
8. D
9. A
10. C
11. B
12. C
13. D
14. A
15. A
16. D
17. D
18. B
19. A
20. B

21. B
22. B
23. A
24. C
25. A
26. B
27. D
28. D
29. A
30. A
31. B

Exercise 2

1. Jugular notch
2. Apices
3. 1. Heart,
   2. Trachea,
   3. Esophagus
4. 1. Very slender.
   2. Organs are longer and narrower.
   3. Organs are located lower in the abdominal cavity.

Exercise 3

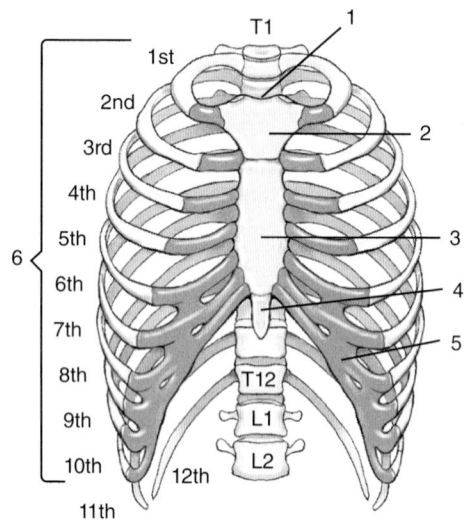

Fig. 16. 1

5. Raised over the head, hands grasping the opposite elbows. If an overhead bar is available, have patient grasp the bar.
6. A chronic lung condition characterized by obstruction of the small airways.
7. 72 inches
8. 1. Demonstrate air-fluid levels
   2. Allows maximum lung expansion
   3. Minimal magnification of the heart
9. 1. Heart
   2. Lungs
   3. Mediastinum
10. Magnification of the heart is reduced.
11. Hypersthenic
12. Rotate the shoulders forward to touch the IR
13. 1.5 to 2 inches
14. Minimize magnification of the heart
15. A collapsed lung
16. In the horizontal position
17. AP axial (lordotic position)

1. Jugular notch

2. Manubrium

3. Body

4. Xiphoid process

5. Costal cartilage

6. Ribs

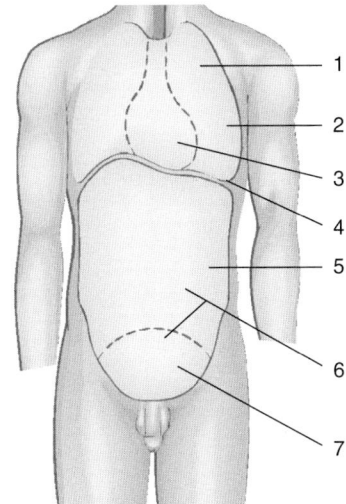

Fig. 16.2

1. Thoracic cavity

2. Pleural cavity

3. Mediastinum

4. Diaphragm

5. Abdominal cavity

6. Abdominopelvic cavity

7. Pelvic cavity

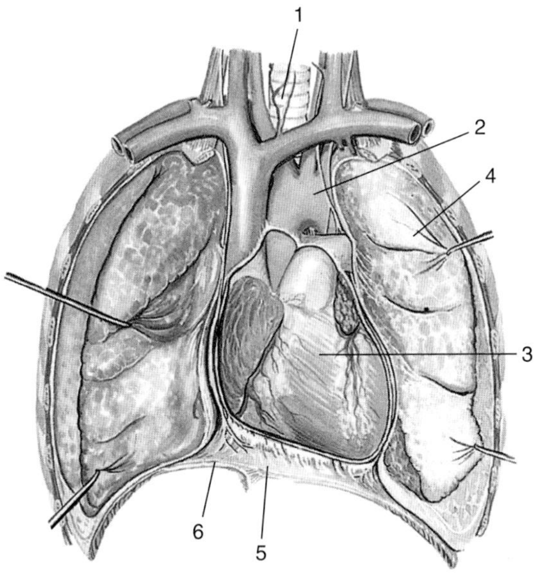

Fig. 16.3

1. Trachea

2. Arch of aorta

3. Heart

4. Left lung

5. Mediastinum (between lungs)

6. Diaphragm muscle

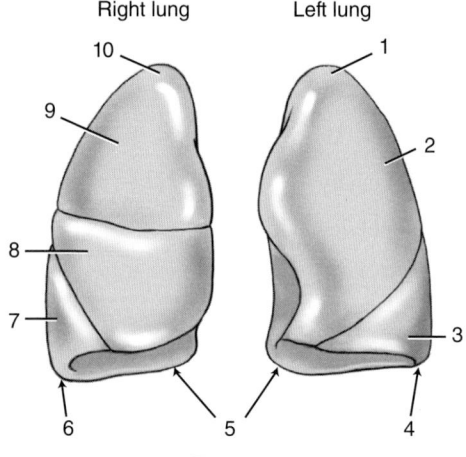

Right lung   Left lung

Fig. 16.4

1. Apex
2. Superior lobe
3. Inferior lobe
4. Costophrenic angle
5. Cardiophrenic angles
6. Costophrenic angle
7. Inferior lobe
8. Middle love
9. Superior lobe
10. Apex

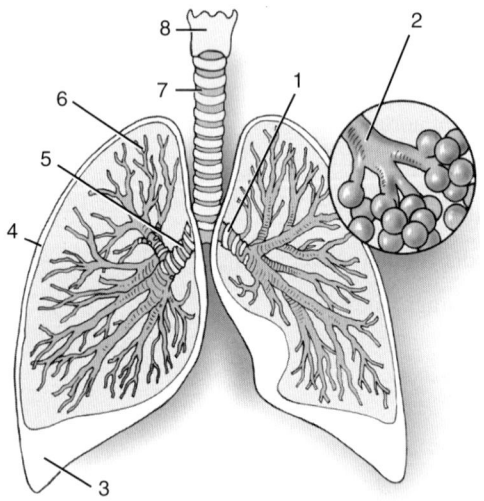

Fig. 16. 5

1. Left primary bronchus
2. Terminal bronchiole
3. Pleural space
4. Pleura
5. Right primary bronchus
6. Bronchioles
7. Trachea
8. Larynx

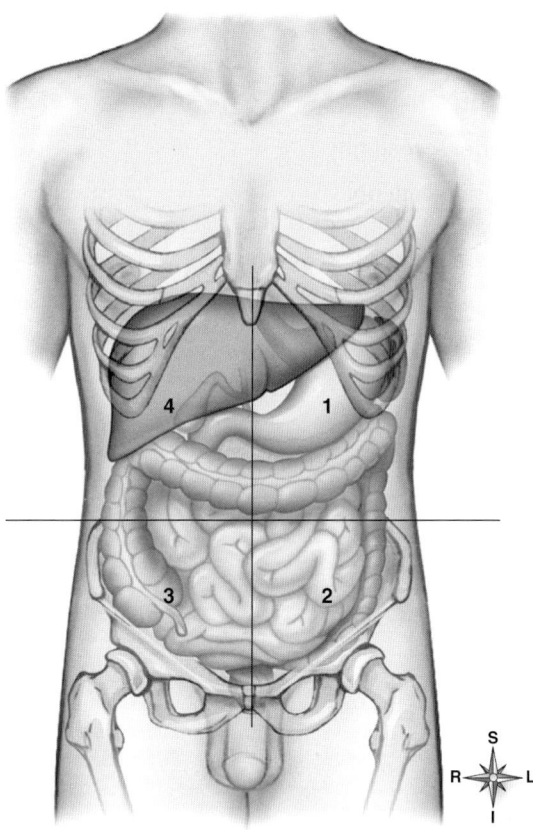

Fig. 16.6

1. Left upper
2. Left lower
3. Right lower
4. Right upper

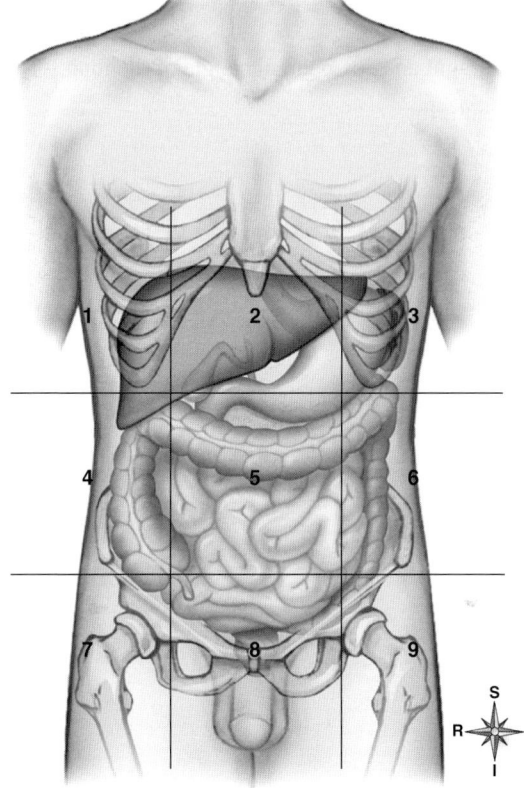

Fig. 16.7

1. Right hypochondriac region
2. Epigastric region
3. Left hypochondriac region
4. Right lumbar region
5. Umbilical region
6. Left lumbar region
7. Right iliac (inguinal) region
8. Hypogastric region
9. Left iliac (inguinal) region

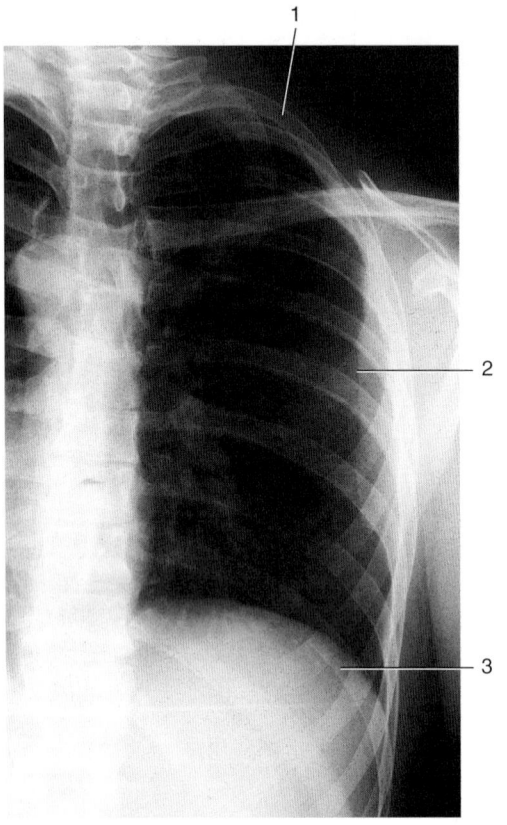

Fig. 16.8

1. First rib
2. Anterior second rib
3. Posterior tenth rib

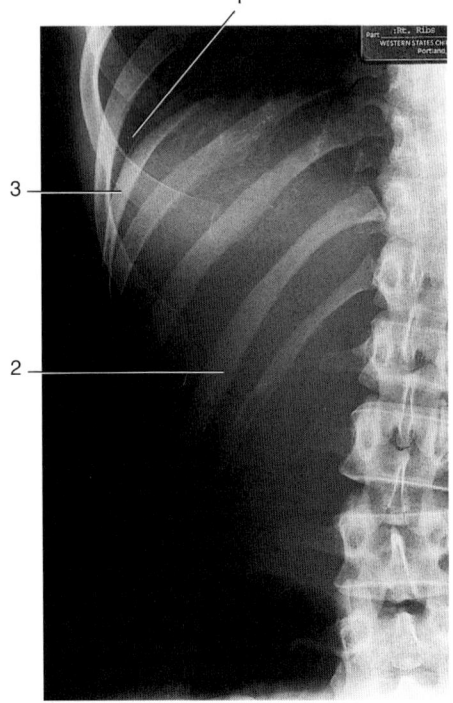

Fig. 16.9

1. Diaphragm and costophrenic angle of the lung
2. Eleventh rib
3. Eighth rib

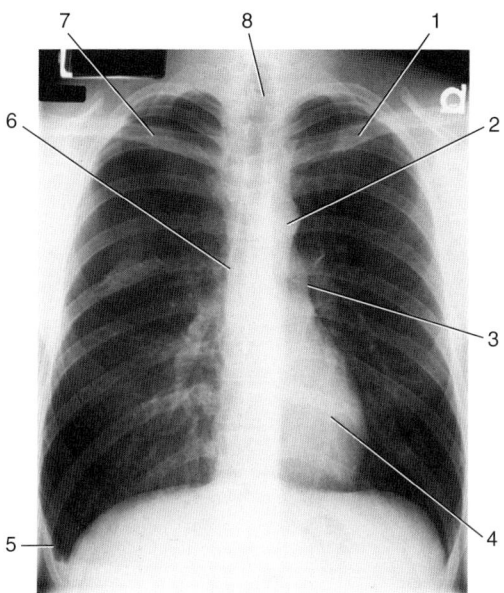

Fig. 16.10

1. Left clavicle
2. Aortic knob
3. Left lung
4. Heart
5. Right costophrenic angle
6. Right lung
7. Right clavicle
8. Trachea

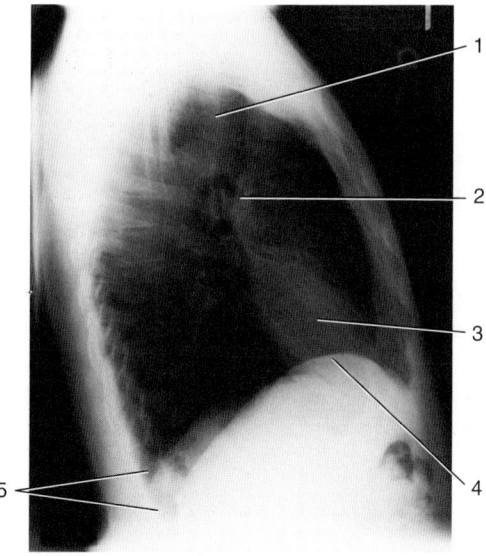

Fig. 16.11

1. Lung apices
2. Heart
3. Dome of diaphragm
4. Costophrenic angles

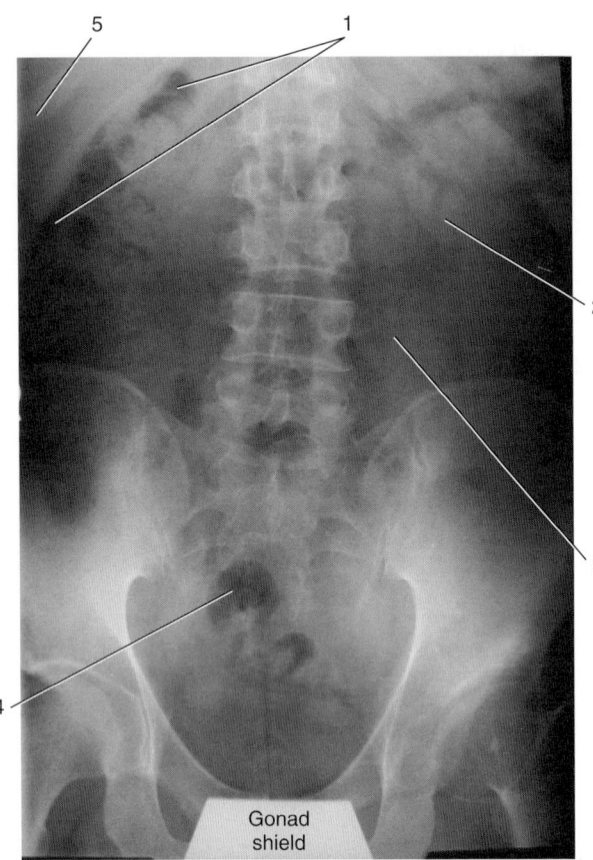

1. Intestinal gas shadows
2. Left kidney
3. Psoas muscle margin
4. Intestinal gas shadows
5. Liver

Gonad shield

Fig. 16.12

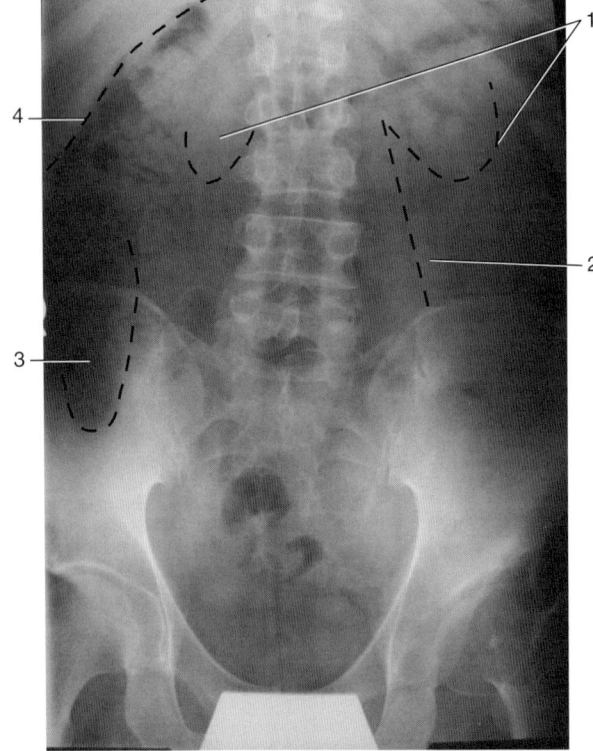

1. Kidneys
2. Psoas muscle margin
3. Gas in colon
4. Liver margin

Fig. 16.13

Challenge Exercise

1. The act of inspiration causes the diaphragm to move caudad. The greater the inspiration is, the greater the depression of the diaphragm will be. Evidence of a full inspiration is seen on a chest radiograph when 10 ribs can be counted superior to the diaphragm.
2. The act of expiration causes the diaphragm to move cephalad.
3. 72 inches
4. Anterior surface of chest is against upright Bucky with coronal plane parallel to IR. Backs of hands are placed on hips, and shoulders are rotated anteriorly. The purpose of arm position is to rotate scapulae out of the way so that they will not be superimposed on lungs. IR is aligned so that upper margin is 1.5 to 2 inches (3.8–5 cm) above level of spinous process of C7.
5. Perpendicular to center of IR. Center point should be at the level of T7.
6. Stop breathing on second deep inspiration.
7. Both arms are raised overhead, with patient grasping opposite elbows. Left side of body is in contact with upright Bucky, and midcoronal plane of thorax is perpendicular to center of IR. IR placement is unchanged from PA projection.
8. Perpendicular to center of IR. Center point should be on the midcoronal plane at the level of T7.
9. Patient is recumbent, lying on side of interest. Midsagittal plane of chest is horizontal. Chest is elevated 2 to 3 inches (5–8 cm) on radiolucent pad. Posterior surface of chest is against a vertical grid device.
10. Patient stands 8 to 12 inches from the IR. Patient arches back to place shoulders against the IR. Backs of hands are on the hips. Shoulders rotated anteriorly. CR is perpendicular or if patient is standing erect, the CR is angled 15 degrees.

CHAPTER 17: SKULL, FACIAL BONES, AND PARANASAL SINUSES

Workbook Answer Keys

Exercise 1

1. C
2. B
3. A
4. C
5. A
6. D
7. C
8. C
9. C
10. C
11. A
12. A
13. C
14. B
15. A
16. D
17. C
18. A
19. A
20. B
21. B
22. B
23. A
24. C
25. C
26. D
27. D
28. A
29. C
30. B
31. D
32. A

Exercise 2

1. The cranium consists of eight bones: frontal, occipital, right and left parietal, right and left temporal, sphenoid, and ethmoid.
2. The temporal bones contain the auditory canals. They are located in the petrous portion.
3. Orbits
4. Frontal bone
5. The cranial base is best demonstrated using the submentovertical (SMV) projection.
6. Coronal suture.
7. The Waters and lateral projections
8. The lateral projection of the nasal bones is done tabletop (non-Bucky), and the lateral projection of the facial bones is done using the Bucky. The radiation field is smaller for the nasal bones than for the lateral projection of the facial bones.
9. An opening in the base of the occipital bone.
10. When the petrous portion is projected over the floor of the maxillary sinuses, more extension of the neck is necessary. Further extension of the neck will project the petrous portion below the maxillary sinuses.
11. Mental protuberance
12. Multiple myeloma
    Osteoma
    Pituitary adenoma
    Paget disease
13. Paranasal sinuses
14. Nasion
15. OML
16. PA and PA axial (Caldwell method)
17. AP axial (Towne method)
18. Cranial base
19. Orbits and zygomas
20. Maxillary and ethmoid
21. Sphenoid and ethmoid
22. Nasal bones

Exercise 3

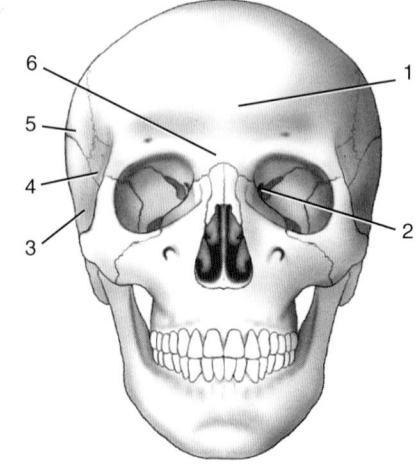

A

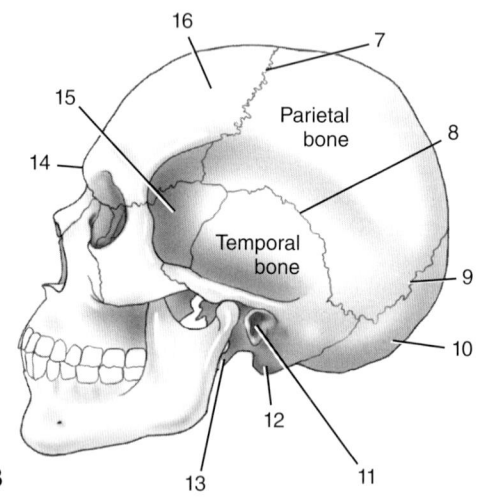

B

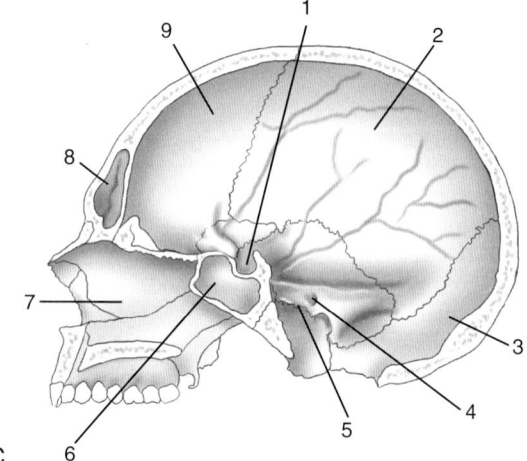

C

Fig. 17. 1

1. Frontal bone
2. Optic foramen
3. Temporal bone
4. Sphenoid bone
5. Parietal bone
6. Glabella
7. Coronal suture
8. Squamosal suture
9. Lambdoidal suture
10. Occipital bone
11. External acoustic meatus
12. Mastoid process
13. Foramen magnum (underside)
14. Glabella
15. Sphenoid bone
16. Frontal bone

1. Sella turcica
2. Parietal bone
3. Occipital bone
4. Internal acoustic meatus
5. Petrous portion of temporal bone
6. Sphenoidal sinus
7. Ethmoid bone
8. Frontal sinus
9. Frontal bone

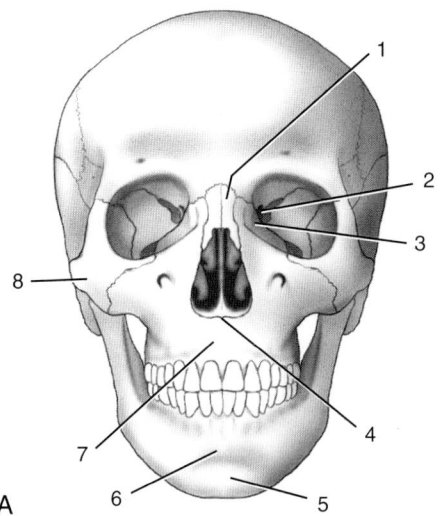

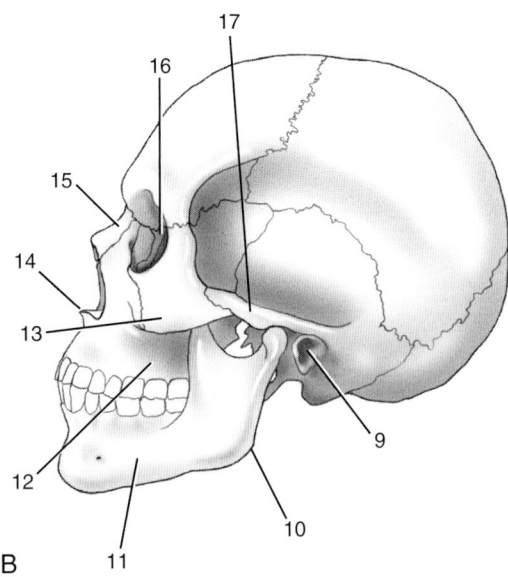

A

B

Fig. 17.2

1. Nasal bone

2. Optic foramen

3. Ethmoid bone

4. Anterior nasal spine (acanthion)

5. Mental protuberance

6. Mandible

7. Maxilla

8. Zygoma

9. External acoustic meatus

10. Angle (gonion)

11. Mandible

12. Maxilla

13. Zygoma

14. Anterior nasal spine (acanthion)

15. Nasal bone

16. Ethmoid bone

17. Zygomatic arch

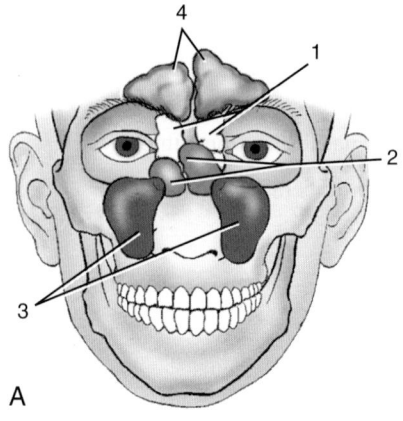

A

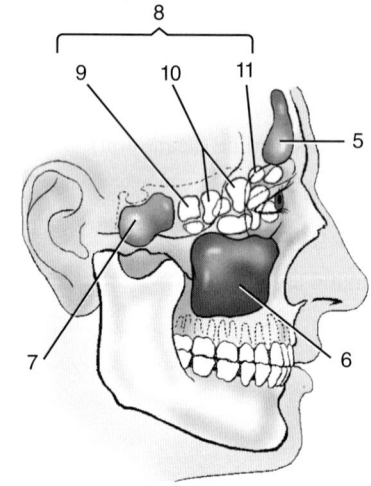

B

Fig. 17. 3

1. Ethmoid sinuses
2. Sphenoid sinuses
3. Maxillary sinuses
4. Frontal sinuses
5. Frontal sinus
6. Maxillary sinus
7. Sphenoid sinus
8. Ethmoid air cells
9. Posterior
10. Middle
11. Anterior

Exercise 4

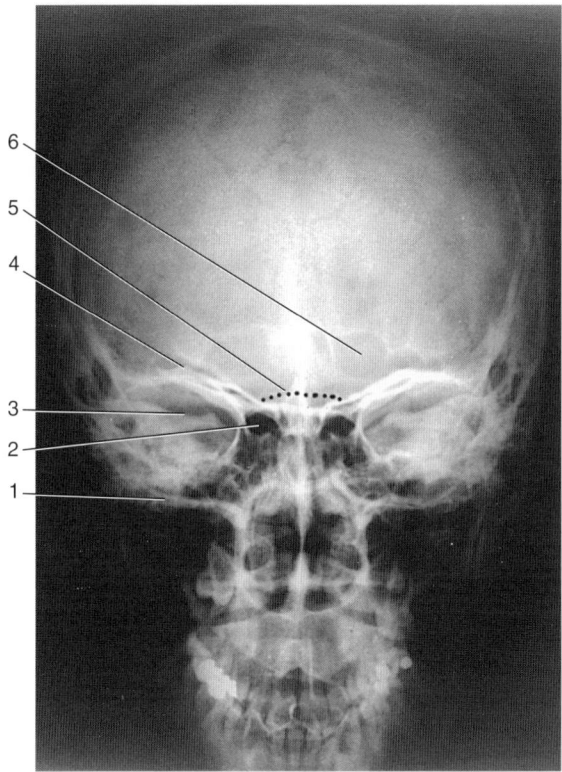

Fig. 17.4

1. Inferior orbital margin
2. Ethmoid sinus
3. Petrous ridge
4. Superior orbital margin
5. Dorsum sellae
6. Frontal sinus

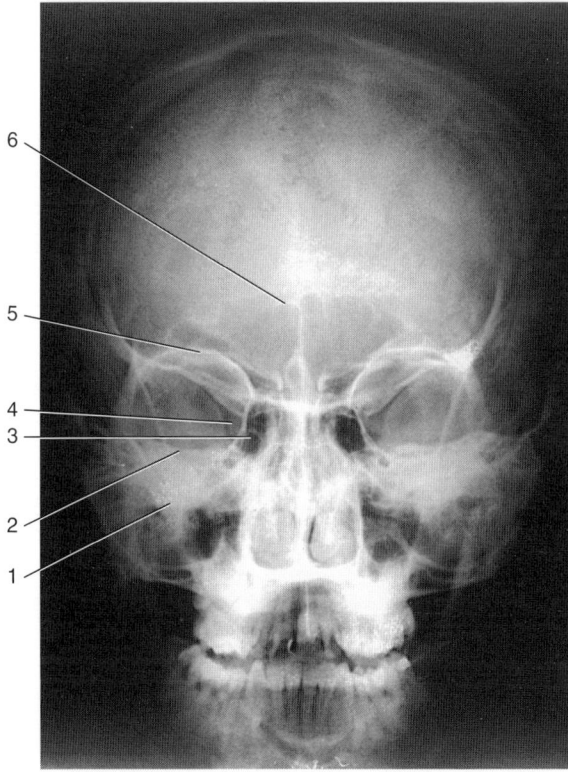

Fig. 17.5

1. Inferior orbital margin
2. Petrous ridge
3. Ethmoid sinus
4. Superior orbital fissure
5. Superior orbital margin
6. Frontal sinus

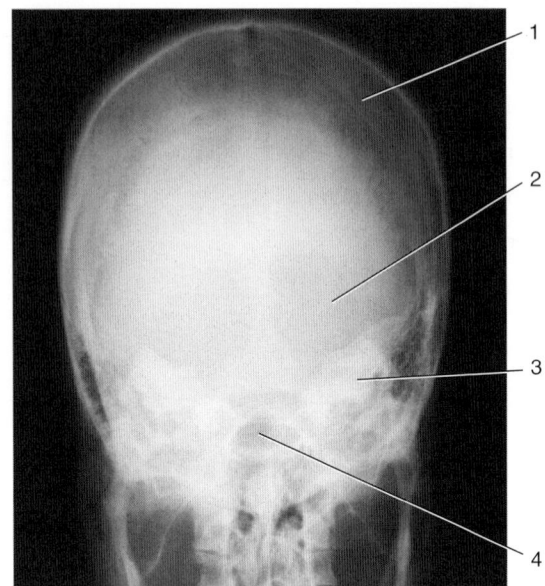

1. Parietal bone
2. Occipital bone
3. Petrous portion of temporal bone
4. Foramen magnum

Fig. 17.6

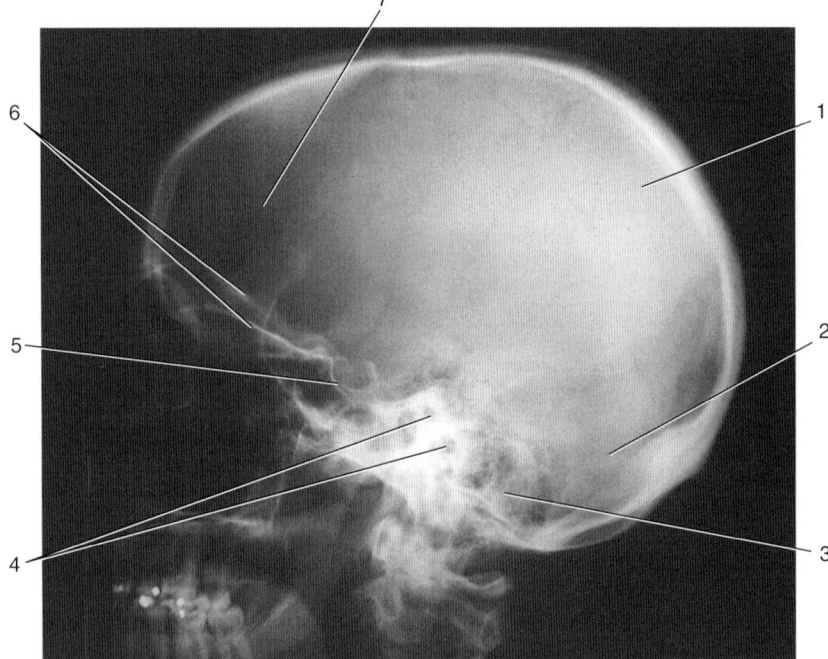

1. Parietal bone
2. Occipital bone
3. Mastoid portion of temporal bone
4. Acoustic meatuses
5. Sella turcica
6. Sphenoid wings
7. Frontal bone

Fig. 17.7

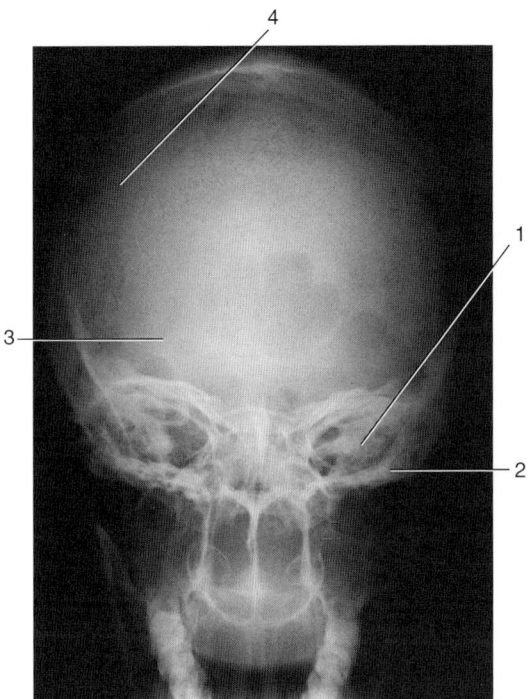

Fig. 17.8

1. Petrous portion of temporal bone
2. Orbit
3. Frontal bone
4. Parietal bone

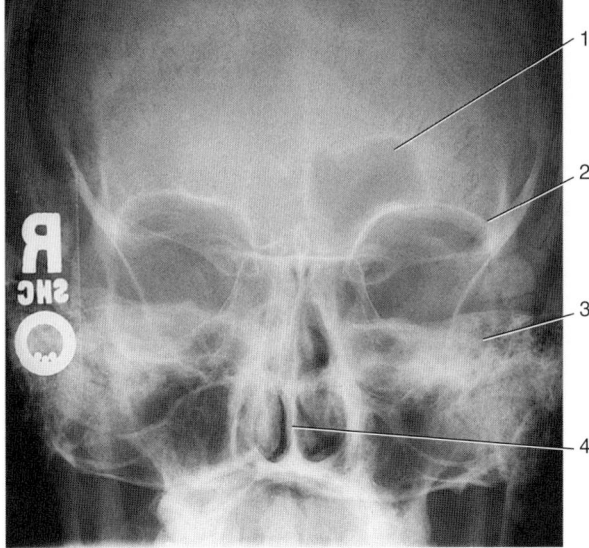

Fig. 17.9

1. Frontal bone
2. Superior orbital rim
3. Petrous portion (ridge)
4. Nasal septum

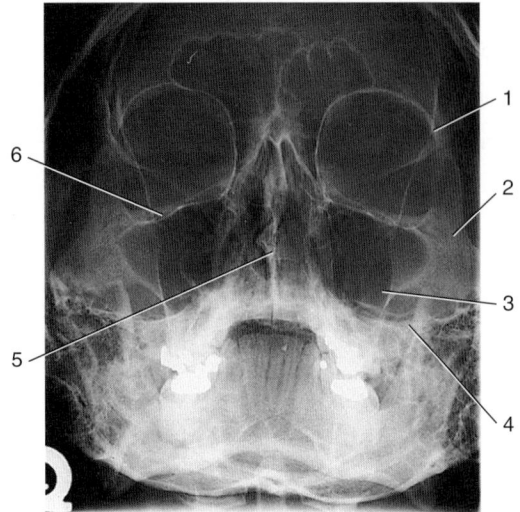

1. Orbit
2. Zygoma
3. Maxillary sinus
4. Petrous portion (ridge)
5. Nasal septum
6. Inferior orbital rim

Fig. 17.10

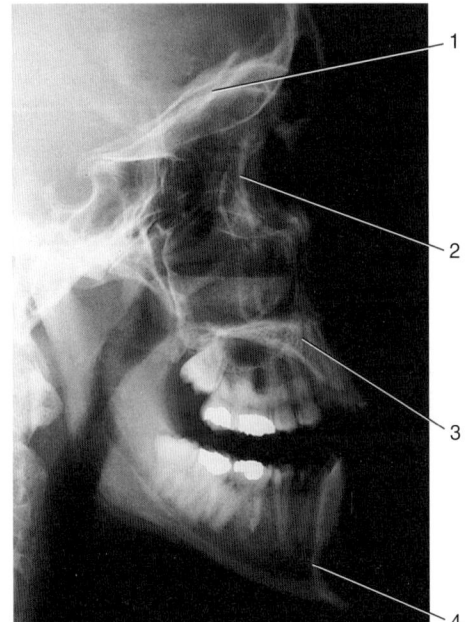

1. Superimposed sphenoid wings
2. Lateral orbital rim
3. Maxilla
4. Mandible

Fig. 17.11

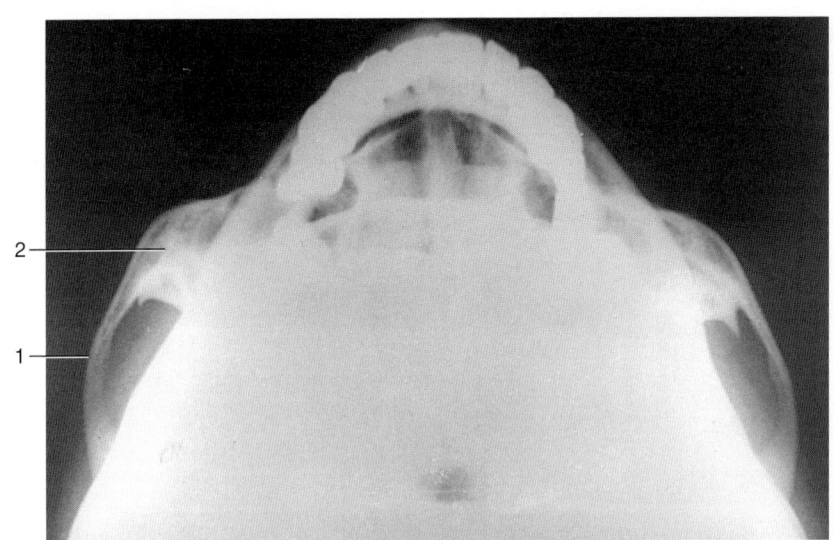

1. Zygomatic arch
2. Temporal process of zygomatic bone

Fig. 17.12

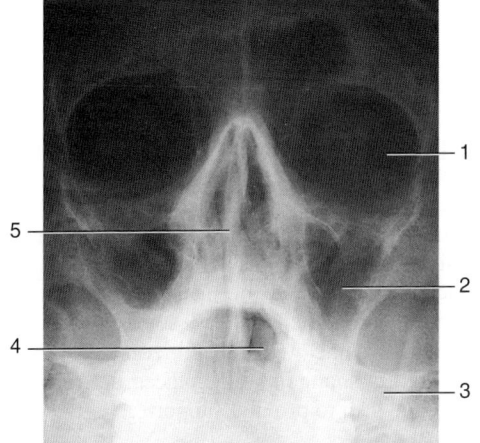

1. Orbit
2. Maxillary sinus
3. Petrous portion (ridge)
4. Sphenoid sinus
5. Nasal septum

Fig. 17.13

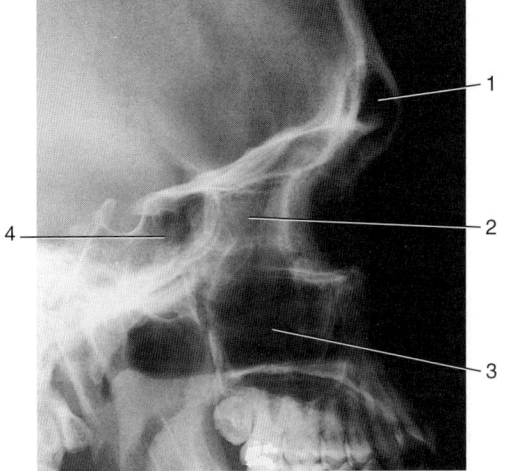

1. Frontal sinus
2. Ethmoid sinuses
3. Maxillary sinuses
4. Sphenoid sinus

Fig. 17. 14

335

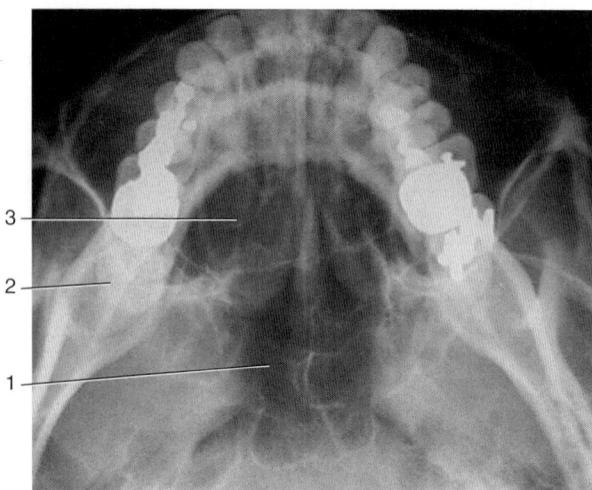

Fig. 17.15

1. Sphenoid sinuses
2. Mandible
3. Ethmoid sinuses

Challenge Exercise

1. The bony prominence on the frontal bone between the eyebrows
2. The anterior depression in the midline of the skull between the orbits
3. The point located at the junction of the nose and the upper lip that corresponds to the anterior nasal spine
4. The prominence in the center of the lower margin of the anterior mandibular body
5. The right angle formed by the contour of the inferior posterior ramus, also called the *angle of the mandible*
6. Sagittal plane of skull is perpendicular to center of IR, with forehead and nose resting on table or against upright Bucky. Neck flexion is adjusted to place OML perpendicular to IR.
7. Angled 15 degrees caudad to center of IR through nasion
8. Sagittal plane of skull is perpendicular to IR with back of head resting on table or against upright Bucky. Neck flexion is adjusted to place OML perpendicular to IR.
9. Angled 30 degrees caudad to center of IR through the foramen magnum at the level of the EAM. Central ray enters skull in midsagittal plane, approximately 2.5 **inches** superior to glabella.
10. If the patient is unable to flex the neck sufficiently to get the OML perpendicular to the IR, the IOML can be placed perpendicular and the central ray angled 37 degrees caudad.
11. Sagittal plane of head is parallel to IR and interpupillary line is perpendicular to it. Support under mandible may assist in maintaining this position. Neck flexion is adjusted to place the IOML parallel to the long axis of the IR.
12. Perpendicular to center of IR through a point approximately 2 **inches** superior to EAM

13. Neck is extended with chin resting on table or upright Bucky. Neck flexion is adjusted so that MML is perpendicular to IR and OML forms a 37-degree angle to IR. Sagittal plane is perpendicular to IR.
14. Perpendicular to IR to exit at the acanthion
15. Perpendicular to center of IR through a point approximately halfway between outer canthus and EAM
16. It is important that all projections be done upright to demonstrate air-fluid levels if they are present.
17. Extend the patient's neck, with the tip of the nose touching the IR and the nasion centered to the IR. Position the patient's head so the OML forms a 15-degree angle with the horizontal central ray. A radiolucent sponge may be placed between the forehead and grid to provide support.

CHAPTER 18: RADIOGRAPHY OF PEDIATRIC AND GERIATRIC PATIENTS

Workbook Answer Keys

Exercise 1

1. Geriatrics
2. Pediatrics
3. 1. Wrap the infant snugly.
   2. Hold the infant gently but firmly; provide gentle motion.
   3. Hold the infant where the infant can see your face.
   4. Talk or sing to the infant softly while you work.
4. True
5. 1. Show disapproval by not smiling and using a calm, firm tone to give instructions.
   2. Praise any attempt to show the right response.
6. A valid choice is one in which both possibilities are acceptable.
7. False
8. True
9. Young adolescence

Exercise 2

1. True
2. False
3. To prevent motion blur on the image from movement of the patient's arms and legs
4. 1. Ossification is incomplete.
    2. The head is larger in proportion to body size.
    3. The spine has a single, C-shaped curvature rather than multiple curves.
    4. Muscle and bone tissues are less dense.
    5. The subcutaneous fat layer is thicker in patients younger than 4 years old.

Exercise 3

1. clavicles, hips
2. True
3. $13\,cm - 8\,cm = 5\,cm$ (difference in size)
   $5\,cm \times 2\,kVp = 10\,kVp$ (kVp change)
   $70\,kVp - 10\,kVp = 60\,kVp$
   $5\,mAs \times 0.8\,(80\%) = 4\,mAs$
   New technique for child would be 4 mAs at 60 kVp, 40 inches SID, nongrid
4. A high mA setting permits the use of shorter exposure times, which helps to prevent motion blur on the image.
5. To demonstrate failure of a lung segment to expand. This helps to identify the location of a bronchial blockage, even when an aspirated object cannot be seen on a radiograph.
6. Greenstick
7. wrist
8. Battered child syndrome or physical child abuse
9. 1. Evidence of chronic or repeated injury with no other explanation
    2. Injuries that are not consistent with the parents' report of the trauma
    3. Failure to seek prompt treatment for serious injury
    4. Bruise marks shaped like hands, fingers, or objects (such as a belt)
    5. Specific patterns of scalding as when a child is immersed in hot water
    6. Burns from hot objects (electric stove, radiator, heater) on the child's hands or buttocks
    7. Cigarette burns on exposed areas or genitals
    8. Black eyes in an infant
    9. Human bite marks
    10. Lash marks
    11. Choke marks around neck
    12. Circular marks around wrists or ankles (twisting)
    13. Separated skull sutures or bulging fontanel on an infant
    14. Unexplained unconsciousness in an infant

Exercise 4

1. Increasing
2. 1. difficulty hearing
    2. failing vision10
    3. loss of mental acuity

3. All of the following are possible answers to this question:
    1. Face the person, preferably with light on your face. Lip reading may be an important supplement to hearing.
    2. Hearing loss is frequently in the upper register, so speak lower and louder. Do not shout.
    3. Speak clearly at a moderate pace.
    4. Avoid noisy background situations.
    5. Rephrase when you are not understood.
    6. Avoid potential misunderstandings by asking open-ended questions.
    7. Validate understanding by asking patients to repeat instructions.
    8. Be patient.
4. Organic brain syndrome
5. Recent events
6. Loss of calcium content in the bones/decreased bone density
7. 1. Muscle atrophy
    2. Loss of subcutaneous fat
    3. Loss of skin elasticity
    4. Vein fragility (tendency to bruise)
8. Decubitus ulcers (or pressure ulcers)
9. Decrease, kVp
10. Diverticulitis
11. Parkinson disease

Challenge Exercise

1. Older adults
2. Density of bone and soft tissue
3. Yes
4. It is an incomplete fracture in which the cortex separates on only one side of the bone.
5. Nonaccidental trauma
6. Osteoporosis or osteopenia
7. Tremors
8. The elderly
9. Nonaccidental trauma, battering, abuse
10. Pressure on bony prominences that restricts circulation and causes tissue necrosis

CHAPTER 19: IMAGE EVALUATION

Workbook Answer Keys

Exercise 1

1. D
2. C
3. A
4. A
5. D
6. C
7. False
8. True
9. A
10. False
11. True
12. A

337

13. C
14. True
15. A
16. A
17. C
18. B
19. True
20. True

Exercise 2

1. I AM ExpERT
2. I Identification (clear and complete, matches requisition)
   A Anatomy (necessary anatomy included and visible)
   M Marking (right or left)
   Exp Exposure (appropriate exposure factors used)
   E Esthetic considerations (artistic merit)
   R Radiation safety (evidence of collimation and shielding)
   T Troubleshooting (identification of problems and ways to improve if repeat radiograph is necessary)
3. The anatomic position is the position in which the patient is standing erect, with the face directed forward, arms extended by the sides with the palms facing forward, and the toes pointing anteriorly.

Challenge Exercise

1. The radiograph will exhibit optimal image brightness, unless the IR was grossly overexposed to the point of pixel saturation.
2. The radiograph will exhibit optimal image contrast, unless the kVp was so low that the part was not adequately penetrated.
3. Patient motion is the most common cause of poor recorded detail, seen as blurring of anatomic structures, in digital images.
4. Image details will be less distinct because of increased magnification distortion.
5. An increase in the SID will counteract the effect of the increased OID.
6. As a general rule, central ray angulation results in shape distortion.
7. The appropriate left or right marker is used to indicate the side for all extremity radiographs; for example, a right marker is placed on the IR when imaging the right wrist. For AP and PA projections that include both sides of the body, a right marker is typically used and placed on the IR to correspond to the patient's right side. For lateral projections of the head and trunk, the side closest to the IR is marked; for example, a left marker is used if the left side is closest.
8. A grainy, mottled, or splotchy appearance on a radiograph is the result of insufficient radiation exposure for the anatomy being imaged. This appearance is corrected by increasing the mAs by at least 50%.
9. All digital images contain an Exposure Indicator number that will be within a specified range of values if the radiation exposure to the IR was sufficient to create a quality image.
10. Unsatisfactory digital images may result from extreme underexposure or extreme overexposure, a kVp that is significantly outside the appropriate range for a particular body part, gross lack of proper collimation, failure to use a grid for body parts that require its use, an SID that is too short, an OID that is too long, patient motion, improper orientation of tube (part, IR), mechanical failure, or presence of artifacts.

CHAPTER 20: ETHICS, LEGAL CONSIDERATIONS, AND PROFESSIONALISM

Workbook Answer Keys

Exercise 1

1. Application of specialized knowledge in a way that benefits others
   a. A high degree of responsibility to the community the profession serves
   b. Organization by the profession to govern itself
   c. Standards of professional behavior, education, and qualification to practice
   d. Enforcement of standards within the profession
   e. Publication of a peer-reviewed journal
2. False
3. True
4. a. Morals: right actions based on religious teachings. *Example:* It is wrong to steal (lie, murder, cheat, etc.).
   b. Values: the priority that is placed on the significance of various moral concepts. *Example:* "Right to life" and "right to choose" are both widely held values with respect to termination of pregnancy.
   c. Ethics: rules that apply values and moral standards to actions. *Example:* It is wrong to gossip (be disloyal, betray a confidence, threaten another, etc.).
5. American Registry of Radiologic Technologists (ARRT) Code of Ethics
6. ARRT Rules of Ethics
7. a. Principle 1: behaves professionally; responds to patient needs; supports colleagues; provides quality patient care
   b. Principle 2: shows respect for human dignity
   c. Principle 3: does not discriminate
   d. Principle 4: practices appropriately
   e. Principle 5: uses careful, responsible judgment
   f. Principle provides information to physicians; does not diagnose or interpret images
   g. Principle 7: meets accepted standards of practice; minimizes radiation exposure
   h. Principle 8: practices ethical conduct; protects the patient's right to quality care
   i. Principle 9: respects confidentiality

    j. Principle 10: participates in professional activities and continuing education

    k. Principle 11: does not use controlled substances that will impair professional judgement or practice

8. True
9. False
10. a. Identify the problem.
    b. Develop alternate solutions.
    c. Select the best solution.
    d. Defend your selection.

Exercise 2

1. False
2. False
3. True
4. Practicing outside the legal requirements may result in fines, loss of credentials, or even imprisonment. Failure to maintain the qualifications required by your employer may result in termination of your employment. Infractions of laws or professional rules may make it impossible for you to obtain professional standing and/or employment as a radiographer in the future.
5. 1. F
    2. B
    3. A
    4. D
    5. C
    6. G
6. Negligence
7. The doctrine of the reasonably prudent person
8. HIPAA
9. Malpractice
10. *Respondeat superior*
11. 1. Identify patients accurately using two sources, usually the patient's full name and birth date, by having the patient state the information or by checking the patient's arm band.
    2. Administer medications accurately.
    3. Comply with all patient safety requirements.
    4. Chart information correctly.

Exercise 3

1. 1. 3
    2. 1
    3. 5
    4. 4
    5. 6
    6. 2
2. Any of the following are acceptable answers to this question:
    1. Stay home and care for yourself when ill or under severe psychological stress.
    2. Ensure proper nutrition.
    3. Get regular exercise.
    4. Develop good sleep habits.
    5. Use good body mechanics when lifting and moving heavy objects.

6. Follow infection control precautions, including getting the hepatitis B vaccination.
7. Follow radiation safety precautions.
3. Any of the following are acceptable answers to this question:
    1. Be a good listener.
    2. Use praise and appreciation as positive reinforcements when work is well done or when others go out of their way to offer assistance.
    3. Demonstrate respect for your co-workers as individuals by avoiding cliques and gossip.
4. Empathy
5. Focus on the needs of the patient.
6. 1. To stay abreast of current trends and technology
    2. To maintain interest in work
    3. To learn new skills and expand knowledge
    4. To qualify for a promotion or a new position
    5. To meet colleagues and share information with them

Exercise 4

1. 1. A smile or pleasant facial expression
    2. Open posture, leaning forward toward another
    3. Positive touch
2. The listener confirmed understanding of the message.
3. Examples from the text: "Would you like a blanket over your knees?" and "Would you like to stop in the restroom before we begin?" Your answer should be something similar.
4. 1. D
    2. E
    3. A
    4. C
    5. B

Exercise 5

1. 1. Does not respond to noises or words spoken out of the range of vision
    2. Uses lip movements without making a sound or speaks in a flat monotone
    3. Points to the ears and mouth while shaking the head in a negative motion
    4. Uses gestures or writing motions to express the need for paper and pencil
2. 1. American Sign Language (ASL)
    2. Lip reading and speech
    3. Reading and writing
3. False
4. False
5. True
6. Eye contact, interpersonal distance, gestures, and speed or tone of speech
7. It brings bad luck to admire or compliment a child without also touching the child.
8. The United States, Hispanic culture, Russian culture
9. Fear or anxiety
10. 1. Direct them to a comfortable waiting area
    2. show interest and concern

339

3. provide practical information such as the length of the procedure and the destination of the patient afterward
4. and direct them to services, such as restrooms and telephones.

Exercise 6

1. Chart
2. The institution in which they are produced
3. Obtain patient's signed consent; record the date and the name and address of the physician requesting the images; send only those images requested; send images by mail or courier, if time permits.

Challenge Exercise

1. A legal document that contains a record of the care and treatment received by a patient
2. The facility in which they are created
3. The facility providing care
4. As the response that would be expected from a reasonably prudent person
5. False imprisonment
6. Invasion of privacy
7. The limited operator provides information to physicians but does not diagnose or interpret images.
8. Professional ethics
9. Ethical analysis
10. The ARRT Code of Ethics

CHAPTER 21: SAFETY AND INFECTION CONTROL

Workbook Answer Keys

Exercise 1

1. Fuel, oxygen, heat
2. False
3. True
4. No smoking
   No open flames
   No use of ungrounded appliances
5. The main evacuation route from your area and at least one alternate route
   A general layout of your facility's floor plan
   The locations of fire extinguishers and fire alarms
   The procedure for reporting a fire
6. RACE
   Rescue
   Alarm
   Contain
   Evacuate/extinguish
7. P: Pull the pin.
   A: Aim the nozzle.
   S: Squeeze the handle.
   S: Sweep. Use a sweeping motion from side to side.
8. Water
9. Limit access to the area.
   Evaluate the risks involved.
   Obtain both the information and the equipment to clean up the spill safely.

Clean up the spill.
If you lack the necessary skill or equipment, call your supervisor.

Exercise 2

1. Body mechanics
2. Bend at the hips and knees.
3. Push it.
4. A. Supine
   B. Prone
   C. Lateral recumbent
   D. Sims
   E. Fowler
   F. Semi-Fowler
   G. Trendelenburg
   H. Knee-chest
   I. Lithotomy
5. Knees
6. Orthopnea
7. Fowler, lateral recumbent
8. Decubitus ulcers (pressure ulcers)
9. Under the shoulders; under the knees
10. Lateral recumbent
11. Orthostatic hypotension
12. Weak side
13. The patient backs into the wheelchair to sit down.
14. True
15. True
16. False. An incident report should be completed for any event that results in injury or potential harm to anyone.

Exercise 3

1. a. Infectious organism
   b. Reservoir of infection
   c. Susceptible host
   d. Means of transmission
2. 1. F
   2. D
   3. G
   4. B
   5. C
   6. H
   7. A
   8. E
3. 1. Fomite: an object that has been in contact with pathogenic organisms; examples in the radiology department include the x-ray table, upright Bucky, cassettes, calipers, and positioning sponges that are contaminated with infectious body fluids.
   2. Vector: an arthropod (insect, spider, or similar form) in whose body an infectious organism develops or multiplies before becoming infective to a new host; examples include the mosquito that spreads malaria and the tick that spreads Lyme disease.
   3. Vehicle: any medium that transports microorganisms; examples include contaminated food, water, drugs, and blood.

4. Airborne contamination: contact with dust containing either endospores or droplet nuclei; examples include the droplet nuclei that spread tuberculosis and chickenpox.

5. Droplet contamination: contact of the mucous membranes of the eyes, nose, or mouth of a susceptible person with droplets containing microorganisms; examples include droplets of mucus that might be spread through coughing or sneezing, spreading colds and flu.

4. Human immunodeficiency virus (HIV)
5. Sexual intercourse, sharing contaminated needles
6. True
7. True
8. False
9. Blood, blood products, or body fluids
10. A, E
11. Hepatitis B virus (HBV)
12. Within 2 hours of the exposure
13. C
14. Virus
15. Airborne droplet nuclei that are generated when an infected person coughs or speaks (the airborne contamination route)
16. False
17. True
18. Tuberculin skin test, also called Mantoux test or purified protein derivative (PPD) test
19. Blood
    All body fluids and wound drainage
    Secretions and excretions (except sweat), regardless of whether they contain visible blood
    Mucous membranes
20. Methicillin-resistant *Staphylococcus aureus* (MRSA)
    Vancomycin-resistant enterococci (VRE)
    Penicillin-resistant *Streptococcus*
    Pseudomonas aeruginosa
    Clostridium difficile

Exercise 4

1. Disinfection
2. Surgical asepsis or sterilization
3. Hand hygiene
4. True
5. False
6. When hands are visibly soiled or contaminated with blood or body fluid or when contamination by endospores is suspected
7. A diluted solution of sodium hypochlorite bleach (Clorox)
8. Biohazard
9. True
10. False. Recapping is a common cause of needle sticks.
11. Sharps container
12. Autoclaving or steam sterilization
13. Gas sterilization
14. Sterile field

15. They are clean, dry, and unopened.
    Their expiration date has not been exceeded.
    Their sterility indicators have changed to a predetermined color, confirming sterilization.
16. Away from you
17. False
18. True
19. True
20. Application

Challenge Exercise

1. Although oxygen does not burn, it supports combustion, making fire more likely and more dangerous.
2. Sims position.
3. Trendelenburg position
4. A person is unable to breathe when lying down.
5. Pathogens
6. On the weak side
7. Tuberculosis; via airborne contamination
8. Sexual intercourse, sharing contaminated needles
9. Standard precautions
10. Hands are visibly soiled or are potentially contaminated with endospores.

CHAPTER 22: ASSESSING PATIENTS AND MANAGING ACUTE SITUATIONS

Workbook Answer Keys

Exercise 1

1. 1. Observation
   2. Evaluation
   3. Assessment
2. 1. Provide ample cover
   2. Display a matter-of-fact attitude
   3. Provide an explanation of the procedure
   4. Your presence is comforting – let the patient know when you will leave the area and when you will return.
3. 1. Use padding for comfort on a hard table if the procedures will be prolonged
   2. Elevate the head if the patient has difficulty lying flat
   3. Inquire if the patient is warm enough; provide a blanket if needed
   4. If the patient is sniffling, provide tissues and place a waste container within reach
4. Incontinence
5. 1. Onset
   2. Duration
   3. Specific location
   4. Quality of pain
   5. What aggravates
   6. What alleviates

Exercise 2

1. Cyanotic
2. Perspiring
3. Fever
4. Higher

5. Lower
6. When the patient has recently taken a hot or cord beverage, is receiving oxygen, or breathes through the mouth.
7. Tachycardia
8. Weak and rapid
9. Systolic
10. High
11. B
12. 1. Inspect emergency supplies to be certain they are current and available for instant use
    2. Never borrow supplies from the emergency set for routine use
    3. Be sure that supplies are replenished and the kit is ready for use before returning it to storage.

Exercise 3

1. Mask
2. 3 to 5 L/min.
3. Less
4. Suction
5. Heart attack

Exercise 4

1. Initiate the "shake and shout" maneuver.
2. Irreparable brain damage.
3. Fibrillation.
4. Intracranial pressure (ICP, pressure within the skull).
5. When a blow to the head causes damage on the side of the head opposite the side of the blow, this is termed a contrecoup injury.
6. 1. Alert and conscious_
    2. Drowsy but responsive
    3. Unconscious bur reactive to painful stimuli
    4. Comatose
7. Compound fracture
8. A hemorrhage
9. Erythema
10. Anaphylaxis or anaphylactic shock
11. A moderate allergic reaction
12. Anaphylaxis is a type of shock caused by drug allergy.
13. Hyperglycemia, an elevated blood glucose level =
14. Insulin
15. Stroke
16. 1) F: Face drooping
    2) A: Arm weakness
    3) S: Speech difficulty
    4) T: Time to call 9-1-1
17. CVA or stroke
18. Keep the patient as safe as possible
19. Seizure
20. Persuade the patient to breathe more slowly or to breathe into a paper bag
21. Fainting
22. Vertigo
23. Epstaxis or nosebleed.

Challenge Exercise

1. Cyanosis
2. Between 60 and 100 beats per minute (bpm)
3. Sphygmomanometer and stethoscope
4. Patients with dyspnea need 3 to 5 L/min, whereas those with emphysema should receive less than 3 L/min because their oxygen blood level controls their respiratory rate and too much oxygen may cause their respiratory rate to brr too slow for adequate ventilation.
5. Brain
6. Anaphylaxis
7. CVA; cerebrovascular accident
8. Diabetes mellitus
9. Blood glucose
10. Fracture fragments protrude through the skin
11. Patient suddenly develops an irregular pulse; appears diaphoretic and pale and is feeling short of breath, faint, weak, or nauseated; or has a sudden onset of pain in the chest, shoulder, or jaw
12. Heart attack

CHAPTER 23: MEDICATIONS AND THEIR ADMINISTRATION

Workbook Answer Keys

Exercise 1

1. Checking the allergy history of the patient
   Preparing medication for administration
   Verifying patient identification
   Assisting the physician
   Monitoring the patient after the medication has been given
2. It is the physician's duty.
3. True
4. False
5. Generic name
6. Proprietary or trade name
7. 1. D
   2. A
   3. E
   4. C
   5. B
8. The US Food and Drug Administration (FDA)
9. Effectiveness
10. Strength

Exercise 2

1. 1. H
   2. C
   3. F
   4. E
   5. A
   6. B
   7. D
   8. G
2. 1. E
   2. A
   3. D
   4. F
   5. B
   6. C
3. Hydration
4. 1. C
   2. B
   3. A
   4. D
5. receptor sites on cells
6. Therapeutic effect
7. controlled
8. opiates, opioids, and benzodiazepines
9. antidote

Exercise 3

1. $40\,lb \times 0.45 = 18\,kg$
2. 3 mL
3. 150 μg
4. True
5. False
6. Vastus lateralis muscle of the thigh
7. True
8. True
9. Date and time, name of drug, dose, route of administration, identification of person charting

CHAPTER 24: MEDICAL LABORATORY SKILLS

Workbook Answer Keys

Exercise 1

1. All pathogens, principally human immunodeficiency virus, hepatitis B virus, and hepatitis C virus
2. All patients' body fluids are potentially infectious.
3. a. Hand hygiene
   b. Barrier techniques
   c. Proper disposal of contaminated waste
4. Biohazardous waste
5. Sharps container

Exercise 2

1. Venipuncture
2. Antecubital fossa (front side of the elbow)
3. the presence or absence of specific additives
4. a. Tubes with additives should be filled after those that have no additives.
   b. Tubes with additives must be gently inverted after filling to ensure adequate mixing.

5. True
6. 21 gauge; 1 or 1 1/2 inches
7. the stopper of the evacuated collection tube; the skin
8. True
9. False
10. Tourniquet
11. Blood cultures; blood alcohol testing
12. False. Shielding is necessary for safety, even with these special tubes.
13. 1. Above the site where intravenous fluids are being infused
    2. Where excess scarring is evident
    3. The arm on the side of a mastectomy
14. Palpation
15. After
16. Before
17. needle is not properly situated in the lumen (channel) of the vein.

Exercise 3

1. Urinalysis
2. 1. Macroscopic examination of physical characteristics
   2. Chemical analysis performed with a urine reagent strip
   3. Microscopic examination of the urine sediment
3. Recap the bottle immediately after a strip is removed, and store the bottle at room temperature.
4. False
5. When the patient awakens in the morning; this is called a first morning specimen.
6. Random specimen
7. Clean-catch midstream specimen (CCMS) technique
8. Anterior to posterior
9. The specimen should be capped, protected from light, and refrigerated until the analysis is performed; before analysis, it should be warmed to room temperature, gently remixed, and transferred to a urinalysis tube.
10. 1. Color
    2. Appearance (clarity)
11. True
12. Send the specimen to a laboratory for analysis by a different method.
13. "Positive for nonhemolyzed blood"
14. The CCMS technique is employed immediately after the insertion of a fresh tampon.
15. Hazy urine (more than slightly hazy); positive results for glucose, protein, blood, nitrite, or leukocyte esterase
16. Centrifuge

CHAPTER 25: ADDITIONAL PROCEDURES FOR ASSESSMENT AND DIAGNOSIS

Workbook Answer Keys

Exercise 1

1. The weights on both calibration bars should be set at zero, and the scale should be in balance.

2. Lower
3. The patient's weight is determined by noting the readings on both calibration bars and adding them together.
4. the patient is not standing still.
5. Before
6. Quarter inch
7. Quarter inch

Exercise 2

1. Myopia: nearsightedness
   Hyperopia: farsightedness
   Presbyopia: farsightedness associated with advancing age
2. Snellen E
3. 20 ft
4. Right eye: OD
   Left eye: OS
5. Ishihara test

Exercise 3

1. Electrocardiogram
2. 1. P wave
   2. P-R segment
   3. S-T segment
   4. T wave
   5. U wave
   6. P-R interval
   7. Q wave
   8. QRS complex
   9. S wave
   10. Q-T interval
3. 1. Standard leads (limb or bipolar leads): I, II, and III
   2. Augmented leads: aVR, aVL, and aVF
   3. Precordial (chest) leads: V1, V2, V3, V4, V5, and V6
4. Wave amplitude
5. Record the ECG at the half-STD setting
6. 25 mm/s
7. Must be connected to a specific electrode
8. 1. B
   2. F
   3. C
   4. D
   5. A
   6. G
   7. E
9. Electrolyte
10. True
11. An exercise tolerance test or an ECG stress test

Exercise 4

1. Spirometry
2. 1. Volume-displacement type
   2. Flow-sensing type
3. 1. Flow-volume spirogram
   2. Time-volume spirogram
4. 1. An immediate forceful start
   2. A maximum effort

3. A smooth continuous exhalation that does not end abruptly
5. Three
6. Eight (After eight attempts, fatigue prevents accurate testing.)
7. 1. Recent abdominal surgery
   2. Recent thoracic surgery
   3. Recent eye surgery, including cataract operations
   4. Hemoptysis (coughing up blood) from an unknown cause
   5. Pneumothorax (collapsed lung)

CHAPTER 26: BONE DENSITOMETRY

Workbook Answer Keys
Exercise 1

1.	D	41.	A
2.	B	42.	B
3.	D	43.	D
4.	A	44.	A
5.	B	45.	A
6.	B	46.	D
7.	C	47.	C
8.	C	48.	D
9.	A	49.	A
10.	B	50.	A
11.	C	51.	C
12.	D	52.	D
13.	B	53.	D
14.	A	54.	B
15.	C	55.	B
16.	A	56.	B
17.	D	57.	A
18.	A	58.	C
19.	B	59.	A
20.	D	60.	B
21.	C	61.	D
22.	A	62.	C
23.	C	63.	A
24.	D	64.	D
25.	B	65.	D
26.	B	66.	B
27.	B	67.	C
28.	A	68.	D
29.	C	69.	A
30.	D	70.	B

31.	C	71.	A
32.	A	72.	C
33.	D	73.	D
34.	D	74.	C
35.	A	75.	D
36.	B	76.	D
37.	A	77.	B
38.	D	78.	A
39.	C	79.	C
40.	B	80.	D

Exercise 2

1. 1. Cortical
   2. Trabecular
2. Bone remodeling
3. Osteoblasts
4. Age 65
5. Fragility fracture
6. 20% of males have osteoporosis
7. Decreased estrogen levels
8. 1. Corticosteroids
   2. Heparin
   3. Anticonvulsants
   4. Thyroid hormone treatment
9. 1. Hip
   2. Spinal vertebrae
   3. Wrist (Colles fracture)
   4. Ribs.
   5. Proximal humerus
10. The mortality rate is 1 in 5.
11. Females: 1200 mg/daily. Males: 1000 mg/daily.
12. 1. Mean
    2. Standard deviation (SD)
    3. Percent of coefficient variation (%CV).
13. A smaller SD.
14. A smaller %CV is preferred.
15. 1. Accuracy.
    2. Precision.
16. Calibration of the scanner
17. 1. Reproduction of positioning.
    2. Anatomic variations that occur over time.
    3. Large weight changes over time
18. Reference population.
19. 1. T-score
    2. Z-score
20. Low bone mass.
21. T-score
22. Discordance.
23. Lower.
24. 1. Pregnant
    2. Recent barium or contrast media examination
    3. Previous fractures or surgery of DXA areas

4. Has a nuclear medicine examination
25. Less than –1
26. 1.5% of the mean from the first 25 measurements done on the scanner
27. Because a patient's BMD changes over time.
28. To reduce the lordotic curve.
29. 1. Spine is straight and centered.
    2. Scan contains a portion of the iliac crest.
    3. Entire scan field is free of external artifacts.
    4. Intervertebral markers are properly placed.
    5. Vertebral levels are properly labeled
    6. Bone edges are correct.
30. It is the best predictor of future hip fracture.
31. It cannot be scanned.
32. 1. Lesser trochanter is small or barely visible.
    2. Midline of the femoral shaft is parallel to the lateral edge of the scan.
    3. Adequate space is present between the ischium and femoral neck.
    4. Midline through the femoral neck is reasonably placed.
    5. Proximal, distal, and lateral edges of the scan field are properly located.
    6. No air is present in the scan field on GE Lunar scans.
33. The nondominant forearm
34. Hyperparathyroidism
35. 1. Forearm is straight and centered in the scan field.
    2. Adequate amounts of soft tissue and air are included.
    3. No motion is present.
    4. Proximal and distal ends of the scan field are properly placed.
    5. Bone edges are properly and consistently placed.
    6. No artifacts or clothing are present in the scan field
36. Capable of showing the lumber and thoracic spine on one continuous image.
37. 0 age
38. Because of the variability in skeletal development
39. "Low bone mineral mass or BMD"
40. Ages 40 to 90

Exercise 3

1. F
2. I
3. A
4. L
5. D
6. H
7. M
8. B
9. K
10. E
11. G
12. C
13. J

Exercise 4

1. Yes. There are six lumbar vertebrae. Based on the densitometric shape, the labeling is correct. It is important for technologists to understand densitometric anatomy and the shape of the individual vertebral bodies. It is imperative to acquire and analyze consistently when obtaining serial scans.

2. A. Compression fracture is seen at L-1. The compression fracture at L-1 will falsely increase the BMD if results for L-1 through L-4 are reported.

   B. Reanalyze excluding L-1 and report on L-2 through L-4 for a comparison of equal area.

2. Greater Trochanter: 4
   Femoral Neck: 6
   Femoral Head: 5
   Pelvic Ischium: 3
   Lesser Trochanter: 1
   Femoral Shaft: 2

3. Ulna: 4
   Radius: 2
   Distal Radius: 1
   Proximal Ulan: 3
   Ulnar Styloid: 5

Introduction

This guide is provided to help you prepare to successfully complete the licensure examination for the limited scope of practice area in which you are or will be working. We have included helpful suggestions for optimizing your study time and a simulated examination to help you identify your areas of strength and weakness. All suggestions and discussions are based on the American Registry of Radiologic Technologists (ARRT) Examination Content Specifications for the **Limited Scope of Practice in Radiography**. We have done this for two reasons: first, this is a comprehensive examination covering all relevant areas of practice, and second, it is likely that the licensure agency in your state uses this examination. If your state does not use this examination, you will still be well prepared if you use the **ARRT Content Specifications** as your study guide. For your convenience, we have included the most recent ARRT Content Specifications in this guide.

If you are using Radiography Essentials for Limited Practice and this accompanying workbook, it is likely that you are participating in an educational program designed to prepare you both to work in a given practice area and to successfully pass the appropriate state licensure examination. This guide should assist you in both these endeavors. Completing the simulated examination will help you identify knowledge that you have already acquired and knowledge that you have yet to master. Because the simulated examination was constructed to assess content identified in the ARRT Content Specifications, it is appropriate to provide an overview of the latter document before moving on to the examination.

ARRT CONTENT SPECIFICATIONS

The ARRT Examination Content Specifications for the Limited Scope of Practice in Radiography covers five practice areas by administering five radiographic procedure modules. These include the chest, extremities, skull/sinuses, spine, and podiatric. The ARRT Content Specifications indicate that there are two components to each practice area licensure examination: a core module that everyone completes and one or more radiographic procedure modules. The core module assesses knowledge in the areas of patient care, safety, and image production.

The patient care area includes questions on patient interactions and management. The safety area includes questions on radiation physics and radiobiology, as well as questions on radiation protection. The image production area includes questions on image acquisition and technical evaluation, as well as questions on equipment operation and quality assurance. According to the Content Specifications document, the ARRT believes that all individuals licensed in limited scope radiography should know this information. Which of the radiographic procedure modules you take will depend on your area of practice. If your practice area is limited to chest radiography, you will complete only the chest module. However, if there is a licensure category in your state that allows radiography in all the procedural areas, you will complete all five modules. Licensure laws differ by state, and each licensure agency has its own procedures and guidelines.

The most valuable component of the AART Content Specifications is the outline of each content area covered on the examination. The numbers in parentheses in this outline indicate how many questions on the examination assess some aspect of knowledge in the designated area. The value to you is that this information will help you determine how much time and effort to spend on certain topics. Without using this information as a guide, you may waste valuable time learning information that is not included on the examination. This guide is to help you prepare for the state licensure examination, not to prepare you to work in your practice area. You will need skills that cannot be directly assessed by a written examination.

SIMULATED EXAMINATION

The limited scope simulated examination is located after the ARRT Content Specifications in this section. You will find a **Core Module** and five **Radiographic Procedure Modules**. You must complete the core module portion of the examination, regardless of your practice area. When you take each exam ensure that you find a quiet space, close your books, and turn off your smart phone. This will simulate what you will have to do when you take the ARRT Limited-Scope exam and it will give you an accurate assessment of your knowledge level.

347

Introduction

After completing the core module, complete the module or modules appropriate for your practice area. You should schedule time to *complete all relevant portions of the examination at the same time*. This will give you experience in completing an examination of that length when you take the ARRT exam and give you some idea of how long it will take you to do so. The core module consists of 100 questions, as prescribed in the ARRT Content Specifications, and contains the appropriate number of questions from each of the content areas: patient interactions and management (18), radiation physics and radiobiology (12), radiation protection (28), image acquisition and technical evaluations (20), and equipment operation and quality assurance (23). The questions are further focused to cover content specified in the outline for each content area. You will see that there are more content topics in each outline than there are questions included in the examination. This means that some content will not be assessed with a question, both on the simulated examination and on your actual state licensure examination. For this reason it is important for you to *review all topics included in each content outline* in the ARRT Content Specifications. You cannot rely only on the simulated examination to prepare you for your state licensure examination.

The five radiographic procedure modules are located after the core module. Each contains the appropriate number of questions prescribed in the ARRT Content Specifications for the five modules: chest (20), extremities (25), skull/sinuses (20), spine (25), and podiatric (20). The questions are further focused to cover content specified in the outline for each module. As mentioned in the previous paragraph, there are more content topics in each outline than there are questions included in the examination. Therefore, some content will not be assessed with a question, both on the simulated examination and on your actual state licensure examination. For this reason, you should review all topics included in each content outline in the ARRT Content Specifications. The answers to all simulated examination questions in each examination module are located after the last question in the module. We have included the correct answer (ANS), as well as the textbook chapter in Radiography Essentials for Limited Practice in which the information is located (REF), the designator for the ARRT Content

Specifications topic outline item (OBJ) that the question is designed to assess, and the topic (TOP) addressed by the question. This information will allow you to easily find and review text material that you have not yet mastered.

Your timeline to prepare for the state licensure examination should be something like the following:

- Participate in the educational course or program.
- Complete all workbook exercises related to the given area of practice. Do not waste time on radiographic procedures chapters outside your licensure area. This activity is especially important if you are not in a formal education program.
- Complete all Challenge Exercises at the end of each relevant workbook chapter.
- Complete the simulated examination.
- Analyze the results of your examination to identify information you have not yet mastered.
- Review information related to questions you missed on the examination. It may be helpful to repeat relevant workbook exercises.
- Complete the simulated examination again and analyze the results. Review additional information as needed.
- Successfully complete the state limited scope licensure examination!

ARRT Content Specifications for the Limited Scope of Practice in Radiography Examination

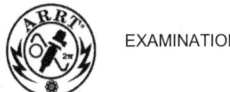

EXAMINATION CONTENT SPECIFICATIONS

ARRT BOARD APPROVED: **JANUARY 2022**
IMPLEMENTATION DATE: **JANUARY 1, 2023**

Limited Scope of Practice in Radiography

The purpose of the *Limited Scope of Practice in Radiography Examination*, which is developed and administered by *The American Registry of Radiologic Technologists (ARRT)* on behalf of state licensing agencies, is to assess the knowledge and cognitive skills underlying the intelligent performance of the tasks typically required of operators of radiographic equipment used to radiograph selected anatomic regions (chest, extremities, etc.). ARRT administers the examination to state approved candidates under contractual arrangement with the state and provides the results directly to the state. This examination is not associated with any type of certification and registration by the ARRT.

The knowledge and skills covered by the examination were determined by administering a comprehensive practice analysis survey to a nationwide sample of radiographers and adopting a subset of the tasks developed for the radiography task inventory as the limited scope task inventory. The task inventory appears in *Attachment C* of this document. The content specifications for the limited scope examination identify the knowledge areas underlying performance of the tasks on the limited scope task inventory. Every content category can be linked to one or more activities on the task inventory.

It is the philosophy of the ARRT that individuals licensed in limited scope radiography possess the same knowledge and cognitive skill, in their specific area of radiography, as radiographers. The modules covered by the examination are outlined below. Subsequent pages describe in detail the topics covered within each module. All candidates take the CORE module of the examination and one or more PROCEDURE modules, depending on the type of license for which they have applied.

Core Module	Number of Scored Questions[1]	Testing Time
Patient Care	18	
Patient Interactions and Management (18)		
Safety	40	
Radiation Physics and Radiobiology (12)		
Radiation Protection (28)		
Image Production	42	
Image Acquisition and Evaluation (20)		
Equipment Operation and Quality Assurance (22)		
Total for Core Module	100	1 hr, 55 min
Procedure Modules		
1. Chest	20	25 min
2. Extremities	25	30 min
3. Skull/Sinuses	20	25 min
4. Spine	25	30 min
5. Podiatric	20	25 min

[1.] The core module includes an additional 15 unscored (pilot) questions. Each of the procedure modules has five additional unscored questions.

ARRT Content Specifications for the Limited Scope of Practice in Radiography Examination

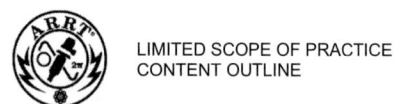
Patient Care

1. Patient Interactions and Management

A. Ethical and Legal Aspects
   1. patients' rights
      a. consent (*e.g., informed, oral, implied)
      b. confidentiality (HIPAA)
      c. American Hospital Association (AHA) Patient Care Partnership (Patients' Bill of Rights)
         1. privacy
         2. extent of care (e.g., DNR)
         3. access to information
         4. living will, health care proxy, advanced directives
         5. research participation
   2. legal issues
      a. verification (e.g., patient identification, compare order to clinical indication)
      b. common terminology (e.g., battery, negligence, malpractice, beneficence)
      c. legal doctrines (e.g., respondeat superior, res ipsa loquitur)
      d. positioning aids used to prevent motion artifact
      e. manipulation of electronic data (e.g., exposure indicator, processing algorithm, brightness and contrast, cropping or masking off anatomy)
      f. documentation (e.g., changes to order)
   3. Professional Ethics

B. Interpersonal Communication
   1. modes of communication
      a. verbal/written
      b. nonverbal (e.g., eye contact, touching)
   2. challenges in communication
      a. interactions with others
         1. language barriers
         2. cultural and social factors
         3. physical, sensory, or cognitive impairments
         4. age
         5. emotional status, acceptance of condition (e.g., stage of grief)
      b. explanation of medical terms
      c. strategies to improve understanding
   3. patient education (e.g., explanation of current procedure purpose, length of time, radiation dose)

C. Ergonomics and Monitoring
   1. body mechanics (e.g., balance, alignment, movement)
      a. patient transfer techniques
      b. safe patient handling devices (e.g., transfer board, gait belt)
   2. assisting patients with medical equipment (e.g., oxygen delivery systems, urinary catheters)
   3. patient monitoring and documentation
      a. vital signs
      b. physical signs and symptoms (e.g., motor control, severity of injury)
      c. fall prevention

D. Medical Emergencies
   1. allergic reactions (e.g., contrast media, latex)
   2. cardiac/respiratory arrest (e.g., CPR, AED)
   3. physical injury or trauma
   4. other medical disorders (e.g., seizures, diabetic reactions)

* The abbreviation "e.g.," is used to indicate that examples are listed in parentheses, but that it is not a complete list of all possibilities.

(Patient Care continues on the following page.)

ARRT Content Specifications for the Limited Scope of Practice in Radiography Examination

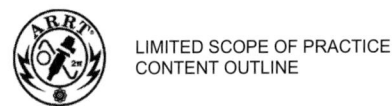

Patient Care (continued)

E. Infection Control
  1. chain of infection (cycle of infection)
     a. pathogen
     b. reservoir
     c. portal of exit
     d. mode of transmission
        1. direct
           a. droplet
           b. direct contact
        2. indirect
           a. airborne
           b. vehicle borne (fomite)
           c. vector borne (mechanical or biological)
     e. portal of entry
     f. susceptible host
  2. asepsis
     a. equipment disinfection
     b. equipment sterilization
     c. medical aseptic technique
     d. sterile technique
  3. CDC Standard Precautions
     a. hand hygiene
     b. use of personal protective equipment (e.g., gloves, gowns, masks)
     c. safe handling of contaminated equipment/surfaces
     d. disposal of contaminated materials
        1. linens
        2. needles
        3. patient supplies
        4. blood and body fluids
  4. transmission-based precautions
     a. contact
     b. droplet
     c. airborne
  5. additional precautions
     a. neutropenic precautions (reverse isolation)
     b. healthcare associated (nosocomial) infections

F. Handling and Disposal of Toxic or Hazardous Material
  1. types of materials
     a. chemicals
  2. safety data sheet (material safety data sheet)

ARRT Content Specifications for the Limited Scope of Practice in Radiography Examination

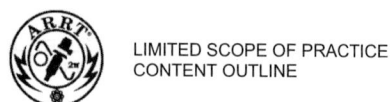
Safety

1. Radiation Physics and Radiobiology

A. Principles of Radiation Physics
   1. x-ray production
     a. source of free electrons
       (e.g., thermionic emission)
     b. acceleration of electrons
     c. focusing of electrons
     d. deceleration of electrons
   2. target interactions
     a. bremsstrahlung
     b. characteristic
   3. x-ray beam
     a. frequency and wavelength
     b. beam characteristics
       1. quality
       2. quantity
       3. primary versus remnant (exit)
     c. inverse square law
     d. fundamental properties
       (e.g., travel in straight lines,
       ionize matter)
   4. photon interactions with matter
     a. photoelectric
     b. Compton
     c. coherent (classical)
     d. attenuation by various tissues
       1. thickness of body part
       2. type of tissue (atomic number)

B. Biological Effects of Radiation
   1. SI units of measurement (NCRP
     Report #160)
     a. absorbed dose (Gy)
     b. dose equivalent (Sv)
     c. exposure (C/kg)
     d. effective dose (Sv)
   2. radiosensitivity
     a. dose-response relationships
     b. relative tissue radiosensitivities
       (e.g., LET, RBE)
     c. cell survival and recovery (LD_{50})
     d. oxygen effect
   3. somatic effects
     a. cells
     b. tissue (e.g., eye, thyroid, breast,
       skin, marrow, gonadal)
     c. embryo and fetus
     d. carcinogenesis
     e. early versus late or acute versus
       chronic
     f. deterministic (tissue reactions)
       versus stochastic
     g. acute radiation syndromes
       1. hemopoietic
       2. gastrointestinal (GI)
       3. central nervous system (CNS)

(Safety continues on the following page.)

4

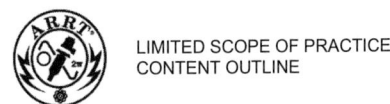
Safety (continued)

2. Radiation Protection

A. Minimizing Patient Exposure
1. exposure factors
   a. kVp
   b. mAs
2. beam restriction
   a. purpose of primary beam restriction
   b. types (e.g., collimators)
3. patient considerations
   a. positioning
   b. communication
   c. pediatric
   d. morbid obesity
4. filtration
   a. effect on skin and organ exposure
   b. effect on average beam energy
   c. NCRP recommendations (NCRP Report #102, minimum filtration in useful beam)
5. radiographic dose documentation
6. image receptors
7. grids
8. dose area product (DAP) meter

B. Personnel Protection (ALARA)*
1. sources of radiation exposure
   a. primary x-ray beam
   b. secondary radiation
      1. scatter
      2. leakage
   c. patient as source
2. basic methods of protection
   a. time
   b. distance
   c. shielding
3. protective devices
   a. types (e.g., aprons, barriers)
   b. attenuation properties
   c. minimum lead equivalent (NCRP Report #102)
4. radiation exposure and monitoring
   a. dosimeters
      1. types
      2. proper use
   b. NCRP recommendations for personnel monitoring (NCRP Report #116)
      1. occupational exposure
      2. public exposure
      3. embryo/fetus exposure
      4. dose equivalent limits
      5. evaluation and maintenance of personnel dosimetry records

* Note: Although it is the responsibility of the individual licensed in limited scope radiography to apply radiation protection principles to minimize bioeffects for both patients and personnel, the ALARA concept is specific to personnel protection and is listed only for that section.

5

353

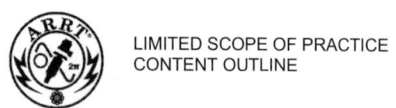
Image Production

1. Image Acquisition and Evaluation

A. Factors Affecting Radiographic Quality
(X indicates topics covered on the examination.)

	1. Receptor Exposure	2. Spatial Resolution	3. Distortion
a. mAs	X		
b. kVp	X		
c. OID		X	X
d. SID	X	X	X
e. focal spot size		X	
f. tube filtration	X		
g. beam restriction	X		
h. motion		X	
i. anode heel effect	X		
j. patient factors (size, pathology)	X	X	X
k. angle (tube, part, or receptor)		X	X

B. Technique Charts
1. anatomically programmed technique
2. fixed versus variable kVp
3. special considerations
   a. casts
   b. pathologic factors
   c. age (e.g., pediatric, geriatric)
   d. body mass index (BMI)
   e. grids
   f. OID

C. Digital Imaging Characteristics
1. spatial resolution
   a. pixel characteristics
      (e.g., size, pitch)
   b. detector element (DEL)
      (e.g., size, pitch, fill factor)
   c. CCD, CMOS (e.g., size, pitch)
   d. sampling frequency (CR)
   e. modulation transfer function (MTF)
2. contrast resolution
   a. bit depth
   b. detective quantum efficiency
      (DQE)
   c. grids
3. image signal
   a. dynamic range
   b. quantum noise (quantum mottle)
   c. signal to noise ratio (SNR)

D. Image Identification
1. methods (e.g., radiographic,
   electronic)
2. legal considerations
   (e.g., patient data, examination data)

E. Criteria for Image Evaluation
1. exposure indicator
2. quantum noise (quantum mottle)
3. gross exposure error (e.g., loss of
   contrast, saturation)
4. spatial resolution
5. distortion (e.g., size, shape)
6. identification markers (e.g.,
   anatomical side, patient, date)
7. image artifacts
8. radiation fog (CR)

(Image Production continues on the following page.)

6

354

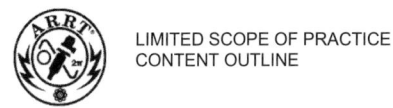
Image Production (continued)

2. Equipment Operation and Quality Assurance

A. Imaging Equipment
1. x-ray generator
   a. basic principles
   b. phase, pulse, and frequency
   c. tube loading
2. components of radiographic unit (fixed or mobile)
   a. operating console
   b. x-ray tube construction
      1. electron source
      2. target materials
      3. induction motor
      4. filtration
   c. automatic exposure control (AEC)
      1. radiation detectors
      2. back-up timer
      3. exposure adjustment (e.g., density, +1 or -2)
      4. minimum response time
   d. manual exposure controls
   e. image receptors
      1. computed radiography
         a. plate (e.g., photo-stimulable phosphor (PSP))
         b. plate reader
      2. digital radiography (DR)
         a. direct conversion
         b. indirect conversion
            1. amorphous silicon (a-Si)
            2. charge coupled device (CCD)
            3. complementary metal oxide semiconductor (CMOS)
   f. beam restriction
3. accessories
   a. stationary grids
   b. Bucky assembly
   c. compensating filters

B. Image Processing and Display
1. raw data (pre-processing)
   a. analog-to-digital converter (ADC)
   b. quantization
   c. corrections (e.g., rescaling, flat fielding, dead pixel correction)
   d. histogram

2. corrected data for processing
   a. grayscale
   b. edge enhancement
   c. equalization
   d. smoothing
3. data for display
   a. values of interest (VOI)
   b. look-up table (LUT)
4. post-processing
   a. brightness
   b. contrast
   c. region of interest (ROI)
   d. electronic cropping or masking
   e. stitching
5. display monitors
   a. viewing conditions (e.g., viewing angle, ambient lighting)
   b. spatial resolution (e.g., pixel size, pixel pitch)
   c. brightness and contrast
6. imaging informatics
   a. information systems (e.g., HIS, RIS, EMR, EHR)
   b. networking
      1. PACS
      2. DICOM
   c. downtime procedures

C. Quality Control of Imaging Equipment and Accessories
1. beam restriction
   a. light field to radiation field alignment
   b. central ray alignment
2. recognition and reporting of malfunctions
3. digital imaging receptor systems
   a. maintenance (e.g., detector calibration, plate reader calibration)
   b. QC tests (e.g., erasure thoroughness, plate uniformity, spatial resolution)
   c. display monitor quality assurance (e.g., grayscale standard display function, luminance)
4. shielding accessories (e.g., testing lead apron, gloves)

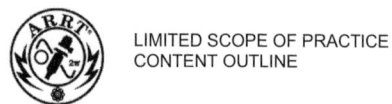
Procedures

The specific positions and projections within each anatomic region that may be covered on the examination are listed in *Attachment A*. A guide to positioning terminology appears in *Attachment B*.

PROCEDURE MODULE [1]		# QUESTIONS PER MODULE [2]	FOCUS OF QUESTIONS [3]
1. Chest			**1. Positioning** (e.g., topographic landmarks, body positions, path of central ray, positioning aids, respiration)
A. Routine		16	
B. Other		4	
	TOTAL	20	emphasis: high
2. Extremities			
A. Lower (toes, foot, calcaneus, ankle, tibia/ fibula, knee/ patella, and femur)		11	**2. Anatomy** (including physiology, basic pathology, and related medical terminology)
B. Upper (fingers, hand, wrist, forearm, elbow, and humerus)		11	emphasis: medium
C. Pectoral Girdle (shoulder, scapula, clavicle, and acromioclavicular joints)		3	**3. Evaluation of displayed anatomical structures** (e.g., patient positioning, tube-part-image receptor alignment)
	TOTAL	25	
3. Skull/Sinuses			
A. Skull		8	emphasis: medium
B. Paranasal Sinuses		8	
C. Facial Bones (orbits, nasal bones)		4	**4. Procedure adaptation** (e.g., body habitus, body mass index, trauma, pathology, age, limited mobility, casts, splints, soft tissue for foreign body, etc.)
	TOTAL	20	
4. Spine			
A. Cervical Spine		8	emphasis: low
B. Thoracic Spine		6	
C. Lumbar Spine		8	**5. Equipment and Accessories** (grids or Bucky, compensating filter, automatic exposure control [AEC], automatic collimation)
D. Sacrum, Coccyx, and Sacroiliac Joints		2	
E. Scoliosis Series		1	emphasis: low
	TOTAL	25	
5. Podiatric			
A. Foot and Toes		14	
B. Ankle		5	
C. Calcaneus (os calcis)		1	
	TOTAL	20	

Notes:

1. Candidates take one or more procedure modules, depending on the type of license they have applied for. Each procedure module has 20 or 25 scored test questions, depending on the module (see chart above). The number of questions <u>within</u> a module should be regarded as approximate values.

2. Each of the procedure modules has five additional unscored questions.

3. The procedure modules may include questions about the five areas listed under *FOCUS OF QUESTIONS* on the right side of the chart. The podiatric module does <u>not</u> include questions from the equipment and accessories section.

8

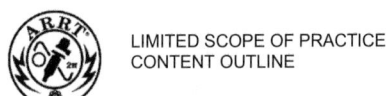

Attachment A
Radiographic Positions and Projections

I. Chest
A. Chest
1. PA or AP upright
2. lateral upright
3. AP Lordotic
4. AP supine
5. lateral decubitus

II. Extremities
A. Toes
1. AP, entire forefoot
2. AP or AP axial toe
3. oblique toe
4. lateral toe
5. sesamoids, tangential
B. Foot
1. AP axial
2. medial oblique
3. lateral oblique
4. lateral
5. AP axial weight bearing
6. lateral weight bearing
C. Calcaneus
1. lateral
2. plantodorsal, axial
3. dorsoplantar, axial
D. Ankle
1. AP
2. mortise
3. lateral
4. medial oblique
5. AP stress
6. AP weight bearing
7. lateral weight bearing
E. Tibia/Fibula
1. AP
2. lateral
F. Knee/patella
1. AP
2. lateral
3. AP weight bearing
4. lateral oblique
5. medial oblique
6. PA axial–intercondylar fossa (Holmblad)
7. PA axial–intercondylar fossa (Camp Coventry)
8. AP axial–intercondylar fossa (Béclère)
9. PA patella
10. Tangential (Merchant)
11. tangential (Settegast)
G. Femur
1. AP
2. lateral
H. Fingers
1. PA entire hand
2. PA finger only
3. lateral
4. medial and/or lateral oblique
5. AP thumb
6. medial oblique thumb
7. lateral thumb
I. Hand
1. PA
2. lateral
3. lateral oblique
J. Wrist
1. PA
2. lateral oblique

3. lateral
4. PA–ulnar deviation
5. PA axial (Stecher)
6. tangential carpal canal (Gaynor-Hart)
K. Forearm
1. AP
2. lateral
L. Elbow
1. AP
2. lateral
3. lateral oblique
4. medial oblique
5. AP partial flexion
6. trauma axial laterals (Coyle)
M. Humerus
1. AP
2. lateral
3. neutral
4. transthoracic lateral
N. Shoulder
1. AP internal and external rotation
2. inferosuperior axial (Lawrence)
3. posterior oblique (Grashey)
4. AP neutral
5. PA oblique (scapular Y)
O. Scapula
1. AP
2. lateral
P. Clavicle
1. AP or PA
2. AP axial
3. PA axial
Q. Acromioclavicular Joints – AP Bilateral With and Without Weights

III. Skull/Sinuses
A. Skull
1. AP axial (Towne)
2. lateral
3. PA axial (Caldwell)
4. PA
5. submentovertex (full basal)
B. Facial Bones
1. lateral
2. parietoacanthial (Waters)
3. PA axial (Caldwell)
4. modified parietoacanthial (modified Waters)
C. Nasal Bones
1. parietoacanthial (Waters)
2. lateral
3. PA axial (Caldwell)
D. Orbits
1. parietoacanthial (Waters)
2. lateral
3. PA axial (Caldwell)
4. modified parietoacanthial (modified Waters)
E. Paranasal Sinuses
1. lateral, horizontal beam
2. PA axial (Caldwell), horizontal beam
3. parietoacanthial (Waters), horizontal beam
4. submentovertex (full basal), horizontal beam

IV. Spine
A. Cervical Spine
1. AP axial
2. AP open mouth
3. lateral
4. PA axial obliques
5. AP axial obliques
6. lateral swimmers
7. lateral flexion and extension
B. Thoracic Spine
1. AP
2. lateral, breathing
3. lateral, expiration
C. Scoliosis Series
1. AP or PA
2. lateral
D. Lumbar Spine
1. AP
2. PA
3. lateral
4. L5-S1 lateral spot
5. posterior oblique
6. anterior oblique
7. AP axial L5-S1
8. AP right and left bending
9. lateral flexion and extension
E. Sacrum and Coccyx
1. AP axial sacrum
2. AP axial coccyx
3. lateral sacrum and coccyx, combined
4. lateral sacrum or coccyx, separate
F. Sacroiliac Joints
1. AP axial
2. posterior oblique
3. anterior oblique

V. Podiatric*
A. Foot and Toes
1. dorsal plantar (DP)
2. medial oblique
3. lateral oblique
4. lateral
5. sesamoidal axial
B. Ankle
1. AP
2. mortise
3. AP medial oblique
4. AP lateral oblique
5. lateral
C. Calcaneus
1. axial calcaneal
2. Harris and Beath (ski-jump)

*weightbearing or non-weightbearing

ARRT Content Specifications for the Limited Scope of Practice in Radiography Examination

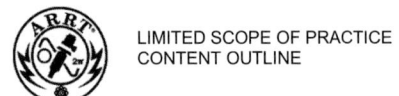
Attachment B
Standard Terminology
for Positioning and Projection

Radiographic View: Describes the body part as seen by the image receptor. Restricted to the discussion of a *radiograph* or *image*.

Radiographic Position: Refers to a specific body position, such as supine, prone, recumbent, erect or Trendelenburg. Restricted to the discussion of the *patient's physical position*.

Radiographic Projection: Restricted to the discussion of the *path of the central ray*.

POSITIONING TERMINOLOGY

A. Lying Down

    1. *supine*   –   lying on the back
    2. *prone*   –   lying face downward
    3. *decubitus*   –   lying down with a horizontal x-ray beam
    4. *recumbent*   –   lying down in any position

B. Erect or Upright

    1. *anterior position*   –   facing the image receptor
    2. *posterior position*   –   facing the radiographic tube

C. Either Upright or Recumbent

    1. oblique torso positions

        a. anterior oblique (facing the image receptor)

           i. *left anterior oblique (LAO)*   body rotated with the left anterior portion closest to the image receptor

           ii. *right anterior oblique (RAO)*   body rotated with the right anterior portion closest to the image receptor

        b. posterior oblique (facing the radiographic tube)

           i. *left posterior oblique (LPO)*   body rotated with the left posterior portion closest to the image receptor

           ii. *right posterior oblique (RPO)*   body rotated with the right posterior portion closest to the image receptor

    2. oblique extremity positions

        a. lateral (external) rotation   outward rotation of the extremity

        b. medial (internal) rotation   inward rotation of the extremity

10

ARRT Content Specifications for the Limited Scope of Practice in Radiography Examination

Anteroposterior Projection

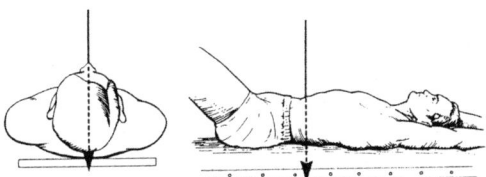

Posteroanterior Projection

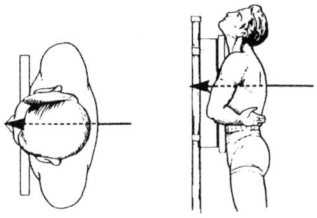

Right Lateral Position

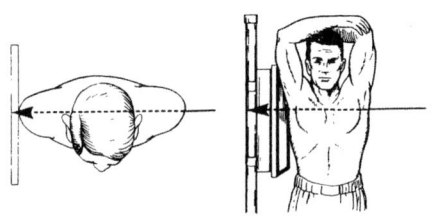

Left Lateral Position

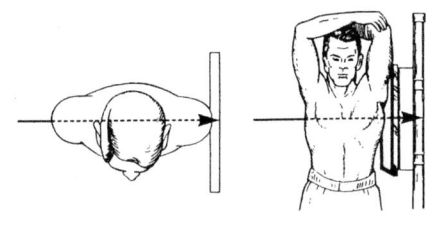

Left Posterior Oblique Position

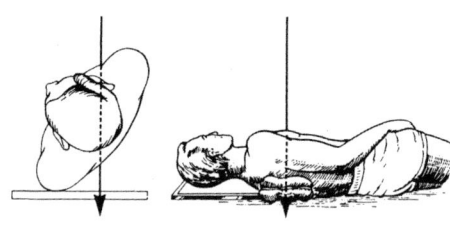

Right Posterior Oblique Position

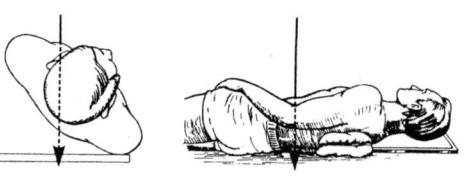

Left Anterior Oblique Position

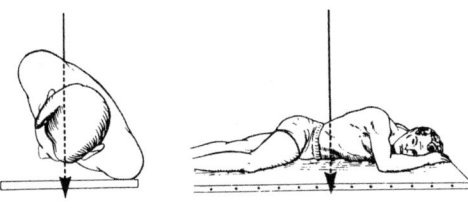

Right Anterior Oblique Position

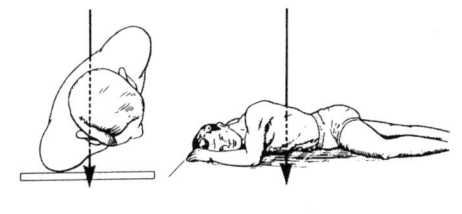

11

359

Simulated Examination for the Limited Scope of Practice in Radiography

CORE MODULE-100 QUESTIONS

Complete this examination in pencil if you plan to take it more than once.

Multiple Choice

Identify the choice that best completes the statement or answers the question.

_____ 1. *Short-term* effects of radiation are typically observed within:
A. 1 day.
B. 3 days.
C. 1 month.
D. 3 months.

_____ 2. Which of the following changes will decrease the patient dose?
A. Using low-mA settings
B. Decreasing the filtration
C. Using high-kVp techniques
D. Using a 36-inch SID

_____ 3. All of the following are true about an individual's personal dosimeter, *except*:
A. should be worn in the region of the collar
B. should be worn inside a lead apron
C. should be worn outside a lead apron
D. should be worn on the anterior surface of the body

_____ 4. What is the primary purpose of using gonad shields during radiography?
A. Reduce the likelihood of genetic effects
B. Reduce the likelihood of somatic effects
C. Protect patient modesty
D. Demonstrate the location of the gonads in the image

_____ 5. Which of the following are types of gonad shields?
1. Aperture
2. Contact
3. Shadow
A. 1 and 2 only
B. 1 and 3 only
C. 2 and 3 only
D. 1, 2, and 3

_____ 6. When should gonad shielding be used?
A. For all patients
B. For all procedures
C. When the gonads are within 10 cm of the radiation field
D. When the gonads are within 5 cm of the radiation field

_____ 7. One of the greatest cause of unnecessary radiation to patients that can be controlled by the limited operator is:
A. patient condition.
B. patient size.
C. repeat exposures.
D. equipment malfunction.

_____ 8. The limited operator can reduce repeat exposures by:
A. accepting marginal images.
B. effective communications
C. increasing the source-image receptor distance (SID).
D. optimizing the kVp.

_____ 9. How does close collimation to only the part of interest minimize patient exposure of x-rays?
A. It increases spatial resolution.
B. It limits the radiation field to the area of interest on the body.
C. It limits the effect of patient motion.
D. It limits repeat exposures.

_____ 10. An equivalent *dose* of 0.350 Sv would be converted to _____ mSv.
A. 3.5
B. 35
C. 350
D. 3500

_____ 11. How does filtration reduce patient exposure?
A. Removes shorter-wavelength photons
B. Removes longer-wavelength photons
C. Reduces the size of the radiation field
D. Reduces the time of exposure

12. What is the National Council on Radiation Protection and Measurements (NCRP) recommendation for the amount of total filtration?
A. 0.5 mm aluminum equivalent (Al equiv)
B. 1.5 mm Al equiv
C. 2.5 mm Al equiv
D. 3.5 mm Al equiv

13. What are the three principal methods used to protect limited operators from unnecessary radiation exposure?
A. Time, distance, and shielding
B. Time, distance, and collimation
C. Distance, collimation, and shielding
D. Time, collimation, and filtration

14. Which of the following is *not* a type of personnel radiation shielding?
A. Apron
B. Glove
C. Thyroid shield
D. Shadow

15. Personnel shielding must be worn on the rare occasion during which the limited operator may need to remain in the radiographic room during an exposure to assist the patient in maintaining the proper position. What is the source of the greatest radiation hazard under this circumstance?
A. Off-focus radiation
B. Leakage radiation
C. Scattered radiation from the patient
D. Backscatter radiation from the IR

16. What is the term for radiation that escapes from the x-ray tube housing?
A. Scattered radiation
B. Off-focus radiation
C. Primary radiation
D. Leakage radiation

17. An *erythema* can develop on a patient if the radiation dose to the skin reaches:
A. 100 mSv.
B. 1000 mSv.
C. 2000 mSv.
D. 2500 mSv.

18. Distance, as a method used to limit operator exposure, means that:
A. the operator should maximize the distance from the source during an exposure.
B. the operator should minimize the distance from the source during an exposure.
C. the operator should maximize the distance from the patient during an exposure.
D. the operator should minimize the distance from the patient during an exposure.

19. Shielding worn for personnel protection is designed to attenuate what source of exposure?
A. Primary radiation
B. Off-focus radiation
C. Leakage radiation
D. Scatter radiation

20. Patient dose in radiography is most often calculated according to the x-ray exposure level at the:
A. skin.
B. gonads.
C. collar.
D. exit of the body part.

21. What is the recommended placement for a personnel dosimeter on the body of the limited operator?
A. Worn in the region of the waist on the anterior surface of the body and outside the lead apron, if worn.
B. Worn in the region of the waist on the posterior surface of the body and inside the lead apron, if worn.
C. Worn in the region of the collar on the posterior surface of the body and inside the lead apron, if worn.
D. Worn in the region of the collar on the anterior surface of the body and outside the lead apron, if worn.

22. What is the NCRP recommended annual effective dose limit for occupational exposure?
A. 0.5 mSv
B. 5 mSv
C. 50 mSv
D. 500 mSv

23. What is the NCRP recommended monthly effective (or equivalent) dose limit to the fetus for a pregnant worker?
A. 0.5 mSv
B. 5 mSv
C. 50 mSv
D. 500 mSv

24. In diagnostic radiology, we are most concerned about which effect of radiation exposure?
A. Somatic effect
B. Genetic effect
C. Long-term effect
D. Short-term effect

25. What is the SI radiation unit used to express radiation intensity in air?
   A. Air kerma
   B. Watt
   C. Ohm
   D. Roentgen

26. The SI unit used to report occupational effective dose to radiation workers is the:
   A. Air kerma
   B. rad.
   C. Gray.
   D. Sievert.

27. What is the SI radiation unit of absorbed dose?
   A. Rad
   B. Sievert
   C. Gray
   D. Air kerma

28. According to the Bergonié-Tribondeau law, which of the following types of cells are most radiosensitive?
   A. Brain cells
   B. Embryonic tissue cells
   C. Cells of the gastric mucosa
   D. Skin cells

29. Which type of x-ray photon interaction with the body is primarily responsible for the radiation dose absorbed by the patient?
   A. Compton
   B. Photoelectric
   C. Coherent
   D. Characteristic

30. What is the NCRP (report #102) recommendation for lead equivalency of aprons used for personnel protection?
   A. 0.05 mm
   B. 0.25 mm
   C. 0.5 mm
   D. 0.75 mm

31. What is erythema, as it relates to radiation exposure?
   A. Loss of hair caused by a high radiation dose
   B. Loss of hair caused by a long-term low radiation dose
   C. Reddening of the skin caused by a high radiation dose
   D. Reddening of the skin caused by a long-term low radiation dose

32. What is the guiding philosophy of radiation protection?
   A. ALARMA-as long as radiographs are made accessible
   B. ALARA-as low as reasonably achievable
   C. ALAIS-as long as ionizations are small
   D. ALAP-as low as possible

33. Which of the following statements reflects current scientific opinion regarding the effects of high levels of ionizing radiation?
   A. It is carcinogenic after a certain number of examinations have been performed.
   B. Spontaneous abortion may occur if the patient is pregnant.
   C. Depression of the white blood cell count is followed by acute gastrointestinal distress.
   D. There is an increased risk of cancer, leukemia, birth defects, and cataracts.

34. Which of the following technique changes will decrease patient dose?
   1. Increasing the mAs by 15%
   2. Increasing the kVp using the 15% rule, while decreasing the mAs to compensate
   3. Using fixed kVp in the technique chart
   A. 1 and 2 only
   B. 1 and 3 only
   C. 2 and 3 only
   D. 1, 2, and 3

35. When radiation exposure occurs during pregnancy, the greatest risk of birth defects occurs when the exposure:
   1. exceeds 150 mGy to the uterus.
   2. occurs within the first trimester of pregnancy.
   3. occurs within the third trimester of pregnancy.
   A. 1 and 2 only
   B. 1 and 3 only
   C. 2 and 3 only
   D. 1, 2, and 3

36. At what kVp levels do Compton interactions occur?
   A. They do not occur with x-ray exposure.
   B. They occur below the diagnostic radiology kVp range.
   C. They occur above the diagnostic radiology kVp range.
   D. They occur throughout the diagnostic radiology kVp range.

_____ 37. What is the principal source of scatter radiation in radiography?
A. The tube housing
B. The patient
C. The IR
D. The collimator

_____ 38. What are the four essential elements required for x-ray production?
A. A target, a vacuum, an electron source, and a high potential difference
B. A target, an electron source, an inert gas environment, and a high potential difference
C. An electron source, a magnetic field, a resistance-free path, and a target
D. An electron source, an electric field, a circuit, and a target

_____ 39. The greatest portion of the x-ray beam is made up of:
A. characteristic radiation.
B. bremsstrahlung radiation.
C. electrons.
D. heat.

_____ 40. The penetrating power of the x-ray beam is controlled by varying the:
A. anode angle.
B. anode speed.
C. milliamperage (mA).
D. kilovoltage (kVp).

_____ 41. Which of the following functions involve the autotransformer?
A. kVp selection
B. mA selection
C. Exposure time selection
D. Automatic exposure control

_____ 42. What is the IR that is used for computed radiography?
A. Direct-conversion flat panel detector
B. Indirect-conversion flat panel detector
C. Rare earth intensifying screen
D. Photostimulable phosphor (PSP) plate

_____ 43. Nearly all new x-ray machines manufactured today use _____ generators.
A. single-phase
B. three-phase, six-pulse
C. three-phase, 12-pulse
D. high-frequency

_____ 44. The target of the x-ray tube is made of:
A. tungsten.
B. glass.
C. stainless steel.
D. fluorescent phosphors.

_____ 45. What is the standard control limit for the field light to radiation field alignment test?
A. Exact alignment
B. ±1% of SID
C. ±2% of SID
D. ±5% of SID

_____ 46. What is the standard control limit for the beam (central ray) alignment test?
A. Exact alignment
B. Within 1 degree of perpendicular
C. Within 2 degrees of perpendicular
D. Within 5 degrees of perpendicular

_____ 47. How often should lead aprons and gloves be checked for cracks or holes?
A. Every 3 months
B. Every 6 months
C. Every 9 months
D. Every 12 months

_____ 48. How can detector fog be prevented when using computed radiography cassettes?
A. Use the maximum SID.
B. Apply close collimation.
C. Protect the cassette before and after exposure.
D. Select the optimum kVp.

_____ 49. Which of the following, if adjusted as a single adjustment by itself, will result in increased image receptor exposure?
1. Increased mA
2. Increased exposure time
3. Increased kVp
A. 1 and 2 only
B. 1 and 3 only
C. 2 and 3 only
D. 1, 2, and 3

_____ 50. If the radiographic image is overexposed (exposure indicator out of range), which of the following changes in exposure factors should be used to correct the problem?
A. Decrease the kVp.
B. Increase the kVp.
C. Adjust the density control using a plus (+) setting
D. Adjust the density control using a minus (−) setting

_____ 51. The relationship between SID and beam intensity is expressed in the:
A. proportional square law.
B. inverse square law.
C. reciprocity law.
D. target-distance law.

363

52. What are the four prime factors of radiographic exposure?
    A. mAs, kVp, SID, and filtration
    B. SID, density, contrast, and mAs
    C. Receptor exposure, contrast, spatial resolution, and distortion.
    D. Receptor exposure, contrast, distortion, and distance

53. Contrast is primarily controlled by the:
    A. mA.
    B. exposure time.
    C. Processing algorithm.
    D. mAs.

54. Scatter radiation fog affects radiographic quality by causing:
    A. underexposure.
    B. decreased contrast.
    C. increased contrast.
    D. decreased density.

55. A change from the small focal spot to the large focal spot will result in:
    A. decreased spatial resolution.
    B. magnification.
    C. distortion.
    D. increased contrast.

56. An increase in object-image receptor distance (OID) will result in:
    A. increased magnification.
    B. increased image sharpness.
    C. loss of contrast.
    D. increased radiographic density.

57. Motion of the patient, the tube, or the IR during the exposure will result in decreased:
    A. contrast.
    B. distortion.
    C. receptor exposure.
    D. spatial resolution.

58. What does quantum mottle (noise) look like on a radiographic image?
    A. Large light and dark spots
    B. Finely speckled or grainy areas
    C. Alternating light and dark lines
    D. Overall grayness

59. Quantum mottle with a digital imaging system is caused by:
    A. not having a fixed kVp technique chart
    B. the mAs or kVp are set too low.
    C. the use of a low ratio grid.
    D. the collimation being set too wide.

60. Which of the following will increase spatial resolution?
    1. Increase in SID
    2. Increase in OID
    3. Decrease in focal spot size
    A. 1 and 2 only
    B. 1 and 3 only
    C. 2 and 3 only
    D. 1, 2, and 3

61. What is the appearance of a high signal-to-noise ratio (SNR) image?
    A. Highly detailed, with very little quantum mottle
    B. Very grainy and poorly detailed
    C. High contrast and very grainy
    D. Very low contrast with few image details seen

62. All of the following are photographic or geometric factors that affect how the x-ray image looks on the monitor, *except*:
    A. kilovoltage
    B. contrast
    C. density
    D. distortion

63. What is the appearance of a low signal-to-noise ratio (SNR) image?
    A. Highly detailed, with very little quantum mottle
    B. Very grainy and poorly detailed
    C. High contrast and very grainy
    D. Very low contrast with few image details seen

64. During digital image processing, electronic masking should *not* be used to replace:
    A. proper kVp selection.
    B. proper mAs selection.
    C. appropriate SID.
    D. proper radiographic collimation.

65. Which of the following is *not* a component of a computed radiography plate reader?
    A. Laser
    B. Analog-to-digital (light to electronic signal) converter
    C. High-intensity eraser light
    D. Developing solution

66. What conditions are most important for optimum viewing of radiographic images?
    A. Low room temperature
    B. High room humidity
    C. Low room light level
    D. Bright room light level

67. Images on a radiograph that are not a part of the intended image (e.g., jewelry, bra hooks, etc.) are called:
    A. fog.
    B. ghosts.
    C. phantoms.
    D. artifacts.

68. If the amount of irradiated tissue increases, what happens to scatter radiation fog?
    A. There is not enough information provided to answer the question.
    B. Scatter radiation fog increases.
    C. Scatter radiation fog decreases.
    D. Scatter radiation fog is not affected by the amount of tissue irradiated.

69. The most effective and practical way to reduce scatter radiation fog on a radiograph is to:
    A. decrease the OID.
    B. decrease the SID.
    C. increase the kVp.
    D. use a grid

70. As a general rule, a grid should be employed when the part thickness is greater than:
    A. 4 cm.
    B. 12 cm.
    C. 18 cm.
    D. 12 inches.

71. Technique charts are based on patient part measurements obtained using an x-ray caliper and are expressed as:
    A. circumference in inches.
    B. thickness in centimeters.
    C. diameter in millimeters.
    D. depth in inches.

72. Which of the following pathologic conditions would require a decrease in exposure?
    1. Multiple myeloma
    2. Emphysema
    3. Osteoporosis
    A. 1 and 2 only
    B. 1 and 3 only
    C. 2 and 3 only
    D. 1, 2, and 3

73. How will the anode heel effect, if present, be seen on an image?
    A. Higher contrast on the anode end than on the cathode end.
    B. Lower contrast on the anode end than on the cathode end.
    C. Darker on the anode end than on the cathode end.
    D. Lighter on the anode end than on the cathode end.

74. Which radiographic quality factor is most affected by angulation of the central ray, part, or IR?
    A. Receptor exposure
    B. Contrast
    C. Spatial resolution
    D. Distortion

75. Which of the following is NOT related to spatial resolution in digital radiography systems?
    A. Pixel size.
    B. Detector element size.
    C. Matrix size.
    D. Bit depth.

76. A characteristic of the imaging plate (IP) is that it will absorb low-energy scatter radiation. This will result in:
    A. deal pixels
    B. unwanted radiation fog on the image
    C. increased contrast in the image
    D. an increased fill factor

77. The SMPTE or AAPM test pattern used to check the x-ray monitor can detect which of the following problems?
    1. dynamic range
    2. geometric distortion
    3. spatial resolution
    A. 1 and 2
    B. 1 and 3
    C. 2 and 3
    D. 1, 2, and 3

78. When viewing a digital image on a monitor, how do you determine if the proper mAs was selected?
    A. Evaluate the image brightness.
    B. Evaluate the image contrast.
    C. Evaluate the image distortion.
    D. Evaluate the exposure index value.

79. Which of the following will result in an image with poor spatial resolution?
    A. IR exposure with collimation wider than needed for the particular anatomic structures
    B. IR exposure with mAs higher than needed for the particular anatomic structures
    C. IR exposure with a kVp higher than needed for the particular anatomic structures
    D. Patient motion

80. Which of the following will result in an image with excessive magnification of image structures?
    A. A kVp higher than needed for the particular anatomic structures
    B. An SID greater than recommended for a particular body part
    C. An OID greater than recommended for a particular body part
    D. A mAs higher than needed for the particular anatomic structures

81. Which of the following will result in an image with excessive distortion of anatomic structures?
    A. Improper central ray angulation for the selected radiographic projection
    B. Use of an 8:1 grid with the mAs set for a 12:1 grid
    C. IR exposure at an SID greater than recommended for a particular body part
    D. IR exposure with the mAs higher than needed for the particular anatomic structures

82. Which of the following is NOT a type of DR image receptor?
    A. Photostimulable phosphor plate
    B. Flat panel detector
    C. Charged coupled device (CCD)
    D. Complementary metal oxide semiconductor (CMOS)

83. What does the acronym PACS stand for?
    A. Patient Archival and Communication System
    B. Picture Archiving and Communication System
    C. Product Advertising and Comparison System
    D. Patient Administration and Counseling System

84. Which of the following would be a violation of patient confidentiality?
    A. A limited operator discusses a patient's existing pathology with a radiographer to get assistance in setting technical factors.
    B. A limited operator talks to his or her friend during lunch about a patient's imaging procedure.
    C. A radiographer asks if a patient is pregnant before an acute abdominal series.
    D. A transporter tells the limited operator that the patient complained of dizziness while riding in the wheelchair to the x-ray department.

85. Which of the following are true regarding informed consent?
    1. Informed consent may be revoked at any time.
    2. The patient must be legally competent to sign.
    3. The patient may sign an incomplete form and the blanks may be filled in later by the physician.
    A. 1 and 2 only
    B. 1 and 3 only
    C. 2 and 3 only
    D. 1, 2, and 3

86. A limited operator innocently commits an error as a result of following the orders of his or her employer, a physician. The employer may be held responsible according to the:
    A. American Society of Radiologic Technologists code of ethics.
    B. rule of professional responsibility.
    C. doctrine of respondeat superior.
    D. doctrine of non compos mentis.

87. Communication has been "validated" when the speaker has:
    A. spoken clearly.
    B. received a response from the listener that demonstrates comprehension.
    C. presented the information accurately.
    D. reviewed the material.

88. Which of the following is *not* a form of nonverbal communication?
    A. Speaking
    B. Touching
    C. Eye contact
    D. Facial expression

89. Mrs. Elizabeth Dunbar is 86 years old and a bit confused. She is most likely to respond appropriately if you address her as:
    A. Betty.
    B. Honey.
    C. Mrs. Dunbar.
    D. Elizabeth.

90. Which of the following are correct statements of proper body mechanics?
    1. Use a broad stance.
    2. Turn and lift using your back muscles.
    3. Carry heavy objects close to your body.
    A. 1 and 2 only
    B. 1 and 3 only
    C. 2 and 3 only
    D. 1, 2, and 3

91. What type of disease transmission is possible when the limited operator does not clean the Bucky device after performing an examination on a patient with influenza?
   A. Vector transmission
   B. Direct contact transmission
   C. Indirect contact or fomite transmission
   D. Airborne transmission

92. Standard precautions involve the use of barriers whenever contact is anticipated with:
   1. blood.
   2. body fluids.
   3. mucous membranes.
   A. 1 and 2 only
   B. 1 and 3 only
   C. 2 and 3 only
   D. 1, 2, and 3

93. The process of reducing the probability that infectious organisms will be transmitted to a susceptible individual is called:
   A. sepsis.
   B. asepsis.
   C. inoculation.
   D. vaccination.

94. A health care worker's single best protection against disease is:
   A. frequent hand washing.
   B. vaccination.
   C. barrier techniques.
   D. protective masks.

95. A limited operator who does not change linens between patients is:
   A. providing an opportunity for fomite transmission.
   B. saving money on laundry expenses.
   C. making wise decisions, as long as there are no stains on the linens.
   D. increasing productivity by saving time between patients.

96. What is anaphylaxis?
   A. The absence of a pain response
   B. A severe allergic reaction
   C. Complete unconsciousness
   D. Inability to breathe

97. What is the basic life support system used to ventilate the lungs and circulate the blood in the event of cardiac or respiratory arrest?
   A. Cardiac tamponade
   B. AED
   C. CPR
   D. ACLS

98. When a patient in cardiac arrest presents with a rapid, weak, and ineffective heartbeat, what device is used to return the heart to a normal rhythm?
   A. Cardiac tamponade
   B. AED
   C. CPR
   D. ACLS

99. Which of the following vital signs can be assessed without touching the patient?
   A. Pulse
   B. Respiration
   C. Blood pressure
   D. Temperature

100. What is the most common site for palpation of a patient's pulse?
   A. Carotid artery
   B. Apex of the heart
   C. Dorsalis pedis
   D. Radial artery at the wrist

Simulated Examination for the Limited Scope of Practice in Radiography–Core Module

Answer Section

Multiple Choice

1.	ANS: D	REF: Ch. 11	OBJ: exam spec Safety	TOP: radiation biology
2.	ANS: C	REF: Ch. 11	OBJ: exam spec Safety	TOP: patient exposure
3.	ANS: B	REF: Ch. 11	OBJ: exam spec Image Production	TOP: imaging equipment
4.	ANS: A	REF: Ch. 11	OBJ: exam spec Safety	TOP: patient exposure
5.	ANS: C	REF: Ch. 11	OBJ: exam spec Safety	TOP: patient exposure
6.	ANS: D	REF: Ch. 11	OBJ: exam spec Safety	TOP: patient exposure

7.	ANS: C	REF: Ch. 11	OBJ: exam spec Safety	TOP: patient exposure
8.	ANS: B	REF: Ch. 11	OBJ: exam spec Safety	TOP: patient exposure
9.	ANS: B	REF: Ch. 11	OBJ: exam spec Safety	TOP: patient exposure
10.	ANS: C	REF: Ch. 2	OBJ: exam spec Safety	TOP: patient exposure
11.	ANS: B	REF: Ch. 5	OBJ: exam spec Safety	TOP: patient exposure
12.	ANS: C	REF: Ch. 5	OBJ: exam spec Safety	TOP: patient exposure
13.	ANS: A	REF: Ch. 11	OBJ: exam spec Safety	TOP: personnel protection
14.	ANS: D	REF: Ch. 11	OBJ: exam spec Safety	TOP: personnel protection
15.	ANS: C	REF: Ch. 11	OBJ: exam spec Safety	TOP: personnel protection
16.	ANS: D	REF: Ch. 11	OBJ: exam spec Safety	TOP: personnel protection
17.	ANS: C	REF: Ch. 11	OBJ: exam spec Safety	TOP: personnel protection
18.	ANS: A	REF: Ch. 11	OBJ: exam spec Safety	TOP: personnel protection
19.	ANS: D	REF: Ch. 11	OBJ: exam spec Safety	TOP: personnel protection
20.	ANS: A	REF: Ch. 11	OBJ: exam spec Safety	TOP: radiation exposure/monitoring
21.	ANS: D	REF: Ch. 11	OBJ: exam spec Safety	TOP: radiation exposure/monitoring
22.	ANS: C	REF: Ch. 11	OBJ: exam spec Safety	TOP: radiation exposure/monitoring
23.	ANS: A	REF: Ch. 11	OBJ: exam spec Safety	TOP: radiation exposure/monitoring
24.	ANS: C	REF: Ch. 11	OBJ: exam spec Safety	TOP: radiation exposure/monitoring
25.	ANS: A	REF: Ch. 11	OBJ: exam spec Safety	TOP: radiation exposure/monitoring
26.	ANS: D	REF: Ch. 11	OBJ: exam spec Safety	TOP: radiation exposure/monitoring
27.	ANS: C	REF: Ch. 11	OBJ: exam spec Safety	TOP: radiation exposure/monitoring
28.	ANS: B	REF: Ch. 11	OBJ: exam spec Safety	TOP: radiation biology
29.	ANS: B	REF: Ch. 11	OBJ: exam spec Safety	TOP: radiation biology
30.	ANS: C	REF: Ch. 11	OBJ: exam spec Safety	TOP: personnel protection
31.	ANS: C	REF: Ch. 11	OBJ: exam spec Safety	TOP: radiation biology
32.	ANS: B	REF: Ch. 11	OBJ: exam spec Safety	TOP: patient exposure
33.	ANS: D	REF: Ch. 11	OBJ: exam spec Safety	TOP: radiation biology
34.	ANS: C	REF: Ch. 11	OBJ: exam spec Safety	TOP: patient exposure
35.	ANS: A	REF: Ch. 11	OBJ: exam spec Safety	TOP: radiation biology
36.	ANS: D	REF: Ch. 9	OBJ: exam spec Safety	TOP: radiation biology
37.	ANS: B	REF: Ch. 9	OBJ: exam spec Safety	TOP: personnel protection
38.	ANS: A	REF: Ch. 5	OBJ: exam spec Image Production	TOP: radiation physics
39.	ANS: B	REF: Ch. 5	OBJ: exam spec Image Production	TOP: radiation physics
40.	ANS: D	REF: Ch. 5	OBJ: exam spec Image Production	TOP: radiation physics
41.	ANS: A	REF: Ch. 6	OBJ: exam spec Image Production	TOP: imaging equipment
42.	ANS: D	REF: Ch. 6	OBJ: exam spec Image Production	TOP: imaging equipment
43.	ANS: D	REF: Ch. 6	OBJ: exam spec Image Production	TOP: imaging equipment
44.	ANS: A	REF: Ch. 6	OBJ: exam spec Image Production	TOP: imaging equipment
45.	ANS: C	REF: Ch. 9	OBJ: exam spec Image Production	TOP: equipment quality control
46.	ANS: B	REF: Ch. 9	OBJ: exam spec Image Production	TOP: equipment quality control
47.	ANS: B	REF: Ch. 11	OBJ: exam spec Image Production	TOP: equipment quality control
48.	ANS: C	REF: Ch. 8	OBJ: exam spec Image Production	TOP: equipment quality control
49.	ANS: D	REF: Ch. 7	OBJ: exam spec Image Production	TOP: technical factor selection
50.	ANS: D	REF: Ch. 7	OBJ: exam spec Image Production	TOP: technical factor selection
51.	ANS: B	REF: Ch. 7	OBJ: exam spec Image Production	TOP: technical factor selection
52.	ANS: A	REF: Ch. 7	OBJ: exam spec Image Production	TOP: technical factor selection
53.	ANS: C	REF: Ch. 7	OBJ: exam spec Image Production	TOP: technical factor selection

54.	ANS: B	REF: Ch. 7	OBJ: exam spec Image Production	TOP: image evaluation
55.	ANS: A	REF: Ch. 7	OBJ: exam spec Image Production	TOP: technical factor selection
56.	ANS: A	REF: Ch. 7	OBJ: exam spec Image Production	TOP: technical factor selection
57.	ANS: D	REF: Ch. 7	OBJ: exam spec Image Production	TOP: technical factor selection
58.	ANS: B	REF: Ch. 7	OBJ: exam spec Image Production	TOP: image evaluation
59.	ANS: B	REF: Ch. 7	OBJ: exam spec Image Production	TOP: technical factor selection
60.	ANS: B	REF: Ch. 7	OBJ: exam spec Image Production	TOP: technical factor selection
61.	ANS: A	REF: Ch. 8	OBJ: exam spec Image Production	TOP: technical factor selection
62.	ANS: A	REF: Ap. H	OBJ: exam spec Image Production	TOP: technical factor selection
63.	ANS: C	REF: Ap. I	OBJ: exam spec Image Production	TOP: technical factor selection
64.	ANS: D	REF: Ch. 8	OBJ: exam spec Image Production	TOP: image processing/quality control
65.	ANS: D	REF: Ch. 8	OBJ: exam spec Image Production	TOP: image processing/quality control
66.	ANS: C	REF: Ch. 8	OBJ: exam spec Image Production	TOP: image processing/quality control
67.	ANS: D	REF: Ap. I	OBJ: exam spec Image Production	TOP: image processing/quality control
68.	ANS: B	REF: Ch. 9	OBJ: exam spec Image Production	TOP: technical factor selection
69.	ANS: D	REF: Ch. 9	OBJ: exam spec Image Production	TOP: technical factor selection
70.	ANS: B	REF: Ch. 9	OBJ: exam spec Image Productionj	TOP: technical factor selection
71.	ANS: B	REF: Ch. 10	OBJ: exam spec Image Production	TOP: technical factor selection
72.	ANS: D	REF: Ch. 10	OBJ: exam spec Image Production	TOP: technical factor selection
73.	ANS: D	REF: Ch. 5	OBJ: exam spec Image Production	TOP: technical factor selection
74.	ANS: D	REF: Ch. 7	OBJ: exam spec Image Production	TOP: technical factor selection
75.	ANS: D	REF: Ch. 19	OBJ: exam spec Image Production	TOP: digital imaging characteristics
76.	ANS: B	REF: Ch. 7	OBJ: exam spec Image Production	TOP: digital imaging characteristics
77.	ANS: C	REF: Ch. 7	OBJ: exam spec Image Production	TOP: digital imaging characteristics
78.	ANS: D	REF: Ch. 9	OBJ: exam spec Image Production	TOP: image evaluation
79.	ANS: D	REF: Ch. 7	OBJ: exam spec Image Production	TOP: image evaluation
80.	ANS: C	REF: Ch. 7	OBJ: exam spec Image Production	TOP: image evaluation
81.	ANS: A	REF: Ch. 7	OBJ: exam spec Image Production	TOP: image evaluation
82.	ANS: A	REF: Ch. 7	OBJ: exam spec Image Production	TOP: components of digital imaging
83.	ANS: B	REF: Ch. 7	OBJ: exam spec Image Production	TOP: components of digital imaging
84.	ANS: B	REF: Ch. 20	OBJ: exam spec Patient Care	TOP: ethics/legal aspects
85.	ANS: A	REF: Ch. 20	OBJ: exam spec Patient Care	TOP: ethics/legal aspects
86.	ANS: C	REF: Ch. 20	OBJ: exam spec Patient Care	TOP: ethics/legal aspects
87.	ANS: B	REF: Ch. 20	OBJ: exam spec Patient Care	TOP: interpersonal communications
88.	ANS: A	REF: Ch. 20	OBJ: exam spec Patient Care	TOP: interpersonal communications
89.	ANS: C	REF: Ch. 20	OBJ: exam spec Patient Care	TOP: interpersonal communications
90.	ANS: B	REF: Ch. 20	OBJ: exam spec Patient Care	TOP: physical assistance/transfer
91.	ANS: C	REF: Ch. 21	OBJ: exam spec Patient Care	TOP: infection control
92.	ANS: D	REF: Ch. 21	OBJ: exam spec Patient Care	TOP: infection control
93.	ANS: B	REF: Ch. 21	OBJ: exam spec Patient Care	TOP: infection control
94.	ANS: A	REF: Ch. 21	OBJ: exam spec Patient Care	TOP: infection control
95.	ANS: A	REF: Ch. 21	OBJ: exam spec Patient Care	TOP: infection control
96.	ANS: B	REF: Ch. 22	OBJ: exam spec Patient Care	TOP: medical emergencies
97.	ANS: C	REF: Ch. 22	OBJ: exam spec Patient Care	TOP: medical emergencies
98.	ANS: B	REF: Ch. 22	OBJ: exam spec Patient Care	TOP: medical emergencies
99.	ANS: B	REF: Ch. 22	OBJ: exam spec Patient Care	TOP: physical assistance/transfer
100.	ANS: D	REF: Ch. 22	OBJ: exam spec Patient Care	TOP: physical assistance/transfer

CHEST MODULE – 20 QUESTIONS

Complete this examination in pencil if you plan to take it
more than once.

Multiple Choice

*Identify the choice that best completes the statement or
answers the question.*

_____ 1. Refer to the diagram. What is the projection?

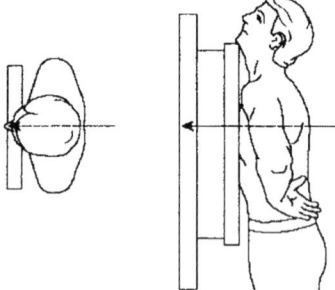

A. Tangential
B. Lateral
C. Posteroanterior (PA)
D. Anteroposterior (AP)

_____ 2. What structure separates the thoracic cavity
from the abdominal cavity?
A. The aortic arch
B. The parietal membrane
C. The visceral membrane
D. The diaphragm

_____ 3. Which of the following organs are found
within the mediastinum?
1. Lungs
2. Heart
3. Trachea
A. 1 and 2 only
B. 1 and 3 only
C. 2 and 3 only
D. 1, 2, and 3

_____ 4. Three lobes are present in which lung(s)?
A. The right lung
B. The left lung
C. Both lungs

_____ 5. What is the name of the upper portion of the
lung?
A. Costophrenic recess
B. Costovertebral angle
C. Apex
D. Base

_____ 6. The inferior lateral corners of the lungs,
visible on a PA chest radiograph, are called
the:
A. hila.
B. apices.
C. cardiophrenic angles.
D. costophrenic angles.

_____ 7. How many ribs can be counted superior to
the diaphragm if a full inspiration has been
achieved?
A. 7 ribs
B. 8 ribs
C. 8 to 10 ribs
D. 10 ribs

_____ 8. What is the purpose of the 72-inch SID
used for chest radiography?
A. Allows more room for accurate patient
positioning
B. Reduces patient dose
C. Minimizes magnification of the heart
shadow
D. Minimizes demonstration of the scapula
in the lungs

_____ 9. Which of the following describe the
importance of using an upright position for
chest radiography?
1. Demonstrates air-fluid levels.
2. Allows maximum lung expansion.
3. Minimizes magnification of the heart.
A. 1 and 2 only
B. 1 and 3 only
C. 2 and 3 only
D. 1, 2, and 3

_____ 10. In chest radiography, which body habitus is
best imaged by placing the 14- × 17-inch
(35- × 43-cm) IR crosswise in the upright
grid cabinet?
A. Sthenic
B. Asthenic
C. Hyposthenic
D. Hypersthenic

_____ 11. Which of the following techniques is
desirable for chest radiography?
A. High kilovoltage (kVp), high
milliamperage (mA), and short exposure
time
B. Low kVp and 40-inch SID
C. Low kVp, long exposure time, and
"breathing technique"
D. High milliampere-seconds (mAs) and
low kVp

12. What is the purpose of rotating the patient's shoulders anteriorly for the PA projection of the chest?
    A. This motion rotates the scapulae out of the lungs.
    B. This motion reduces magnification of the heart shadow.
    C. This motion makes the position more comfortable for the patient.
    D. This motion places the coronal plane parallel to the upright grid cabinet.

13. Where does the central ray enter the patient for the upright, PA projection of the chest?
    A. Midsagittal plane at the level of T7
    B. Midcoronal plane at the level of T7
    C. Midsagittal plane at the level of the iliac crests
    D. Midcoronal plane at the level of the iliac crests

14. What is the proper placement of the arms for the upright lateral projection of the chest?
    A. Backs of the hands on the hips with the shoulders rolled anteriorly
    B. Arms raised over the head with the hands grasping opposite elbows
    C. Arms abducted from the thorax
    D. Arms adducted from the thorax

15. What are the proper patient instructions for the PA projection of the chest?
    A. Stop breathing after the second deep inspiration.
    B. Stop breathing after deep inspiration.
    C. Stop breathing after expiration.
    D. Breathe slowly and evenly.

16. Lateral projections of the chest are taken with the left side against the IR because:
    A. lung pathology is more common on the left side.
    B. it is conventional to have a routine standard, and the left has been established as the standard.
    C. magnification of the cardiac silhouette is reduced with the left side nearer the IR.
    D. the right hilum provides high-contrast details that may be confusing.

17. How much should the central ray be angled cephalad for an AP axial projection of the chest if the patient cannot assume the lordotic position?
    A. No angle is needed
    B. 10 degrees
    C. 15 degrees
    D. 25 degrees

18. Which chest projection and position are needed to demonstrate free pleural fluid along the lung or pleura??
    A. AP, upright
    B. PA, recumbent
    C. AP, lordotic
    D. AP, lateral decubitus

19. Pulmonary effusion is:
    A. a bacterial infection of the lung
    B. inhalation of irritating dust
    C. a collection of fluid in the pleural cavity
    D. air escaping from a collapsed lung

20. Why is a grid used for routine chest radiography?
    A. To reduce scatter fog caused by use of a high kVp
    B. To reduce the patient dose by filtration
    C. To reduce magnification caused by an increased SID
    D. To increase the recorded detail

Simulated Examination for the Limited Scope of Practice in Radiography–Chest Module

Answer Section

Multiple Choice

1. ANS: C   REF: Ch. 12   OBJ: exam spec 1. Chest   TOP: routine chest positioning
2. ANS: D   REF: Ch. 16   OBJ: exam spec 1. Chest   TOP: chest anatomy
3. ANS: C   REF: Ch. 16   OBJ: exam spec 1. Chest   TOP: chest anatomy
4. ANS: A   REF: Ch. 16   OBJ: exam spec 1. Chest   TOP: chest anatomy
5. ANS: C   REF: Ch. 16   OBJ: exam spec 1. Chest   TOP: chest anatomy
6. ANS: D   REF: Ch. 16   OBJ: exam spec 1. Chest   TOP: chest anatomy
7. ANS: D   REF: Ch. 16   OBJ: exam spec 1. Chest   TOP: routine chest positioning
8. ANS: C   REF: Ch. 16   OBJ: exam spec 1. Chest   TOP: routine chest positioning
9. ANS: D   REF: Ch. 16   OBJ: exam spec 1. Chest   TOP: routine chest positioning
10. ANS: D   REF: Ch. 16   OBJ: exam spec 1. Chest   TOP: routine chest positioning
11. ANS: A   REF: Ch. 16   OBJ: exam spec 1. Chest   TOP: routine chest technical factors
12. ANS: A   REF: Ch. 16   OBJ: exam spec 1. Chest   TOP: routine chest positioning
13. ANS: A   REF: Ch. 16   OBJ: exam spec 1. Chest   TOP: routine chest positioning
14. ANS: B   REF: Ch. 16   OBJ: exam spec 1. Chest   TOP: routine chest positioning
15. ANS: A   REF: Ch. 16   OBJ: exam spec 1. Chest   TOP: routine chest positioning
16. ANS: C   REF: Ch. 16   OBJ: exam spec 1. Chest   TOP: routine chest positioning
17. ANS: C   REF: Ch. 16   OBJ: exam spec 1. Chest   TOP: other chest positioning
18. ANS: D   REF: Ch. 16   OBJ: exam spec 1. Chest   TOP: other chest positioning
19. ANS: C   REF: Ch. 16   OBJ: exam spec 1. Chest   TOP: other chest positioning
20. ANS: A   REF: Ch. 16   OBJ: exam spec 1. Chest   TOP: routine chest equipment

SIMULATED EXAMINATION FOR THE LIMITED SCOPE OF PRACTICE IN RADIOGRAPHY

EXTREMITIES MODULE– 25 QUESTIONS

Complete this examination in pencil if you plan to take it more than once.

Multiple Choice

Identify the choice that best completes the statement or answers the question.

_____ 1. Which of the following bones are in the hindfoot portion of the foot?
1. Cuneiforms
2. Calcaneus
3. Talus
A. 1 and 2 only
B. 1 and 3 only
C. 2 and 3 only
D. 1, 2, and 3

_____ 2. The anatomic name for the bone commonly known as the *kneecap* is the:
A. fibula.
B. tibia.
C. patella.
D. fabella.

_____ 3. The palpable portion at the distal end of the tibia is called the:
A. lateral malleolus.
B. medial malleolus.
C. medial condyle.
D. lateral condyle.

_____ 4. When the ankle is flexed to raise the foot, the movement is termed:
A. plantar flexion.
B. eversion.
C. inversion.
D. dorsiflexion.

_____ 5. What device may help provide an even density on a radiograph of an anteroposterior (AP) axial projection of the foot?
A. Lead shield
B. Wedge compensating filter
C. Wedge positioning sponge
D. Sandbag

_____ 6. Which of the following is true regarding the correct positioning of the ankle for a lateral projection?
A. The medial surface of the ankle joint is in contact with the image receptor (IR).
B. The sagittal plane of the foot and leg is perpendicular to the IR.
C. The central ray enters perpendicular to the medial malleolus.
D. The ankle joint is extended so that the foot is 15 to 20 degrees from the IR.

_____ 7. When the leg is extended in the supine position, the ankle is maximally dorsiflexed, and the central ray is directed 40 degrees cephalad through the plantar surface of the foot, the resulting image will demonstrate:
A. an axial projection of the calcaneus.
B. a medial oblique position of the tarsals and metatarsals.
C. the ankle mortise, especially the talofibular articulation.
D. the cuboid and the third cuneiform.

_____ 8. Which of the following are true regarding the correct position for an AP projection of the lower leg?
1. The leg should be extended and resting on the IR.
2. The ankle should be dorsiflexed so that the foot forms a 90-degree angle with the lower leg.
3. The sagittal plane of the leg is placed parallel to the IR.
A. 1 and 2 only
B. 1 and 3 only
C. 2 and 3 only
D. 1, 2, and 3

_____ 9. Where should the central ray enter the patient for the AP projection of the knee?
A. 0.5 inch below the apex of the patella
B. 0.5 inch below the base of the patella
C. 1 inch distal to the medial epicondyle of the femur
D. 1 inch proximal to the medial epicondyle of the femur

_____ 10. When a lateral projection of the knee is taken, flexion of the knee joint should be limited to 10 degrees when there is suspicion of:
A. a loose fragment within the joint.
B. collateral ligament injury.
C. damage to the medial meniscus cartilage.
D. a fracture of the patella.

_____ 11. What change in technical factors is required when an ankle in a dry plaster cast must be radiographed?
A. Measure the cast size and set the technique based on the technique chart.
B. Decrease mAs by 50%.
C. Increase mAs by three times.
D. Decrease mAs by 25%.

_____ 12. The bones that are located in the palm of the hand are called:
A. carpals.
B. phalanges.
C. metacarpals.
D. digits.

_____ 13. The bones of the forearm are the:
A. radius and ulna.
B. tibia and fibula.
C. humerus and radius.
D. clavicle and scapula.

_____ 14. The coronal plane of the body is turned how many degrees for the AP oblique (Grashey) projection of the shoulder?
A. 15 degrees
B. 20 degrees
C. 20 to 30 degrees
D. 35 to 45 degrees

_____ 15. Which surface of the hand should be in contact with the IR for the posteroanterior (PA) projection?
A. Lateral
B. Medial
C. Posterior (dorsal)
D. Anterior (palmar)

_____ 16. What is the center point of the central ray for the PA projection of the hand?
A. Third metacarpophalangeal joint
B. Second metacarpophalangeal joint
C. Third proximal interphalangeal joint
D. Base of the third metacarpal

373

17. Which surface of the hand should be in contact with the IR for the lateral projection of the fifth digit (pinky)?
    A. The medial surface
    B. The lateral surface
    C. The anterior (palmar) surface
    D. The posterior (dorsal) surface

18. What is the position of the wrist for the PA oblique projection in lateral rotation?
    A. Hand and wrist flat with the anterior surface in contact with the IR
    B. Fingers flexed with the anterior surface of the wrist in contact with the IR
    C. Coronal plane of the wrist at a 45-degree angle to the IR with the anteromedial surface on the IR
    D. Medial surface of the wrist on the IR with the coronal plane perpendicular to the IR

19. What is the proper patient position for the AP projection of the forearm?
    A. Elbow extended, wrist and elbow parallel to the IR, hand supinated
    B. Elbow extended, wrist and elbow parallel to the IR, hand pronated
    C. Elbow flexed, wrist and elbow perpendicular to the IR, hand in the lateral position
    D. Elbow flexed, wrist and elbow perpendicular to the IR, hand pronated

20. Which of the following describes the proper method for positioning the humerus for an AP projection?
    A. Upper limb adducted, elbow flexed, humeral epicondyles perpendicular to the IR
    B. Upper limb abducted, elbow extended, humeral epicondyles parallel to the IR
    C. Upper limb adducted, elbow extended, humeral epicondyles parallel to the IR
    D. Upper limb abducted, elbow flexed, humeral epicondyles perpendicular to the IR

21. What specific anatomy is demonstrated without superimposition in the AP oblique projection in 45-degree lateral rotation?
    A. Radial head and capitulum
    B. Superimposed humeral epicondyles and open elbow joint
    C. Olecranon process in profile
    D. Coronoid process of the ulna and the trochlea

22. The projection that would benefit from the use of a compensating filter is the?
    A. AP shoulder
    B. PA hand
    C. AP humerus
    D. Lateral hand

23. Where is the central ray entrance point for the AP projections of the shoulder?
    A. 1 inch superior to the coracoid process
    B. 1 inch inferior to the coracoid process
    C. 1 inch medial and inferior to the acromion
    D. 1 inch superior to the acromion

24. Where is the CR center point for the PA projection of the second digit?
    A. Proximal IP joint
    B. Distal IP joint
    C. MCP joint
    D. Base of the 3rd metacarpal

25. What is the name of the large, rounded projection that can be felt on the superior lateral surface of the shoulder?
    A. Coracoid process
    B. Lateral epicondyle
    C. Acromion
    D. Inferior angle of the scapula

Simulated Examination for the Limited Scope of Practice in Radiography–Extremities Module

Answer Section

Multiple Choice

1.	ANS: C	REF: Ch. 14	OBJ: exam spec 2. Extremities	TOP: lower extremity anatomy
2.	ANS: C	REF: Ch. 14	OBJ: exam spec 2. Extremities	TOP: lower extremity anatomy
3.	ANS: B	REF: Ch. 14	OBJ: exam spec 2. Extremities	TOP: lower extremity anatomy
4.	ANS: D	REF: Ch. 14	OBJ: exam spec 2. Extremities	TOP: lower extremity positioning
5.	ANS: B	REF: Ch. 14	OBJ: exam spec 2. Extremities	TOP: lower extremity accessory equipment

6.	ANS: C	REF: Ch. 14	OBJ: exam spec 2. Extremities	TOP: lower extremity positioning
7.	ANS: A	REF: Ch. 14	OBJ: exam spec 2. Extremities	TOP: lower extremity positioning
8.	ANS: A	REF: Ch. 14	OBJ: exam spec 2. Extremities	TOP: lower extremity positioning
9.	ANS: A	REF: Ch. 14	OBJ: exam spec 2. Extremities	TOP: lower extremity positioning
10.	ANS: D	REF: Ch. 14	OBJ: exam spec 2. Extremities	TOP: lower extremity positioning
11.	ANS: A	REF: Ch. 10	OBJ: exam spec 2. Extremities	TOP: lower extremity technical factors
12.	ANS: C	REF: Ch. 13	OBJ: exam spec 2. Extremities	TOP: upper extremity anatomy
13.	ANS: A	REF: Ch. 13	OBJ: exam spec 2. Extremities	TOP: upper extremity anatomy
14.	ANS: D	REF: Ch. 13	OBJ: exam spec 2. Extremities	TOP: upper extremity anatomy
15.	ANS: D	REF: Ch. 13	OBJ: exam spec 2. Extremities	TOP: upper extremity positioning
16.	ANS: A	REF: Ch. 13	OBJ: exam spec 2. Extremities	TOP: upper extremity positioning
17.	ANS: A	REF: Ch. 13	OBJ: exam spec 2. Extremities	TOP: upper extremity positioning
18.	ANS: C	REF: Ch. 13	OBJ: exam spec 2. Extremities	TOP: upper extremity positioning
19.	ANS: A	REF: Ch. 13	OBJ: exam spec 2. Extremities	TOP: upper extremity positioning
20.	ANS: B	REF: Ch. 13	OBJ: exam spec 2. Extremities	TOP: upper extremity positioning
21.	ANS: A	REF: Ch. 13	OBJ: exam spec 2. Extremities	TOP: upper extremity positioning
22.	ANS: A	REF: Ch. 10	OBJ: exam spec 2. Extremities	TOP: upper extremity technical factors
23.	ANS: B	REF: Ch. 13	OBJ: exam spec 2. Extremities	TOP: shoulder positioning
24.	ANS: A	REF: Ch. 13	OBJ: exam spec 2. Extremities	TOP: shoulder positioning
25.	ANS: C	REF: Ch. 13	OBJ: exam spec 2. Extremities	TOP: shoulder anatomy

SIMULATED EXAMINATION FOR THE LIMITED SCOPE OF PRACTICE IN RADIOGRAPHY

SKULL/SINUS MODULE – 20 QUESTIONS

Complete this examination in pencil if you plan to take it more than once.

Multiple Choice

Identify the choice that best completes the statement or answers the question.

_____ 1. Which of the following cranial bones are paired (right and left)?
   1. Frontal
   2. Parietal
   3. Temporal
   A. 1 only
   B. 1 and 2 only
   C. 2 and 3 only
   D. 1, 2, and 3

_____ 2. What structure serves as the passageway for the spinal cord to exit the skull and pass into the spinal canal of the vertebral column?
   A. External auditory meatus (EAM)
   B. Foramen magnum
   C. Sella turcica
   D. Crista galli

_____ 3. When taking a posteroanterior (PA) axial projection (Caldwell method) of the skull, the central ray is directed:
   A. 15 degrees cephalad.
   B. 15 degrees caudad.
   C. 30 degrees cephalad.
   D. 30 degrees caudad.

_____ 4. Which radiographic baseline is used to position the PA axial projection (Caldwell method) of the cranium?
   A. Either the orbitomeatal line (OML) or the infraorbitomeatal line (IOML) can be used
   B. The mentomeatal line
   C. The IOML
   D. The OML

_____ 5. Which cranial projection best demonstrates the occipital bone?
   A. PA
   B. PA axial (Caldwell method)
   C. Anteroposterior (AP) axial (Towne method)
   D. Lateral

6. The patient is in a prone oblique position with the midsagittal plane of the head parallel to the IR and the interpupillary line perpendicular to the IR. The CR is directed perpendicularly to enter 2 inches superior to the EAM. What projection of the cranium will be demonstrated on the radiograph?
   A. Lateral
   B. AP axial (Towne method)
   C. PA axial (Caldwell method)
   D. PA

7. The patient is positioned supine with the midsagittal plane and OML perpendicular to the IR. The central ray is angled 30 degrees caudad and enters the midsagittal plane at approximately 2.5 inches superior to the glabella. What projection will be imaged on the radiograph?
   A. Lateral
   B. PA axial (Caldwell method)
   C. PA
   D. AP axial (Towne method)

8. What positioning accessory can be used to assist the patient in holding the correct position for an AP axial projection of the skull?
   A. A lead mask
   B. A wedge sponge
   C. A wedge filter
   D. An Angiliner

9. Air-filled cavities located in some bones of the face and cranium are called:
   A. cranial sutures.
   B. zygomatic prominences.
   C. paranasal sinuses.
   D. paranasal foramina.

10. Which of the following bones contain paranasal sinuses?
    1. Frontal
    2. Ethmoid
    3. Temporal
    A. 1 and 2 only
    B. 1 and 3 only
    C. 2 and 3 only
    D. 1, 2, and 3

11. What is the purpose of performing sinus radiography with the patient in the upright position?
    A. To demonstrate air-fluid levels
    B. For ease of patient positioning
    C. To prevent superimposition of the cranial structures on the paranasal sinuses
    D. Sinus radiography does not have to be performed with the patient upright

12. Which paranasal sinuses are best demonstrated in the PA axial projection (Caldwell method)?
    1. Maxillary
    2. Frontal
    3. Ethmoid
    A. 1 and 2 only
    B. 1 and 3 only
    C. 2 and 3 only
    D. 1, 2, and 3

13. Which of the following projections will demonstrate the sphenoid sinus?
    A. Parietoacanthial (Waters method)
    B. Lateral
    C. AP axial (Towne method)
    D. PA axial (Caldwell method)

14. Which projection best demonstrates the maxillary sinuses?
    A. Parietoacanthial (Waters method)
    B. Submentovertex (SMV)
    C. PA axial (Caldwell method)
    D. AP axial (Towne method)

15. Which paranasal sinuses are demonstrated by the SMV projection?
    1. Sphenoid
    2. Ethmoid
    3. Maxillary
    A. 1 and 2 only
    B. 1 and 3 only
    C. 2 and 3 only
    D. 1, 2, and 3

16. Which projection will demonstrate all of the paranasal sinuses?
    A. PA axial (Caldwell method)
    B. Parietoacanthial (Waters method)
    C. Lateral
    D. SMV

_____ 17. A blowout fracture involves the:
A. nasal bones.
B. occipital bone.
C. mandible.
D. Floor of the orbit.

_____ 18. A lateral projection of the face using a nongrid is used to demonstrate the:
A. mandible.
B. zygoma.
C. orbits.
D. nasal bones.

_____ 19. Which projection of the facial bones requires the central ray to exit the acanthion?
A. AP axial (Towne method)
B. PA axial (Caldwell method)
C. Lateral
D. Parietoacanthial (Waters method)

_____ 20. Which projection of the cranium demonstrates the petrous ridges within the orbits?
A. PA axial (Caldwell method)
B. PA
C. AP axial (Towne method)
D. SMV

Simulated Examination for the Limited Scope of Practice in Radiography–Skull/Sinuses Module

Answer Section

Multiple Choice

1.	ANS: C	REF: Ch. 17	OBJ: exam spec 3. Skull/sinuses	TOP: skull anatomy
2.	ANS: B	REF: Ch. 17	OBJ: exam spec 3. Skull/sinuses	TOP: skull anatomy
3.	ANS: B	REF: Ch. 17	OBJ: exam spec 3. Skull/sinuses	TOP: skull anatomy
4.	ANS: D	REF: Ch. 17	OBJ: exam spec 3. Skull/sinuses	TOP: skull positioning
5.	ANS: C	REF: Ch. 17	OBJ: exam spec 3. Skull/sinuses	TOP: skull positioning
6.	ANS: A	REF: Ch. 17	OBJ: exam spec 3. Skull/sinuses	TOP: skull positioning
7.	ANS: D	REF: Ch. 17	OBJ: exam spec 3. Skull/sinuses	TOP: skull positioning
8.	ANS: C	REF: Ch. 17	OBJ: exam spec 3. Skull/sinuses	TOP: skull positioning accessory
9.	ANS: C	REF: Ch. 17	OBJ: exam spec 3. Skull/sinuses	TOP: sinus anatomy
10.	ANS: A	REF: Ch. 17	OBJ: exam spec 3. Skull/sinuses	TOP: sinus anatomy
11.	ANS: A	REF: Ch. 17	OBJ: exam spec 3. Skull/sinuses	TOP: sinus technique
12.	ANS: C	REF: Ch. 17	OBJ: exam spec 3. Skull/sinuses	TOP: sinus positioning
13.	ANS: B	REF: Ch. 17	OBJ: exam spec 3. Skull/sinuses	TOP: sinus positioning
14.	ANS: A	REF: Ch. 17	OBJ: exam spec 3. Skull/sinuses	TOP: sinus positioning
15.	ANS: A	REF: Ch. 17	OBJ: exam spec 3. Skull/sinuses	TOP: sinus positioning
16.	ANS: C	REF: Ch. 17	OBJ: exam spec 3. Skull/sinuses	TOP: sinus positioning
17.	ANS: D	REF: Ch. 17	OBJ: exam spec 3. Skull/sinuses	TOP: facial bones anatomy
18.	ANS: D	REF: Ch. 17	OBJ: exam spec 3. Skull/sinuses	TOP: facial bones positioning
19.	ANS: D	REF: Ch. 17	OBJ: exam spec 3. Skull/sinuses	TOP: facial bones positioning
20.	ANS: A	REF: Ch. 17	OBJ: exam spec 3. Skull/sinuses	TOP: facial bones positioning

SPINE MODULE – 25 QUESTIONS

Complete this examination in pencil if you plan to take it more than once.

Multiple Choice

Identify the choice that best completes the statement or answers the question.

_____ 1. How many vertebrae are located in the cervical region of the spine?
A. 5
B. 12
C. 7
D. 9

_____ 2. What is the odontoid process and where is it located?
A. A sharp process on the inferior surface of C1
B. A toothlike projection on the superior surface of C2
C. A rounded prominence on the posterior aspect of C7
D. A palpable landmark on the mandible

_____ 3. When taking an anteroposterior (AP) axial projection of the cervical spine, the central ray is directed:
A. 15 degrees caudad.
B. 15 degrees cephalad.
C. 25 degrees caudad.
D. 25 degrees cephalad.

_____ 4. What is the rationale for using a 72-inch source-image receptor distance (SID) for the lateral projection of the cervical spine?
A. This SID enables the limited operator to use a technique with lower kilovoltage (kVp).
B. This SID reduces the patient dose.
C. This SID helps to overcome the magnification caused by the increased object-image receptor distance (OID) of the position.
D. This SID provides more room for the limited operator to assist the patient in getting into the proper position.

_____ 5. What anatomic structures of the cervical spine are best demonstrated by the lateral projection?
A. Intervertebral disks
B. Intervertebral foramina
C. Zygapophyseal joints
D. Pedicles

_____ 6. What is the proper central ray angle and direction for the AP oblique projections of the cervical spine?
A. 15 degrees cephalad
B. 15 degrees caudad
C. 45 degrees cephalad
D. 45 degrees caudad

_____ 7. What is the proper patient position for an AP oblique projection of the cervical spine?
A. 45-degree posterior oblique position
B. 45-degree anterior oblique position
C. Coronal plane positioned parallel to the image receptor (IR)
D. Supine with the base of the skull aligned with the edges of the front teeth

_____ 8. What anatomic structures are best demonstrated by the posteroanterior (PA) oblique projections of the cervical spine?
A. Zygapophyseal joints closer to the IR
B. Zygapophyseal joints farther from the IR
C. Intervertebral foramina closer to the IR
D. Intervertebral foramina farther from the IR

_____ 9. How many vertebrae make up the thoracic spine?
A. 5
B. 7
C. 12
D. 22

_____ 10. Which vertebrae have special facets for articulation with the ribs?
A. Cervical
B. Thoracic
C. Lumbar
D. Sacral

_____ 11. The "breathing technique" is used to advantage when taking a lateral projection of the:
A. cervical spine.
B. thoracic spine.
C. lumbar spine.
D. sacrum.

12. The patient is positioned with the coronal plane of the body perpendicular to the IR, the midsagittal plane parallel to the IR, and the arm closest to the IR raised over the head. The CR is perpendicular and centered to the level of the C7 to T1 interspace. What projection and anatomy will be demonstrated in this image?
    A. A lateral projection of the cervicothoracic region
    B. An AP projection of the lower cervical spine
    C. A lateral projection of the lower cervical spine
    D. An AP projection of the cervicothoracic region

13. What device(s) may be used to improve visualization of the spinous processes of the thoracic spine on the lateral projection?
    A. A piece of lead placed behind the shadow of the patient's back
    B. A wedge filter placed with the thicker end on the upper thoracic spine
    C. A sandbag placed near the patient's shoulders and another put near the patient's hips
    D. A positioning sponge used to elevate the patient's waist

14. Which structures should be seen on the lateral projection of the thoracic spine?
    A. C7 through L1
    B. T3 through T12
    C. C5 through T7
    D. C6 through L2

15. What is the number of vertebrae in the normal lumbar spine?
    A. 4
    B. 5
    C. 7
    D. 8

16. Which portion of the spine is made up of five vertebrae and has a lordotic curve?
    A. Cervical
    B. Thoracic
    C. Lumbar
    D. Sacral

17. When using a 14- × 17-inch (35- × 43-cm) IR, where should the central ray enter the patient for an AP projection of the lumbar spine?
    A. At the level of the iliac crest in the midline of the patient
    B. At a level 1.5 inches superior to the iliac crest in the midline of the patient
    C. At the level of the sacrum along the coronal plane of the patient
    D. An IR of this size is not appropriate for lumbar spine images.

18. When using a 10- × 12-inch (30- × 35-cm) IR, where should the central ray enter the patient for an AP projection of the lumbar spine?
    A. At the level of the iliac crest in the midline of the patient
    B. At a level 1.5 inches superior to the iliac crest in the midline of the patient
    C. At the level of the sacrum along the coronal plane of the patient
    D. An IR of this size is not appropriate for lumbar spine images

19. What positioning maneuver is used to improve patient comfort and reduce the lordotic curve of the lumbar spine when positioning a recumbent patient for an AP projection of the lumbar spine?
    A. Raising the patient's arms above the head
    B. Crossing the patient's arms across the chest
    C. Flexing the knees and using a support under them
    D. Having the patient distribute his or her weight equally on both feet

20. Which projection of the lumbar spine demonstrates open intervertebral foramina?
    A. AP
    B. PA
    C. Lateral
    D. AP oblique

21. Which of the following body positions will demonstrate the left zygapophyseal joints of the lumbar spine?
    A. Left lateral
    B. 45 degrees right posterior oblique (RPO)
    C. 45 degrees left anterior oblique (LAO)
    D. 45 degrees left posterior oblique (LPO)

22. What specific anatomy is best demonstrated on the AP oblique projection of the lumbar spine if the patient is positioned in a 45-degree RPO position?
    A. Right intervertebral foramina
    B. Right zygapophyseal joints
    C. Left intervertebral foramina
    D. Left zygapophyseal joints

23. What is the central ray angle and direction for the AP axial projection of the sacrum?
    A. 10 degrees cephalad
    B. 10 degrees caudad
    C. 15 degrees cephalad
    D. 15 degrees caudad

24. What portion of the spine is commonly called the *tailbone?*
    A. Thoracic spine
    B. Lumbar spine
    C. Sacrum
    D. Coccyx

25. Which of the following statements is *true* regarding spine radiography to evaluate scoliosis?
    A. The AP projection is preferred.
    B. No patient shielding should be used.
    C. The IR should extend from the top of the patient's ear to the level of the greater trochanter.
    D. A 30-inch SID is recommended.

Simulated Examination for the Limited Scope of Practice in Radiography–Spine Module

Answer Section

Multiple Choice

1. ANS: C   REF: Ch. 15   OBJ: exam spec 4. Spine   TOP: cervical spine anatomy
2. ANS: B   REF: Ch. 15   OBJ: exam spec 4. Spine   TOP: cervical spine anatomy
3. ANS: B   REF: Ch. 15   OBJ: exam spec 4. Spine   TOP: cervical spine positioning
4. ANS: C   REF: Ch. 15   OBJ: exam spec 4. Spine   TOP: cervical spine technique
5. ANS: C   REF: Ch. 15   OBJ: exam spec 4. Spine   TOP: cervical spine positioning
6. ANS: A   REF: Ch. 15   OBJ: exam spec 4. Spine   TOP: cervical spine positioning
7. ANS: A   REF: Ch. 15   OBJ: exam spec 4. Spine   TOP: cervical spine positioning
8. ANS: C   REF: Ch. 15   OBJ: exam spec 4. Spine   TOP: cervical spine positioning
9. ANS: C   REF: Ch. 15   OBJ: exam spec 4. Spine   TOP: thoracic spine anatomy
10. ANS: B   REF: Ch. 15   OBJ: exam spec 4. Spine   TOP: thoracic spine anatomy
11. ANS: B   REF: Ch. 15   OBJ: exam spec 4. Spine   TOP: thoracic spine positioning
12. ANS: A   REF: Ch. 15   OBJ: exam spec 4. Spine   TOP: thoracic spine positioning
13. ANS: A   REF: Ch. 15   OBJ: exam spec 4. Spine   TOP: thoracic spine positioning accessories
14. ANS: B   REF: Ch. 15   OBJ: exam spec 4. Spine   TOP: thoracic spine positioning
15. ANS: B   REF: Ch. 15   OBJ: exam spec 4. Spine   TOP: lumbar spine anatomy
16. ANS: C   REF: Ch. 15   OBJ: exam spec 4. Spine   TOP: lumbar spine anatomy
17. ANS: A   REF: Ch. 15   OBJ: exam spec 4. Spine   TOP: lumbar spine positioning
18. ANS: B   REF: Ch. 15   OBJ: exam spec 4. Spine   TOP: lumbar spine positioning
19. ANS: C   REF: Ch. 15   OBJ: exam spec 4. Spine   TOP: lumbar spine positioning
20. ANS: C   REF: Ch. 15   OBJ: exam spec 4. Spine   TOP: lumbar spine positioning
21. ANS: D   REF: Ch. 15   OBJ: exam spec 4. Spine   TOP: lumbar spine positioning
22. ANS: B   REF: Ch. 15   OBJ: exam spec 4. Spine   TOP: lumbar spine positioning
23. ANS: C   REF: Ch. 15   OBJ: exam spec 4. Spine   TOP: sacrum positioning
24. ANS: D   REF: Ch. 15   OBJ: exam spec 4. Spine   TOP: coccyx anatomy
25. ANS: C   REF: Ch. 15   OBJ: exam spec 4. Spine   TOP: scoliosis spine positioning

PODIATRIC MODULE – 20 QUESTIONS

Complete this examination in pencil if you plan to take it more than once.

Multiple Choice

Identify the choice that best completes the statement or answers the question.

_____ 1. The bones of the forefoot include the:
   A. phalanges and tarsals.
   B. tarsals and metatarsals.
   C. phalanges and metatarsals.
   D. cuneiforms and cuboid.

_____ 2. The bones of the midfoot are called the:
   A. metatarsals.
   B. tarsals.
   C. phalanges.
   D. cuneiforms.

_____ 3. Small, flat, oval bones in the region of the first metatarsophalangeal (MTP) joint are called the:
   A. phalanges.
   B. tarsals.
   C. metatarsals.
   D. sesamoid bones.

_____ 4. What tarsal is commonly referred to as the *heel bone*?
   A. Talus
   B. Cuneiforms
   C. Navicular
   D. Calcaneus

_____ 5. Which of the following bones are tarsal bones?
      1. Cuneiforms
      2. Cuboid
      3. Calcaneus
   A. 1 and 2 only
   B. 1 and 3 only
   C. 2 and 3 only
   D. 1, 2, and 3

_____ 6. When taking a dorso-plantar (DP) projection of the foot, the central ray is directed:
   A. 10 degrees toward the toes.
   B. 10 to 15 degrees toward the heel.
   C. 25 degrees toward the heel.
   D. perpendicular to the image receptor (IR).

_____ 7. Where does the central ray enter the patient for the dorso-plantar (DP) projection of the foot?
   A. At the third MTP joint
   B. At the first MTP joint
   C. At the base of the third metatarsal
   D. At the head of the third metatarsal

_____ 8. Which surface of the foot should be in contact with the IR for the lateral projection of the foot?
   A. Medial
   B. Lateral
   C. Dorsal
   D. Plantar

_____ 9. Which of the following is true regarding the lateral projection of the foot?
   A. The ankle does not have a specific position when a lateral projection of the foot is performed.
   B. The ankle should be dorsiflexed so that the long axis of the foot forms a 45-degree angle with the tibia.
   C. The ankle should be extended so that the plantar surface of the foot forms a 45-degree angle with the IR.
   D. The ankle should be dorsiflexed so that the long axis of the foot is perpendicular to the tibia.

_____ 10. How much is the plantar surface of the foot elevated from the IR for the AP oblique projection of the foot?
   A. 45 degrees
   B. 30 degrees
   C. 10 degrees
   D. 25 degrees

_____ 11. Which foot projection and position will demonstrate the metatarsals without superimposition?
   A. AP axial projection with the plantar surface of the foot in contact with the IR
   B. AP oblique projection in 45-degree lateral rotation
   C. AP oblique projection in 45-degree medial rotation
   D. Lateral projection with the MTP joints perpendicular to the IR

12. Which foot projection and position will demonstrate the medial and intermediate cuneiforms without superimposition?
    A. AP axial projection with the plantar surface of the foot in contact with the IR
    B. AP oblique projection in 45-degree lateral rotation
    C. AP oblique projection in 45-degree medial rotation
    D. Lateral projection with the MTP joints perpendicular to the IR

13. The AP oblique projections of the ankle require the foot to be angled:
    A. 30 degrees
    B. 35 degrees
    C. 45 degrees
    D. 15 to 20 degrees

14. Which foot projection and position will demonstrate the entire foot in near anatomic position?
    A. Dorso-plantar (DP) projection with the plantar surface of the foot in contact with the IR
    B. AP oblique projection in 45-degree lateral rotation
    C. AP oblique projection in 30-degree medial rotation
    D. Lateral projection with the 45 MTP joints perpendicular to the IR

15. What is the name given to the distal end of the fibula?
    A. Talus
    B. Medial malleolus
    C. Lateral malleolus
    D. Astragalus

16. Which of the following are the bones that articulate to form the ankle mortise?
    A. Talus, tibia, and fibula
    B. Tibia, fibula, and calcaneus
    C. Talus and tibia
    D. Calcaneus and tibia

17. When the leg is extended, the ankle is dorsiflexed to form an angle of 90 degrees between the foot and leg, the leg is rotated medially approximately 15 degrees, and the central ray is perpendicular to the IR through the midpoint between the malleoli, the resulting image will demonstrate:
    A. an axial projection of the calcaneus.
    B. an AP projection of the tarsals and metatarsals.
    C. the ankle mortise, especially the talofibular articulation.
    D. the cuboid and the third cuneiform.

18. Where should the central ray enter the patient for the AP projection of the ankle joint?
    A. Perpendicular to a point midway between the malleoli
    B. Perpendicular to the base of the third metatarsal
    C. Angled 10 degrees cephalad to a point midway between the malleoli
    D. Angled 10 degrees cephalad to the base of the third metatarsal

19. Which surface of the ankle is placed in contact with the IR for the lateral projection of the ankle?
    A. Medial surface
    B. Lateral surface
    C. Anterior surface
    D. Posterior surface

20. What is the central ray angle and direction for the axial calcaneal projection of the calcaneus?
    A. 10 degrees cephalad
    B. 40 degrees cephalad
    C. 10 degrees caudad
    D. 40 degrees caudad

Simulated Examination for the Limited Scope of Practice in Radiography–Podiatric Module

Answer Section

Multiple Choice

1.	ANS: C	REF: Ch. 14	OBJ: exam spec 5. Podiatric	TOP: foot anatomy
2.	ANS: B	REF: Ch. 14	OBJ: exam spec 5. Podiatric	TOP: foot anatomy
3.	ANS: D	REF: Ch. 14	OBJ: exam spec 5. Podiatric	TOP: foot anatomy
4.	ANS: D	REF: Ch. 14	OBJ: exam spec 5. Podiatric	TOP: foot anatomy
5.	ANS: A	REF: Ch. 14	OBJ: exam spec 5. Podiatric	TOP: foot anatomy
6.	ANS: B	REF: Ch. 14	OBJ: exam spec 5. Podiatric	TOP: foot positioning
7.	ANS: C	REF: Ch. 14	OBJ: exam spec 5. Podiatric	TOP: foot positioning
8.	ANS: A	REF: Ch. 14	OBJ: exam spec 5. Podiatric	TOP: foot positioning
9.	ANS: D	REF: Ch. 14	OBJ: exam spec 5. Podiatric	TOP: foot positioning
10.	ANS: B	REF: Ch. 14	OBJ: exam spec 5. Podiatric	TOP: foot positioning
11.	ANS: C	REF: Ch. 14	OBJ: exam spec 5. Podiatric	TOP: foot positioning
12.	ANS: B	REF: Ch. 14	OBJ: exam spec 5. Podiatric	TOP: foot positioning
13.	ANS: C	REF: Ch. 14	OBJ: exam spec 5. Podiatric	TOP: foot positioning
14.	ANS: A	REF: Ch. 14	OBJ: exam spec 5. Podiatric	TOP: foot positioning
15.	ANS: C	REF: Ch. 14	OBJ: exam spec 5. Podiatric	TOP: ankle anatomy
16.	ANS: A	REF: Ch. 14	OBJ: exam spec 5. Podiatric	TOP: ankle anatomy
17.	ANS: C	REF: Ch. 14	OBJ: exam spec 5. Podiatric	TOP: ankle positioning
18.	ANS: A	REF: Ch. 14	OBJ: exam spec 5. Podiatric	TOP: ankle positioning
19.	ANS: A	REF: Ch. 14	OBJ: exam spec 5. Podiatric	TOP: ankle positioning
20.	ANS: B	REF: Ch. 14	OBJ: exam spec 5. Podiatric	TOP: calcaneus positioning

Introduction

This guide is provided to help you prepare to successfully complete the licensure examination for the limited scope of practice area in which you are or will be working. We have included helpful suggestions for optimizing your study time and a simulated practice examination to help identify your areas of strength and weakness. All suggestions and discussions are based on the American Registry of Radiologic Technologists (ARRT) Content Specifications for the **Bone Densitometry Equipment Operators Examination**. We have done this for two reasons: first, this is a comprehensive examination covering all relevant areas of practice, and, second, it is likely that the licensure agency in your state uses this examination. If your state does not use this examination, you will still be well prepared if you use the **ARRT Content Specifications** as your study guide. For your convenience, we have included the most recent ARRT Content Specifications in this guide.

If you are using Radiography Essentials for Limited Practice and this accompanying workbook, it is likely that you are participating in an educational program designed to prepare you to both work in the practice area and to successfully pass the appropriate state licensure examination. This guide should assist you in both of these areas. Completing the simulated examination will help identify knowledge you have already acquired and knowledge that you have yet to master. Because the simulated examination was constructed to assess content identified in the ARRT Content Specifications, it is appropriate to provide an overview of this document before moving on to the examination.

ARRT CONTENT SPECIFICATIONS

The ARRT Content Specifications for the Bone Densitometry Equipment Operators Examination covers six content areas. These include basic concepts, equipment operation radiation safety, and dual-energy x-ray absorptiometry (DXA) scanning of the forearm, lumbar spine, and proximal femur.

The most valuable component of the Content Specifications is the outline of each content area covered on the examination. The numbers in parentheses indicate how many questions on the examination assess some aspect of that knowledge area. The value to you is

that this information will help you determine how much time and effort to spend on certain topics. Without using this information as a guide, you may waste valuable time learning information that is not included in the examination. This guide is to help you prepare for the state licensure examination, not to prepare you to work in your practice area. You will need skills that cannot be directly assessed on a written examination.

SIMULATED EXAMINATION

The Simulated Examination for Bone Densitometry Equipment Operators Licensure is located after the ARRT Content Specifications in this section. You should schedule enough time to complete the entire examination at one sitting. This will give you experience in completing an examination of the length of the simulated examination and will also give you some idea of how much time you will need for this examination.

The simulated examination consists of 60 questions, as prescribed in the ARRT Content Specifications, and contains the appropriate number of questions from each of the four content areas: patient care (12); safety (8); image production (12); procedures (25). The questions are further focused to cover content topics specified in the outline for each content area. You will see that there are more content topics in each outline than there are questions included in the examination. This means that some content will not be assessed with a question on both the simulated examination and your actual state licensure examination. For this reason, it is important for you to *review all topics included in each content outline* in the ARRT Content Specifications. You cannot rely only on the simulated examination to prepare you for your state licensure examination.

The answers to all simulated examination questions are located after the last question. We have included the correct answer (ANS), as well as the Radiography Essentials for Limited Practice textbook chapter (REF) where the information is located, the ARRT Content Specifications topic outline designator (OBJ) that the question is designed to assess, and the topic (TOP) assessed by each question. This information will allow you to easily find and review text material that you have not yet mastered.

385

Introduction

Your timeline to prepare for the state licensure examination should be something like this:

- Participate in the bone densitometry educational course or program.
- Complete all workbook exercises related to bone densitometry. Do not waste time on radiographic procedures chapters outside of this area. This activity is especially important if you are not in a formal education program.
- Complete the simulated examination.
- Analyze the results of your examination to identify information you have not yet mastered.
- Successfully complete the state bone densitometry licensure examination!

ARRT Content Specifications for the Bone Densitometry Equipment Operator Examination

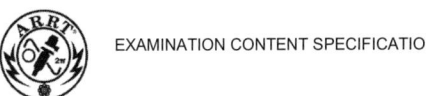

EXAMINATION CONTENT SPECIFICATIONS

ARRT BOARD APPROVED: **JULY 2021**
IMPLEMENTATION DATE: **JANUARY 1, 2023**

Bone Densitometry Equipment Operator

The purpose of the bone densitometry equipment operator examination, which is developed and administered by The American Registry of Radiologic Technologists (ARRT) on behalf of state licensing agencies, is to assess the knowledge and cognitive skills underlying the intelligent performance of the tasks typically required of operators of bone densitometry equipment at entry into the profession. ARRT administers the examination to state approved candidates under contractual arrangement with the state and provides the results directly to the state. This examination is not associated with any type of certification and registration by the ARRT.

The knowledge and skills covered by the examination were determined by administering a comprehensive practice analysis survey to a nationwide sample of bone densitometrists and adopting a list of tasks for bone densitometry equipment operators as the task inventory. The task inventory appears in Attachment A of this document.[1]

The content specifications identify the knowledge areas underlying performance of the tasks on the bone densitometry equipment operator task inventory. Every content category can be linked to one or more activities on the task inventory.

The table below presents the major categories covered on the examination, along with the number of test questions in each category. The remaining pages of this document list the Specific topics addressed within each category are addressed in the remaining pages of the content specifications.

Section	Number of Scored Questions[2]
Patient Care	12
Safety	8
Image Production	15
Procedures	<u>25</u>
Total	**60**

[1] A special debt of gratitude is due to the hundreds of professionals participating in the project as committee members, survey respondents, and reviewers.

[2] The exam includes an additional 25 unscored (pilot) questions.

1

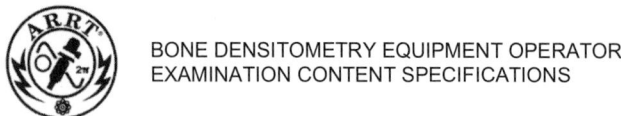
Patient Care

1. Osteoporosis
A. World Health Organization (WHO) Definition
B. Primary
C. Secondary

2. Bone Physiology
A. Functions of Bone
   1. structural support and protection
   2. storage of essential minerals
B. Structural Anatomy
C. Types of Bone
   1. cortical bone
   2. trabecular bone
D. Bone Remodeling Cycle
   1. resorption/formation
   2. osteoblasts/osteoclasts
   3. factors affecting remodeling (e.g., age, hormones, pathology)

3. Bone Health and Patient Education
A. Prevention and Treatment
   1. exercise
   2. nutrition
   3. smoking cessation
   4. fall prevention
B. Risk Factors
   1. controllable (*e.g., smoking, alcohol, calcium, vitamin D, hormone therapy, medications)
   2. uncontrollable (genetics, race, gender, age, medical conditions)

4. Patient Preparation
A. Patient Instructions and Explanation of Procedure
B. Patient History
   1. medical history (e.g., bone disorder, hyperparathyroidism, prosthesis, peak height)
   2. medications use (e.g., long term steroid use, hormone therapy, osteoporosis treatment)
   3. current height and weight
   4. contraindications (e.g., recent contrast agents, calcium supplements,)
   5. possible pregnancy
   6. clinical indications and guidelines (Bone Mass Measurement Act)
C. Patient Factors
   1. limited mobility or mental impairment
   2. unusual anatomy, pathology, or body habitus
   3. removable artifacts
   4. pediatric patients
D. Operator Ergonomics
   1. body mechanics (e.g., balance, alignment, movement)
   2. patient transfer techniques
E. Infection Control (e.g., disinfect work area and equipment)

* The abbreviation "e.g.," is used to indicate that examples are listed in parenthesis, but that it is not a complete list of all possibilities.

Safety

1. Fundamental Principles
A. ALARA
B. Basic Methods of Protection
   1. time
   2. distance
   3. shielding

2. Biological Effects of Radiation
A. Long-Term Effects
B. Radiosensitive Tissues/Organs

3. Units of Measurement
A. Absorbed Dose (e.g., mGy)
B. Dose Equivalent (e.g., mSv)

4. Radiation Protection
A. General Protection Issues
   1. radiation signs posted
   2. door closed
   3. limit unnecessary people in room
B. Occupational Protection
   1. scanner-operator distance
   2. personnel monitoring
   3. exposure records
C. Patient Protection
   1. comparison levels of radiation
      a. peripheral DXA
      b. axial DXA
      c. natural background radiation
   2. strategies to minimize patient exposure
      a. patient instructions
      b. correct exam performance

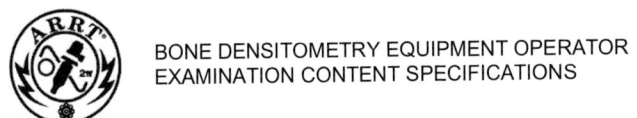
Image Production

1. Fundamentals of X-ray Production
A. Properties of X-ray Beam (e.g., scatter, mass, wavelength, frequency)
B. X-ray Energy Production

2. DXA Systems
A. Dual Photon Energies
B. DXA Components
   1. x-ray production
      a. k-edge filtration
      b. energy switching
   2. radiation detector system
C. Fan Beam
   1. mechanics of fan beam
   2. geometry of fan beam

3. Quality Control
A. Equipment Safety (electrical, pinch points, emergency stop)
B. Use of Phantoms
   1. frequency
   2. types
C. Calibration
   1. recalibration (e.g., relocation)
   2. cross-calibration (e.g., new scanner, software upgrade)
D. Troubleshooting and Actions
   1. shift or drift
   2. pass/fail criteria
   3. need for service
E. Record Maintenance

4. Measuring BMD
A Scan Analysis Algorithm
   1. bone edge detection
   2. definition and calculation of BMC, area, and BMD
B. Basic Statistical Concepts
   1. mean
   2. standard deviation
   3. coefficient of variation
C. Reporting Patient Results
   1. Z-score
   2. T-score
   3. WHO diagnostic criteria
D. FRAX® (WHO Fracture Risk Assessment Tool)
E. Vertebral Fracture Assessment (VFA)
F. Pediatric/Adolescent Scanning (ages 5-19)

5. Determining Quality in BMD
A. Precision
B. Accuracy
C. Factors Related to Accuracy and Precision
   1. scanner (e.g., speed/mode)
   2. operator
      a. in vivo precision study
      b. positioning
   3. patient variables (e.g., body habitus, variant anatomy)

6. File and Database Management
A. Storage and Retrieval of Data
B. Back-up and Archiving

ARRT Content Specifications for the Bone Densitometry Equipment Operator Examination

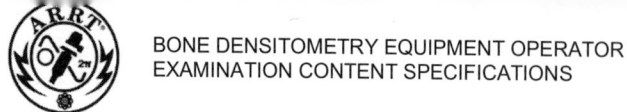
Procedures

1. DXA Scanning of Lumbar Spine
A. Anatomy
1. regions of interest
2. bony landmarks
3. radiographic appearance
4. significant adjacent structures (e.g., pelvis, ribs, T12)

B. Scan Acquisition
1. patient instructions
2. patient positioning
3. compensation for variations in anatomy, body habitus, pathology, or low bone density

C. Common Problems and Potential Causes
1. poor bone edge detection
2. nonremovable artifacts
3. variant anatomy
4. fractures or pathology
5. aortic and other calcifications

D. Scan Analysis
1. accurate ROI placement
2. BMC, area, and BMD
3. T-score, Z-score
4. graphical display
5. exclusion of vertebrae

E. Follow-Up Scans
1. unit of comparison
   a. BMD
   b. T-score
2. reproduce baseline study

2. DXA Scanning of Proximal Femur
A. Anatomy
1. regions of interest
2. bony landmarks
3. radiographic appearance
4. significant adjacent structures (e.g., pelvis)

B. Scan Acquisition
1. patient instructions
2. femur selection (right versus left or dual)
3. patient positioning
   a. femoral neck rotation
   b. femoral shaft placement
4. compensation for variations in anatomy, body habitus, pathology, or low bone density

C. Common Problems and Potential Causes
1. poor bone edge detection
2. nonremovable artifacts

3. variant anatomy (e.g., short femoral neck, inadequate space between ischium and femur)
4. fractures or pathology

D. Scan Analysis
1. accurate ROI placement
2. BMC, area, and BMD
3. T-score, Z-score
4. graphical display

E. Follow-Up Scans
1. unit of comparison
   a. BMD
   b. T-score
2. reproduce baseline study

3. DXA Scanning of Forearm
A. Anatomy
1. regions of interest
2. bony landmarks
3. radiographic appearance
4. significant adjacent structures (e.g., carpal bones, soft tissue)

B. Scan Acquisition
1. patient instructions
2. selection (right versus left)
3. forearm length
4. patient positioning
5. compensation for variations in anatomy, body habitus, pathology, or low bone density

C. Common Problems and Potential Causes
1. poor bone edge detection
2. nonremovable artifacts
3. variant anatomy
4. fractures or pathology

D. Scan Analysis
1. accurate ROI placement
2. BMC, area, and BMD
3. T-score, Z-score
4. graphical display

V 2021.07.28

ARRT Content Specifications for the Bone Densitometry Equipment Operator Examination

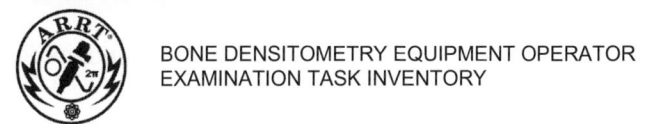
Attachment A
Task Inventory for Bone Densitometry Equipment Operator

Content Categories

Legend: PC = Patient Care
S = Safety, IP = Image
Production, P = Procedures

	Activity	
1.	Perform routine QC tests on scanning equipment according to manufacturer guidelines.	IP.3.
2.	Record results of QC tests in binder, chart, or database.	IP.3.E.
3.	Inspect and interpret results of routine QC tests and determine need for corrective action.	IP.3.
4.	Arrange for corrective action or repairs based on the results of the QC tests as needed.	IP.3.D.3.
5.	Coordinate software upgrades with manufacturer when recommended.	IP.3.C.2.
6.	Troubleshoot equipment errors (e.g., contact manufacturer for guidance) if needed.	IP.3.D.
7.	Troubleshoot computer software errors (e.g., contact manufacturer for guidance) as needed.	IP.3.D.
8.	Inspect equipment to make sure it is safe and operable (*e.g., cables, cords, table pads).	IP.3.A.
9.	Ensure that cross-calibration between new/existing machines is performed as needed.	IP.3.C.2.
10.	Clean and disinfect work area facilities and equipment.	PC.4.E.
11.	Verify current clinical indications meet specifications of CMS billing and coding guidelines if appropriate.	PC.4.B.6.
12.	Import previously archived or baseline studies for direct comparison.	IP.6.A.
13.	Educate new residents, staff technologists, ancillary staff, or students regarding bone densitometry.	PC.1., PC.2., PC.3.
14.	Answer basic questions put forth by the patient, patient's family, or authorized representative (or refer them to the appropriate resources) concerning bone health, fall prevention, exercise, and nutrition.	PC.3., PC.4.
15.	Direct patients to where they can find more information about low bone density.	PC.1., PC.2., PC.3.
16.	Provide assistance to patients with disabilities or limited mobility.	PC.4.C.
17.	Use proper body mechanics and/or ergonomic devices to promote personnel safety.	PC.4.D.
18.	Explain procedure of DXA exam including positioning, duration, and notification policy of results.	PC.4.A.

* The abbreviation "e.g.," is used to indicate that examples are listed in parenthesis, but that it is not a complete list of all possibilities.

ARRT Content Specifications for the Bone Densitometry Equipment Operator Examination

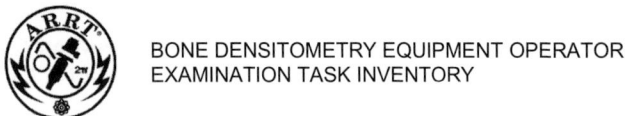
Content Categories

Legend: PC = Patient Care
S = Safety, IP = Image
Production, P = Procedures

	Activity	
19.	Review patient records and provider's request to determine appropriate anatomical sites to scan.	PC.4.B.
20.	Record patient history relevant to bone densitometry.	PC.4.B.
21.	Ask patients about their peak height, maximum height, or height loss.	PC.4.B.1.
22.	Measure and record patient's current height.	PC.4.B.3.
23.	Measure and record patient's current weight.	PC.4.B.3.
24.	Determine if patient has recently received a radiopaque contrast agent or radionuclide.	PC.4.B.4.
25.	Determine if patient has recently ingested contraindicated medications or supplements (e.g., calcium).	PC.4.B.2., PC.4.B.4.
26.	Screen female patients of childbearing age about possibility of pregnancy.	PC.4.B.5.
27.	Enter accurate patient data necessary to initiate scan to utilize correct reference data.	P.1.B., P.2.B., P.3.B.
28.	Review prior scans and reproduce patient positioning during follow-up scan appointments.	P.1.E., P.2.E.
29.	Ensure that artifact-producing objects (e.g., zippers, buttons, jewelry, medical devices) within scan area have been removed from the patient when possible.	PC.4.C.3.
30.	Determine if patient anatomy, pathology, or other limitations require special consideration in patient positioning.	PC.4.C., P.1.B, P.2.B., P.3.B.
31.	Position patient to scan desired region of interest (ROI) using bony landmarks and surface anatomical features.	P.1.A., P.2.A., P.3.A.
32.	Use positioning aids as needed to reduce patient movement and/or promote patient safety.	IP.5.
33.	Record positioning details in patient records to ensure consistency.	P.1.E., P.2.E.
34.	Take appropriate precautions to minimize occupational radiation exposure.	S.4.B.
35.	Take appropriate precautions to minimize radiation exposure to the patient.	S.
36.	Keep all unnecessary persons out of the immediate area during radiation exposure.	S.4.B.
37.	Select appropriate exam modes and perform necessary scans.	IP.1., P.
38.	Perform bone densitometry scans using a fan beam system.	IP.2.
39.	Perform and analyze bone densitometry scans of the lumbar spine - PA utilizing DXA equipment.	P.1.

ARRT Content Specifications for the Bone Densitometry Equipment Operator Examination

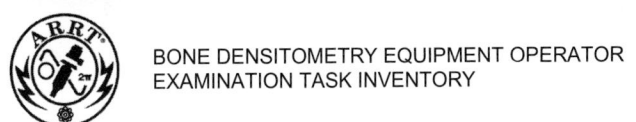
Content Categories

Legend: PC = Patient Care
S = Safety, IP = Image
Production, P = Procedures

	Activity	
40.	Perform and analyze bone densitometry scans of the proximal femur utilizing DXA equipment.	P.2.
41.	Perform and analyze bone densitometry scans of the forearm utilizing DXA equipment.	P.3.
42.	Perform bone densitometry scans of the spine – VFA (vertebral fracture assessment) utilizing DXA equipment.	IP.4.E.
43.	Perform and analyze bone densitometry scans on pediatric patients (ages 5-19) utilizing DXA equipment.	PC.4.C.4., IP.4.F.
44.	Enhance or modify image appearance.	P.1.D., P.2.D., P.3.D.
45.	Evaluate automatic placement of region of interest (ROI) and modify if necessary (e.g., vertebral body exclusions, hardware).	IP.4.A.
46.	Review scan results to identify bone density measurements that may be inaccurate due to artifacts, unusual anatomy, pathology, or positioning errors and rescan if necessary.	IP.4.A.
47.	Evaluate scan results for technical problems (e.g., incorrect scan mode or site) and take corrective action.	IP.5.
48.	Review scan results to determine if scanning an additional site is required in order to obtain more precise bone density measurements.	IP.4.
49.	Evaluate accuracy of vertebral labels and intervertebral markers for scan of lumbar spine and modify if necessary.	P.1.D.
50.	Compare bone density measurements from two different occasions (for same patient) to assess changes over time.	P.1.E., P.2.E.
51.	Identify bone density measurements that require interpreting provider's attention (e.g., low T-score, unreliable results).	IP.5.
52.	Identify exam-limiting patient anatomy or pathology that requires interpreting provider's attention (e.g., scoliosis, severe arthritis).	P.1.C., P.2.C., P.3.C.
53.	Perform an in vivo precision study.	IP.5.C.2.A.
54.	Operate electronic digital imaging devices and record keeping information technology system devices including PACS and medical information systems.	IP.6.
55.	Conduct system backup and archive as recommended by the manufacturer (e.g., external hard drive, DVD).	IP.6.A.
56.	Utilize FRAX® tool to assess 10-year fracture risk.	IP.4.D.

ARRT Content Specifications for the Bone Densitometry Equipment Operator Examination

Simulated Examination for Bone Densitometry Equipment Operator Licensure

Complete this examination in pencil if you plan to take it more than once. If you are not sure of the answer to a question, skip it and return to it after completing the entire examination.

Multiple Choice

Identify the choice that best completes the statement or answers the question.

PATIENT CARE (12)

_____ 1. According to the World Health Organization (WHO), what T-score level indicates osteoporosis?
A. +1 to −1
B. −1 to −2.5
C. −2.5 or less
D. −1 or greater

_____ 2. Primary type I osteoporosis is classified as:
A. premenopausal.
B. postmenopausal.
C. senile.
D. rheumatoid.

_____ 3. Which of the following is an uncontrollable risk factor for osteoporosis?
A. Gender
B. Estrogen deficiency
C. Low calcium intake
D. Smoking

_____ 4. What are the two basic types of bone?
A. Cortical and trabecular
B. Cortical and compact
C. Trabecular and cancellous
D. Trabecular and os calcis

_____ 5. Which of the following cells are responsible for building bone?
A. Osteotytes
B. Osteolytes
C. Osteoclasts
D. Osteoblasts

_____ 6. Bone health requires adequate intake and absorption of what two substances?
A. Calcium and potassium
B. Calcium and vitamin D
C. Potassium and vitamin D
D. Vitamin D and vitamin E

_____ 7. Two common conditions known to cause secondary osteoporosis are:
A. hyperparathyroidism and rheumatoid arthritis.
B. hyperlipidemia and rheumatoid arthritis.
C. hyperlipidemia and hyperparathyroidism.
D. rheumatoid arthritis and osteoarthritis.

_____ 8. Two weight-bearing types of exercise important for building and maintaining bone mass are:
A. swimming and jogging.
B. swimming and dancing.
C. dancing and jogging.
D. dancing and bicycling.

_____ 9. Three controllable risk factors for osteoporosis include:
A. smoking, alcohol, and calcium.
B. smoking, alcohol, and age.
C. smoking, gender, and calcium.
D. smoking, gender, and alcohol.

_____ 10. Trabecular bone accounts for what percentage of the skeletal mass?
A. 10%
B. 20%
C. 30%
D. 40%

_____ 11. Contraindications for a DXA scan include:
A. Elevated cholesterol
B. Hypertension
C. Pregnancy
D. Fatigue

_____ 12. Cortical bone accounts for what percentage of the skeletal mass?
A. 20%
B. 40%
C. 60%
D. 80%

_____ 13. What does the radiation protection principle ALARA stand for?
   A. As long as reasonably allowed
   B. As long as realistically achievable
   C. As low as reasonably achievable
   D. As low as realistically allowed

_____ 14. What are the three basic methods of minimizing radiation exposure?
   A. Time, distance, and shielding
   B. Time, distance, and monitoring
   C. Time, exposure, and monitoring
   D. Time, exposure, and shielding

_____ 15. What is the unit of absorbed dose, in addition to rad?
   A. Rem
   B. Sievert
   C. Gray
   D. Roentgen

_____ 16. What is the unit of dose equivalent that replaces the "rem"?
   A. Rad
   B. Sievert
   C. Gray
   D. Roentgen

_____ 17. Which of the following will be the highest radiation source?
   A. Posteroanterior (PA) chest radiograph
   B. Round-trip cross-country airline flight
   C. Daily natural background radiation
   D. DXA scan of the forearm

_____ 18. Which of the following will be the lowest radiation source?
   A. PA chest radiograph
   B. Round-trip cross-country airline flight
   C. Daily natural background radiation
   D. DXA scan of the forearm

_____ 19. Which of the following is a potential long-term effect of radiation exposure?
   A. Cancer
   B. Skin reddening
   C. Significant, rapid hair loss
   D. Sudden intestinal bleeding

_____ 20. For maximum radiation protection, the suggested distance between an array or fan-beam scanner source and the operator is:
   A. 3 feet.
   B. 6 feet.
   C. 9 feet.
   D. 12 feet.

_____ 21. Which BMD testing method is considered the "gold standard" for diagnosis and monitoring of osteoporosis?
   A. QUS
   B. RA
   C. SXA
   D. DXA

_____ 22. What does BMD stand for, as it relates to osteoporosis testing?
   A. Body mass determination
   B. Bone mineral density
   C. Bone muscle distribution
   D. Biomass density

_____ 23. Which BMD measurement score indicates the number of standard deviations (SDs) from the average BMD of young, normal, gender-matched individuals with peak bone mass?
   A. T-score
   B. W-score
   C. V-score
   D. Z-score

_____ 24. Which BMD measurement score indicates the number of SDs from the average BMD for the patient's respective age group and gender group?
   A. T-score
   B. W-score
   C. V-score
   D. Z-score

_____ 25. Which prime factor of x-ray production controls the quality or penetrating property?
   A. mA
   B. mAs
   C. S
   D. kVp

_____ 26. Which prime factor of x-ray production controls the quantity or intensity property?
   A. mA
   B. S
   C. kVp
   D. Filtration

_____ 27. DXA bone densitometry requires how many photon energy levels?
   A. One
   B. Two
   C. Three
   D. Four

28. Which quantitative performance measure is most important in following a patient's BMD over time?
   A. Stability
   B. Accuracy
   C. Geometry
   D. Precision

29. Scanner quality control to detect shift or drift is accomplished by imaging what object?
   A. Phantom
   B. Filter
   C. Grid
   D. Patient

30. On a normal functioning scanner, when should daily scanner quality control be performed?
   A. Before the first patient
   B. Between every patient
   C. Between every fifth and sixth patient
   D. After the last patient only

31. In order to adequately preserve scan files and data, which daily computer procedures are recommended?
   A. Locate and restore
   B. Locate and backup
   C. Backup and archive
   D. Backup and restore

32. In how many directions does an array or fan-beam DXA scanner system travel?
   A. One
   B. Two
   C. Three
   D. Four

33. What is the formula for determining BMD?
   A. BMD = BMC/Area
   B. BMD = BMD/BMC
   C. BMD = Area/BMD
   D. BMD = BMC/BMD

34. What is the purpose of the FRAX tool?
   A. Monitor phantom scan
   B. Monitor bone mass
   C. Evaluate 10-year machine accuracy
   D. Evaluate 10-year fracture risk

35. Vertebral fracture assessment (VFA) is performed for what purpose?
   A. Detect bone mass
   B. Detect fractures
   C. Detect osteoporosis
   D. Detect osteopenia

DXA SCANNING OF THE LUMBAR SPINE (10)

36. What are the regions of interest for a lumbar spine DXA scan?
   A. T12 through L3
   B. L1 through L4
   C. L1 through L5
   D. L2 through L5

37. What positioning aid is typically used during lumbar spine DXA scanning?
   A. Positioning leg block
   B. Positioning spine block
   C. Gonad shielding
   D. Measuring calipers

38. Which vertebra has an H or X appearance on a lumbar spine DXA scan?
   A. L2
   B. L3
   C. L4
   D. L5

39. Which of the following variant anatomic conditions can result in a falsely elevated bone mass density (BMD) measurement on lumbar spine DXA scans?
   A. Scoliosis
   B. Kyphosis
   C. Lordosis
   D. Spina bifida

40. Which lumbar vertebra commonly has the widest transverse process?
   A. L1
   B. L2
   C. L3
   D. L4

41. Which of the following can falsely elevate the BMD measurement in a lumbar spine scan?
   A. Compression fracture
   B. Motion
   C. Obesity
   D. Spina bifida

42. When analyzing a lumbar spine scan in which more than five vertebral bodies have been imaged, always analyze by:
   A. locating L1 and counting down.
   B. locating L5 and counting up.
   C. locating L2 and counting down.
   D. locating L3 and counting up.

_____ 43. When scanning the lumbar spine, what is one of the external landmarks used for placement of the central ray?
A. 2 cm below the greater trochanter
B. 2 cm below the iliac crest
C. 2 cm above the greater trochanter
D. 2 cm above the xiphoid process

_____ 44. To which scan should a serial scan of the lumbar spine be compared?
A. Second scan
B. Third scan
C. Baseline scan
D. Do not compare

_____ 45. What is the least number of vertebrae that can be used for diagnostic BMD interpretation?
A. One
B. Two
C. Three
D. Four

SCANNING OF THE PROXIMAL FEMUR (10)

_____ 46. When positioning the proximal femur, the femoral shaft is:
A. abducted 5 to 15 degrees.
B. abducted 15 to 25 degrees.
C. adducted 5 to 15 degrees.
D. adducted 15 to 25 degrees.

_____ 47. Name the two regions of interest (ROIs) for the proximal femur.
A. Femoral neck and total hip
B. Greater trochanter and total hip
C. Lesser trochanter and total hip
D. Femoral head and total hip

_____ 48. When positioning the proximal femur, the femoral neck is also:
A. lateral with the tabletop.
B. oblique with the tabletop.
C. perpendicular to the tabletop.
D. parallel with the tabletop.

_____ 49. To which scan should a serial scan of the proximal femur be compared?
A. Baseline scan
B. Second scan
C. Third scan
D. Do not compare

_____ 50. Name one contraindication to scanning the proximal femur.
A. Hyperlipidemia
B. Fracture of the proximal femur
C. Fracture of the proximal humerus
D. Appendectomy

_____ 51. Name one of the landmarks used for placement of the central ray when scanning the proximal femur.
A. Perpendicular to the xiphoid process
B. Perpendicular to the iliac crest
C. 7 to 8 cm below the greater trochanter
D. 7 to 8 cm below the lesser trochanter

_____ 52. Why is the proximal femur scan one of the most important skeletal scans in central densitometry?
A. Best predictor of future hip fractures
B. Best predictor of future wrist fractures
C. Best predictor of future vertebral fractures
D. Best predictor of future knee fractures

_____ 53. Which of the following conditions can falsely elevate the BMD in a proximal femur scan?
A. Osteoporosis
B. Osteoarthritis
C. Osteopenia
D. Osteogenesis imperfecta

_____ 54. Image analysis of a proximal femur scan must include adequate space between:
A. greater trochanter and femoral neck.
B. ischium and femoral neck.
C. lesser trochanter and femoral neck.
D. femoral head and femoral neck.

_____ 55. Image analysis of a proximal femur scan that shows a prominent lesser trochanter may indicate:
A. osteoporosis.
B. osteopenia.
C. poor rotation.
D. artifacts.

DXA SCANNING OF THE FOREARM (5)

_____ 56. Which forearm is recommended for scanning?
A. Left
B. Right
C. Dominant
D. Nondominant

_____ 57. The preferred region of interest (ROI) when analyzing the forearm is:
A. ultradistal ulna.
B. ultradistal radius.
C. one-third (33%) region of the ulna.
D. one-third (33%) region of the radius.

397

58. What is the most common problem in scanning a forearm?
    A. Artifacts
    B. Motion
    C. Poor edge detection
    D. Poor positioning

59. When doing a forearm scan, the same chair should be used to ensure consistency over time. Name a necessary characteristic of the chair.
    A. No wheels
    B. No padding
    C. No back
    D. No metal

60. When positioning a forearm for scanning:
    A. forearm must be straight and centered.
    B. forearm must be straight and not centered.
    C. forearm must be obliqued and centered.
    D. forearm must be obliqued and not centered.

SIMULATED EXAMINATION FOR BONE DENSITOMETRY EQUIPMENT OPERATOR LICENSURE

Answer Section

Multiple Choice

1. **ANS: C**	REF. Chapter 26	OBJ: exam spec 1.A	TOP: Patient Care
2. **ANS: B**	REF. Chapter 26	OBJ: exam 1.B	TOP: Patient Care
3. **ANS: A**	REF. Chapter 26	OBJ: exam 3. 2	TOP: Patient Care
4. **ANS: A**	REF. Chapter 26	OBJ: exam 2.B.	TOP: Patient Care
5. **ANS: D**	REF. Chapter 26	OBJ: exam spec 2.C.2	TOP: Patient Care
6. **ANS: B**	REF. Chapter 26	OBJ: exam 3.A	TOP: Patient Care
7. **ANS: A**	REF. Chapter 26	OBJ: exam 1. B	TOP: Patient Care
8. **ANS: C**	REF. Chapter 26	OBJ: exam 3.B	TOP: Patient Care
9. **ANS: A**	REF. Chapter 26	OBJ: exam spec 3.C.1	TOP: Patient Care
10. **ANS: B**	REF. Chapter 26	OBJ: exam spec 2.B.2	TOP: Patient Care
11. **ANS: C**	REF. Chapter 26	OBJ: exam 4.B.2	TOP: Patient Care
12; **ANS: D**	REF. Chapter 26	OBJ: exam B.B.1	TOP: Patient Care

SAFETY

13. **ANS: C**	REF. Chapter 26	OBJ: exam 1.A	TOP: Safety
14. **ANS: A**	REF. Chapter 26	OBJ: exam 1.B	TOP: Safety
15. **ANS: C**	REF. Chapter 26	OBJ: exam 3.A	TOP: Safety
16. **ANS: B**	REF. Chapter 26	OBJ: exam 3.B	TOP: Safety
17. **ANS: B**	REF. Chapter 26	OBJ: exam C.1.c	TOP: Safety
18. **ANS: D**	REF. Chapter 26	OBJ: exam C.1.c	TOP: Safety
19. **ANS: A**	REF. Chapter 26	OBJ: exam 2.A	TOP: Safety
20. **ANS: C**	REF. Chapter 26	OBJ: exam spec 4.B.1	TOP: Safety

IMAGE PRODUCTION

21. **ANS: D**	REF. Chapter 26	OBJ: exam spec 3.A	TOP: Image Production
22. **ANS: B**	REF. Chapter 26	OBJ: exam spec 3.B.1	TOP: Image Production
23. **ANS: A**	REF. Chapter 26	OBJ: exam spec 3.B.3	TOP: Image Production
24. **ANS: D**	REF. Chapter 26	OBJ: exam spec 3.B.2	TOP: Image Production
25. **ANS: D**	REF. Chapter 26	OBJ: exam spec 1.A.1	TOP: Image Production

26. **ANS: A**	REF. Chapter 26	OBJ: exam spec 1.A.2	TOP: Image Production
27. **ANS: B**	REF. Chapter 26	OBJ: exam 1.C	TOP: Image Production
28. **ANS: D**	REF. Chapter 26	OBJ: exam 4.A	TOP: Image Production
29. **ANS: A**	REF. Chapter 26	OBJ: exam spec 2.D.1	TOP: Image Production
30. **ANS: A**	REF. Chapter 26	OBJ: exam 2.B	TOP: Image Production
31. **ANS: C**	REF. Chapter 26	OBJ: exam 5.B	TOP: Image Production
32. **ANS: A**	REF. Chapter 26	OBJ: exam 1.D	TOP: Image Production
33. **ANS: A**	REF. Chapter 26	OBJ: exam spec 3.B.1	TOP: Image Production
34. **ANS: D**	REF. Chapter 26	OBJ: exam 3.C	TOP: Image Production
35. **ANS: B**	REF. Chapter 26	OBJ: exam 3.D	TOP: Image Production
36. **ANS: B**	REF. Chapter 26	OBJ: exam 1.B.1	TOP: Procedures (Spine) (10)
37. **ANS: B**	REF. Chapter 26	OBJ: exam 1.B.2	TOP: Procedures (Spine) (10)
38. **ANS: C**	REF. Chapter 26	OBJ: exam 1.A.2	TOP: Procedures (Spine) (10)
39. **ANS: A**	REF. Chapter 26	OBJ: exam 1.D.3	TOP: Procedures (Spine) (10)
40. **ANS: C**	REF. Chapter 26	OBJ: exam spec 1.A.2	TOP: Procedures (Spine) (10)
41. **ANS: A**	REF. Chapter 26	OBJ: exam 1.D.4	TOP: Procedures (Spine)
42. **ANS: B**	REF. Chapter 26	OBJ: exam 1.C.1	TOP: Procedures (Spine) (10)
43. **ANS: B**	REF. Chapter 26	OBJ: exam 1.B.1	TOP: Procedures (Spine) (10)
44. **ANS: C**	REF. Chapter 26	OBJ: exam 1.E.1	TOP: Procedures (Spine) (10)
45. **ANS: B**	REF. Chapter 26	OBJ: exam 1.E.1	TOP: Procedures (Spine) (10)
46. **ANS: D**	REF. Chapter 26	OBJ: exam 2.B.2	TOP: Procedures (Hip) (10)
47. **ANS: A**	REF. Chapter 26	OBJ: exam 2.C.1	TOP: Procedures (Hip) (10)
48. **ANS: D**	REF. Chapter 26	OBJ: exam 2.B.2	TOP: Procedures (Hip) (10)
49. **ANS: A**	REF. Chapter 26	OBJ: exam 2.E.2	TOP: Procedures (Hip) (10)
50. **ANS: B**	REF. Chapter 26	OBJ: exam 2.B.1	TOP: Procedures (Hip) (10)
51. **ANS: C**	REF. Chapter 26	OBJ: exam 2.A.2	TOP: Procedures (Hip) (10)
52. **ANS: A**	REF. Chapter 26	OBJ: exam	TOP: Procedures (Hip) (10)
53. **ANS: B**	REF. Chapter 26	OBJ: exam 2.D.4	TOP: Procedures (Hip) (10)
54. **ANS: B**	REF. Chapter 26	OBJ: exam 2.C.1	TOP: Procedures (Hip) (10)
55. **ANS: C**	REF. Chapter 26	OBJ: exam 2.B.2	TOP: Procedures (Hip) (10)
56. **ANS: D**	REF. Chapter 26	OBJ: exam 3.B.4	TOP: Procedures (Forearm) (5)
57. **ANS: D**	REF. Chapter 26	OBJ: exam 3.C.1	TOP: Procedures (Forearm) (5)
58. **ANS: B**	REF. Chapter 26	OBJ: exam 3.D.2	TOP: Procedures (Forearm) (5)
59. **ANS: A**	REF. Chapter 26	OBJ: exam 3.B.2	TOP: Procedures (Forearm) (5)
60. **ANS: A**	REF. Chapter 26	OBJ: exam 3.B.2	TOP: Procedures (Forearm) (5)